Role of Natural Compounds in Inflammation and Inflammatory-Related Diseases

Role of Natural Compounds in Inflammation and Inflammatory-Related Diseases

Special Issue Editor

Francesco Maione

MDPI • Basel • Beijing • Wuhan • Barcelona • Belgrade

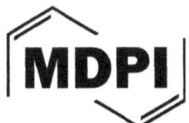

Special Issue Editor
Francesco Maione
University of Naples Federico II
Italy

Editorial Office
MDPI
St. Alban-Anlage 66
4052 Basel, Switzerland

This is a reprint of articles from the Special Issue published online in the open access journal *Molecules* (ISSN 1420-3049) from 2018 to 2019 (available at: https://www.mdpi.com/journal/molecules/special_issues/NaturalProducts_Inflammation).

For citation purposes, cite each article independently as indicated on the article page online and as indicated below:

LastName, A.A.; LastName, B.B.; LastName, C.C. Article Title. *Journal Name* **Year**, *Article Number*, Page Range.

ISBN 978-3-03921-552-2 (Pbk)
ISBN 978-3-03921-553-9 (PDF)

© 2019 by the authors. Articles in this book are Open Access and distributed under the Creative Commons Attribution (CC BY) license, which allows users to download, copy and build upon published articles, as long as the author and publisher are properly credited, which ensures maximum dissemination and a wider impact of our publications.

The book as a whole is distributed by MDPI under the terms and conditions of the Creative Commons license CC BY-NC-ND.

Contents

About the Special Issue Editor vii

Preface to "Role of Natural Compounds in Inflammation and Inflammatory-Related Diseases" ix

Yun-Da Yao, Xiu-Yu Shen, Jorge Machado, Jin-Fang Luo, Yi Dai, Chon-Kit Lio, Yang Yu, Ying Xie, Pei Luo, Jian-Xin Liu, Xin-Sheng Yao, Zhong-Qiu Liu and Hua Zhou
Nardochinoid B Inhibited the Activation of RAW264.7 Macrophages Stimulated by Lipopolysaccharide through Activating the Nrf2/HO-1 Pathway
Reprinted from: *Molecules* 2019, 24, 2482, doi:10.3390/molecules24132482 1

Francesco Maione, Paola Minosi, Amalia Di Giannuario, Federica Raucci, Maria Giovanna Chini, Simona De Vita, Giuseppe Bifulco, Nicola Mascolo and Stefano Pieretti
Long-Lasting Anti-Inflammatory and Antinociceptive Effects of Acute Ammonium Glycyrrhizinate Administration: Pharmacological, Biochemical, and Docking Studies
Reprinted from: *Molecules* 2019, 24, 2453, doi:10.3390/molecules24132453 17

Xueying Liu, Xiaoku Ran, Muhammad Riaz, Haixue Kuang, Deqiang Dou and Decheng Cai
Mechanism Investigation of *Tagetes patula* L. against Chronic Nonbacterial Prostatitis by Metabolomics and Network Pharmacology
Reprinted from: *Molecules* 2019, 24, 2266, doi:10.3390/molecules24122266 36

Hye Soo Wang, Yoon Jeong Hwang, Jun Yin and Min Won Lee
Inhibitory Effects on NO Production and DPPH Radicals and NBT Superoxide Activities of Diarylheptanoid Isolated from Enzymatically Hydrolyzed Ehtanolic Extract of *Alnus sibirica*
Reprinted from: *Molecules* 2019, 24, 1938, doi:10.3390/molecules24101938 51

Aline Boveto Santamarina, Giovana Jamar, Laís Vales Mennitti, Daniel Araki Ribeiro, Caroline Margonato Cardoso, Veridiana Vera de Rosso, Lila Missae Oyama and Luciana Pellegrini Pisani
Polyphenols-Rich Fruit (*Euterpe edulis* Mart.) Prevents Peripheral Inflammatory Pathway Activation by the Short-Term High-Fat Diet
Reprinted from: *Molecules* 2019, 24, 1655, doi:10.3390/molecules24091655 59

Palanivel Ganesan, Byungwook Kim, Prakash Ramalaingam, Govindarajan Karthivashan, Vishnu Revuri, Shinyoung Park, Joon Soo Kim, Young Tag Ko and Dong-Kug Choi
Antineuroinflammatory Activities and Neurotoxicological Assessment of Curcumin Loaded Solid Lipid Nanoparticles on LPS-Stimulated BV-2 Microglia Cell Models
Reprinted from: *Molecules* 2019, 24, 1170, doi:10.3390/molecules24061170 73

Yasuhisa Ano, Rena Ohya, Masahiro Kita, Yoshimasa Taniguchi and Keiji Kondo
Theaflavins Improve Memory Impairment and Depression-Like Behavior by Regulating Microglial Activation
Reprinted from: *Molecules* 2019, 24, 467, doi:10.3390/molecules24030467 84

Yufeng Cao, Fu Li, Yanyan Luo, Liang Zhang, Shuya Lu, Rui Xing, Bingjun Yan, Hongyin Zhang and Weicheng Hu
20-Hydroxy-3-Oxolupan-28-Oic Acid Attenuates Inflammatory Responses by Regulating PI3K–Akt and MAPKs Signaling Pathways in LPS-Stimulated RAW264.7 Macrophages
Reprinted from: *Molecules* 2019, 24, 386, doi:10.3390/molecules24030386 97

Vafa Baradaran Rahimi, Hassan Rakhshandeh, Federica Raucci, Benedetta Buono, Reza Shirazinia, Alireza Samzadeh Kermani, Francesco Maione, Nicola Mascolo and Vahid Reza Askari
Anti-Inflammatory and Anti-Oxidant Activity of *Portulaca oleracea* Extract on LPS-Induced Rat Lung Injury
Reprinted from: *Molecules* **2019**, *24*, 139, doi:10.3390/molecules24010139 110

Yasuhisa Ano, Yuta Takaichi, Kazuyuki Uchida, Keiji Kondo, Hiroyuki Nakayama and Akihiko Takashima
Iso-α-Acids, the Bitter Components of Beer, Suppress Microglial Inflammation in rTg4510 Tauopathy
Reprinted from: *Molecules* **2018**, *23*, 3133, doi:10.3390/molecules23123133 124

Chao Zhang, Jianjun Deng, Dan Liu, Xingxia Tuo, Yan Yu, Haixia Yang and Nanping Wang
Nuciferine Inhibits Proinflammatory Cytokines via the PPARs in LPS-Induced RAW264.7 Cells
Reprinted from: *Molecules* **2018**, *23*, 2723, doi:10.3390/molecules23102723 133

Ana-Maria Dull, Marius Alexandru Moga, Oana Gabriela Dimienescu, Gabriela Sechel, Victoria Burtea and Costin Vlad Anastasiu
Therapeutic Approaches of Resveratrol on Endometriosis via Anti-Inflammatory and Anti-Angiogenic Pathways
Reprinted from: *Molecules* **2019**, *24*, 667, doi:10.3390/molecules24040667 144

About the Special Issue Editor

Francesco Maione graduated in Pharmacy in 2005 from the University of Naples Federico II and trained in Pharmacology at the Department of Experimental Pharmacology of the Faculty of Pharmacy. During his PhD in Pharmacology (2005–2008), he studied the role of N-formyl-peptides (fMLF and FTM) in different models of pain and inflammation. During these studies, Dr. Francesco Maione demonstrated that these endogenous (fMLF) and synthetic peptides (FTM) have a remarkable in vivo inflammatory and painful activity. Dr Maione extended this research path after beginning his post-doctoral training in the laboratory of Prof. Mauro Perretti and Prof Fulvio D'acquisto, at William Harvey Research Institute, Queen Mary University of London (2008–2010). During this time, he expanded his knowledge on inflammation by focusing on immune-mediated inflammatory diseases and investigated the role of Annexin-1 (ANX-1) and interleukin-17A (IL-17A) in different models of inflammation. Since 2010, he has been a member of Prof. Nicola Mascolo's laboratory where he has re-activated his long-term interest in natural compound biology, charting an unexplored path in the role of natural molecules in the inflammatory response and cardiovascular system. In 2013 Dr Francesco Maione obtained the Specialization in Clinical Pharmacy at University of Naples Federico II. Actually, Dr Francesco Maione is Assistant Professor and leader of the ImmunoPharmaLab at Department of Pharmacy, University of Naples Federico II.

Preface to "Role of Natural Compounds in Inflammation and Inflammatory-Related Diseases"

Inflammation is a complex biological response to injury as a result of different stimuli such as pathogens, damaged cells, or irritants. Inflammatory injuries induce the release of a variety of systemic mediators, cytokines, and chemokines, that orchestrate the cellular infiltration that consequentially bring about the resolution of inflammatory responses and the restoration of tissue integrity. However, persistent inflammatory stimuli or the disregulation of mechanisms of the resolution phase can lead to chronic inflammation and inflammatory-based diseases.

Nowadays, commercially approved anti-inflammatory drugs are represented by nonsteroidal anti-inflammatory drugs (NSAID); glucocorticoids (SAID); and, in some cases, immunosuppressant and/or biological drugs. These agents are effective for the relief of the main inflammatory symptoms. However, they induce severe side effects, and most of them are inadequate for chronic use.

Starting from these premises, the demand for new, effective, and safe anti-inflammatory drugs has led research in new therapeutic directions. The recent and emerging scientific community slant is oriented towards natural products/compounds that could represent a boon for the discovery of new active molecules and for the development of new drugs and potentially useful therapeutic agents in different inflammatory-related diseases.

Francesco Maione
Special Issue Editor

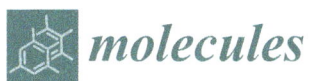

Article

Nardochinoid B Inhibited the Activation of RAW264.7 Macrophages Stimulated by Lipopolysaccharide through Activating the Nrf2/HO-1 Pathway

Yun-Da Yao [1,2], Xiu-Yu Shen [3], Jorge Machado [4], Jin-Fang Luo [1,2], Yi Dai [5], Chon-Kit Lio [1,2], Yang Yu [5], Ying Xie [1,2], Pei Luo [1,2], Jian-Xin Liu [6], Xin-Sheng Yao [3,5], Zhong-Qiu Liu [7,*] and Hua Zhou [1,2,7,*]

1. Faculty of Chinese Medicine, Macau University of Science and Technology, Taipa, Macao 999078, China
2. State Key Laboratory of Quality Research in Chinese Medicine, Macau University of Science and Technology, Taipa, Macao 999078, China
3. College of Traditional Chinese Materia Medica, Shenyang Pharmaceutical University, Shenyang 110016, China
4. ICBAS-Laboratory of Applied Physiology, Abel Salazar Institute of Biomedical Sciences, University of Porto, Rua de Jorge Viterbo Ferreira, 228, 4050-313 Porto, Portugal
5. Institute of Traditional Chinese Medicine and Natural Products, College of Pharmacy, Jinan University, Guangzhou 510632, China
6. College of Pharmacy, Hunan University of Chinese Medicine, Changsha 418000, China
7. Joint Laboratory for Translational Cancer Research of Chinese Medicine of the Ministry of Education of the People's Republic of China, Guangzhou University of Chinese Medicine, Guangzhou 510006, China
* Correspondence: liuzq@gzucm.edu.cn (Z.-Q.L.); hzhou@must.edu.mo (H.Z.); Tel.: +86-20-3935-8061 (Z.-Q.L.); +853-8897-2458 (H.Z.)

Academic Editor: Francesco Maione
Received: 15 May 2019; Accepted: 5 July 2019; Published: 6 July 2019

Abstract: Nardochinoid B (NAB) is a new compound isolated from *Nardostachys chinensis*. Although our previous study reported that the NAB suppressed the production of nitric oxide (NO) in lipopolysaccharide (LPS)-activated RAW264.7 cells, the specific mechanisms of anti-inflammatory action of NAB remains unknown. Thus, we examined the effects of NAB against LPS-induced inflammation. In this study, we found that NAB suppressed the LPS-induced inflammatory responses by restraining the expression of inducible nitric oxide synthase (iNOS) proteins and mRNA instead of cyclooxygenase-2 (COX-2) protein and mRNA in RAW264.7 cells, implying that NAB may have lower side effects compared with nonsteroidal anti-inflammatory drugs (NSAIDs). Besides, NAB upregulated the protein and mRNA expressions of heme oxygenase (HO)-1 when it exerted its anti-inflammatory effects. Also, NAB restrained the production of NO by increasing HO-1 expression in LPS-stimulated RAW264.7 cells. Thus, it is considered that the anti-inflammatory effect of NAB is associated with an induction of antioxidant protein HO-1, and thus NAB may be a potential HO-1 inducer for treating inflammatory diseases. Moreover, our study found that the inhibitory effect of NAB on NO is similar to that of the positive drug dexamethasone, suggesting that NAB has great potential for developing new drugs in treating inflammatory diseases.

Keywords: *Nardostachys chinensis*; nardochinoid B; nitric oxide; inducible nitric oxide synthase; heme oxygenase-1

---

1. Introduction

Inflammation is a kind of defensive reaction of living organisms with vascular systems to harmful factors such as pathogens, damaged cells, and irritants [1]. The inflammation may happen in a number of diseases, such as arthritis, arthrophlogosis, asthma, and so on [2]. The nonsteroidal anti-inflammatory drugs (NSAIDs) are widely used for fighting against inflammation diseases in clinical conditions. Restraining the cyclooxygenases (COXs) to inhibit prostaglandins is the main mechanism by which NSAIDs produce their anti-inflammatory effect [3]. However, many critical side effects, such as the increasing risk of serious and even fatal stomach and intestinal adverse reactions [4], myocardial infarction [5], stroke [6], systemic and pulmonary hypertension [7], and heart failures [8], happen during COX inhibition. Therefore, NSAIDs are not ideal for treating every inflammatory disease because of their side effects in the clinic. Thus, it is necessary to develop new, safer drugs to treat inflammation diseases better.

Macrophages play important roles in the innate immune response. They protect cells from injury induced by exogenous factors such as bacteria and viruses and endogenous factors such as other damaged cells. Also, macrophages promote the repair processes of tissue injury [9]. Proinflammatory mediators, such as interleukin-1β (IL-1β), interleukin-6 (IL-6), tumor necrosis factor alpha (TNF-α), prostaglandin E_2 (PGE_2), and nitric oxide (NO) [10–14], are produced by the activated macrophages and then promote the development of inflammation [15]. Thus, in our study, the LPS-stimulated RAW264.7 cells, a classical inflammatory cell model [16], was chosen to study the anti-inflammatory mechanism of NAB.

In recent years, there has been growing interest in the anti-inflammatory effects of natural components present in commonly used traditional herbal medicines. *Nardostachys chinensis* is one of the traditional Chinese medicines that was reported to have an anti-inflammatory effect [17]. The extracts of the plant roots and rhizomes of *N. chinensis* have been used for the treatment of blood disorders, disorders of the circulatory system, and herpes infection [18]. Recently, some compounds isolated from *N. chinensis* were reported to inhibit the protein expression of inducible nitric oxide synthase (iNOS) and cyclooxygenase-2 (COX-2) in LPS-activated RAW264.7 macrophages [18–20]. Nardochinoid B (NAB) is a compound isolated from *N. chinensis*. Our previous research has proved that NAB inhibits the production of NO in the LPS-induced RAW264.7 macrophages [20]. However, the mechanisms of the anti-inflammatory action of NAB have not been identified clearly. In this study, the mechanisms of anti-inflammatory activity and the antioxidant effect of nardochinoid B (NAB) were for the first time investigated in LPS-stimulated RAW264.7 cells.

The progression of inflammation could be inhibited through activating the nuclear factor erythroid 2-related factor 2 (Nrf2) pathway, meaning that activating the Nrf2 pathway could be a potential therapeutic strategy in anti-inflammatory disorders [21]. The translocation of Nrf2 protein into the cell nucleus induces the expression of heme oxygenase (HO)-1. Then, followed by the overexpression of HO-1, the production of inflammatory mediators is reduced and the inflammatory process is modulated [22]. Yet, few Nrf2 activators have been validated and used in the clinic. Tecfidera (dimethyl fumarate) is one of the Nrf2 activators that have been approved for the treatment of multiple sclerosis [23]. However, the long-term use of it causes several side effects [24]. Therefore, the discovery of new, safer Nrf2 activators for the clinic has become an essential and urgent matter.

In the present study, we have focused on these certain aspects of NAB: (1) whether NAB has the ability to suppress the LPS-induced inflammatory responses in RAW264.7 cells, and (2) whether NAB upregulates HO-1 to promote its anti-inflammatory effects by activating the Nrf2 signaling pathway. The results in this study revealed that NAB exerted its anti-inflammatory effects in LPS-induced RAW264.7 cells in a manner related to the activation of the Nrf2/HO-1 pathway, rather than the inhibition of the nuclear factor-κB (NF-κB) pathway and mitogen-activated protein kinase (MAPK) pathway.

2. Results

2.1. Anti-Inflammatory Activities of NAB on LPS-Activated RAW264.7 Macrophages

2.1.1. NAB Reduced the Release of NO in LPS-Stimulated RAW264.7 Macrophages

The results from the MTT assay show that NAB (Figure 1) had no significant cytotoxicity to LPS-stimulated RAW264.7 cells at the concentrations lower than 20 µM (Figure 2A,B). The nitrite level (evaluated through the stable oxidized product of NO) and the production of PGE$_2$ in the culture medium of the RAW264.7 cells were significantly increased ($P < 0.01$) after 18 h of LPS stimulation. The pretreatment with NAB markedly decreased the LPS-induced NO production in a concentration-dependent manner (Figure 2C), while it did not inhibit the production of PGE$_2$ (Figure 2D). Dexamethasone (DEX) was selected to serve as the positive control. The results show that DEX markedly reduced the production of both NO and PGE$_2$ in LPS-stimulated RAW264.7 cells (Figure 2C,D).

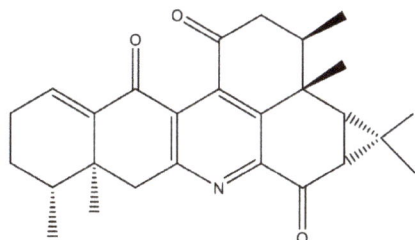

Figure 1. Chemical structure of nardochinoid B (NAB).

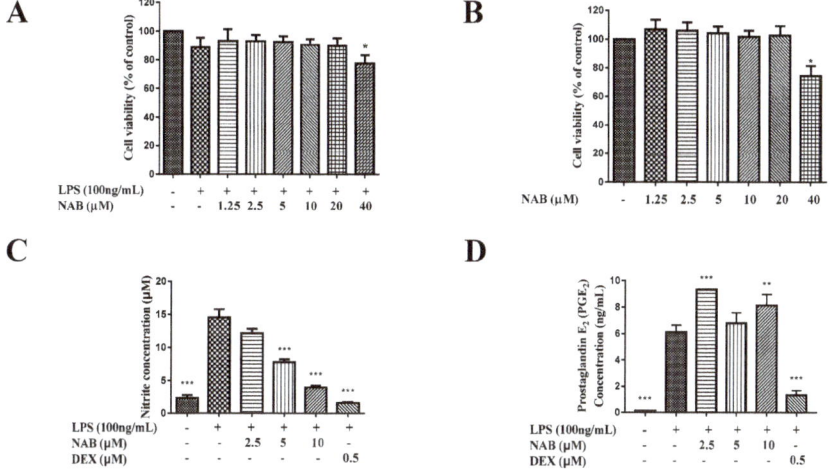

Figure 2. The effect of NAB on the release of nitric oxide (NO) and prostaglandin E$_2$ (PGE$_2$) in lipopolysaccharide (LPS)-induced RAW264.7 macrophages. (**A**) Cytotoxicity of NAB to LPS-stimulated RAW264.7 cells. (**B**) Cytotoxicity of NAB to normal RAW264.7 cells. Cells were treated with NAB at multiple concentrations (1.25, 2.5, 5, 10, 20, and 40 µM) for 1 h and then incubated with or without LPS stimulation (100 ng/mL) for 18 h. Cell viability was analyzed with the MTT method. (**C**) Effect of NAB on the production of NO by the LPS-stimulated RAW264.7 cells. (**D**) Effect of NAB on the production of PGE$_2$ by the LPS-stimulated RAW264.7 cells. Cells were pretreated with NAB or the positive control drug (dexamethasone, DEX) for 1 h and then stimulated with or without LPS (100 ng/mL) for 18 h. Culture medium was collected, and the NO concentration was analyzed by the Griess reagent. The PGE$_2$ concentration was measured by the ELISA method. The density ratio of the control group (blank control) in the cytotoxicity test was set to 1. In other tests, the variances were compared with the LPS group. Results are expressed as the mean ± SEM of three independent experiments. * $P < 0.05$, ** $P < 0.01$, and *** $P < 0.001$ vs. normal cells (**A**,**B**) or LPS-stimulated cells (**C**,**D**).

2.1.2. NAB Inhibited the Expression of iNOS Rather Than COX-2 in LPS-Stimulated RAW264.7 Macrophages

The mRNA and protein expression of iNOS and COX-2 in the cells were significantly increased after stimulation with LPS (100 ng/mL) for 18 h (Figure 3). NAB markedly downregulated the protein expression level of iNOS in the LPS-stimulated RAW264.7 cells in a concentration-dependent manner (Figure 3A) and decreased the mRNA expression of iNOS at the concentration of 10 μM (Figure 3C). However, NAB did not significantly downregulate the mRNA and protein expression levels of COX-2 in the same conditions (Figure 3B,D).

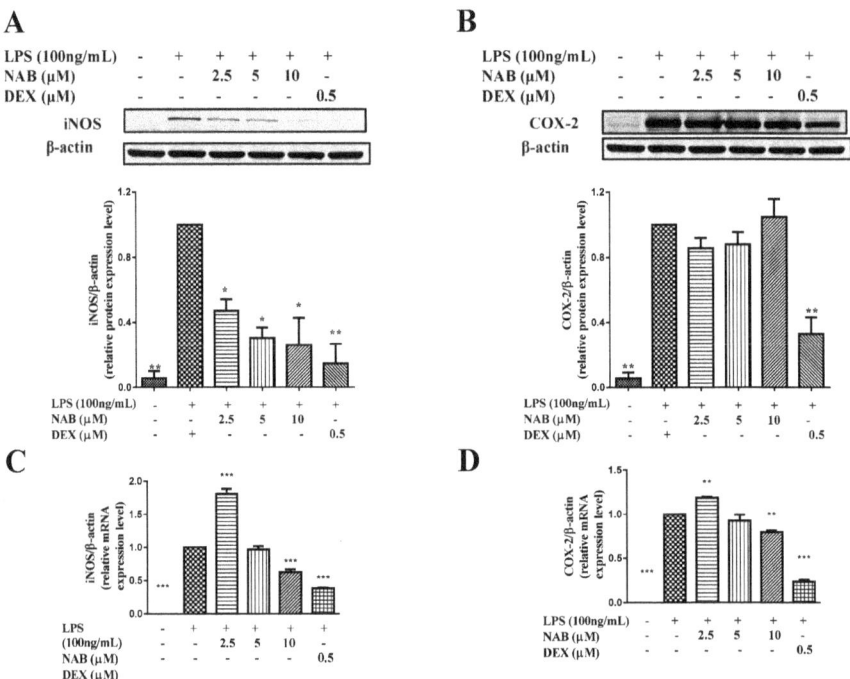

Figure 3. The effect of NAB on the expression levels of inducible nitric oxide synthase (iNOS) and cyclooxygenase-2 (COX-2) in LPS-induced RAW264.7 macrophages. (**A,B**) Effect of NAB on the expression levels of iNOS and COX-2 in LPS-stimulated RAW264.7 cells. Cells were pretreated with NAB or positive control drug (dexamethasone, DEX) for 1 h and then stimulated with LPS (100 ng/mL) for 18 h. The total protein of the cells was collected, and the expression levels of iNOS (**A**) and COX-2 (**B**) were analyzed with Western blotting; (**C,D**) Effect of NAB on the mRNA expression levels of iNOS and COX-2 in LPS-stimulated RAW264.7 cells. Cells were pretreated with NAB or positive control drug (dexamethasone, DEX) for 1 h and then stimulated with LPS (100 ng/mL) for 18 h. The total RNA was prepared, and the mRNA expression levels of iNOS (**C**) and COX-2 (**D**) were analyzed with qRT-PCR. The density ratio of the LPS group (model control) was set to 1. Results are expressed as the mean ± SEM of three independent experiments. * $P < 0.05$, ** $P < 0.01$, and *** $P < 0.001$ vs. LPS-stimulated cells.

2.2. Potential Anti-Inflammatory Mechanisms of NAB on LPS-Induced RAW264.7 Macrophages

2.2.1. NAB Increased the mRNA and Protein Expression Levels of HO-1 in LPS-Stimulated RAW264.7 Cells

The results (Figure 4) show that the expression level of HO-1 was increased after stimulation with LPS (100 ng/mL) for 6 h. Sulforaphane (SFN), a confirmed Nrf2 activator, was selected as an alternate positive control drug to DEX in the following mechanism study. NAB significantly increased the mRNA (Figure 4A) and protein (Figure 4B) expression levels of HO-1 in LPS-stimulated RAW264.7 cells.

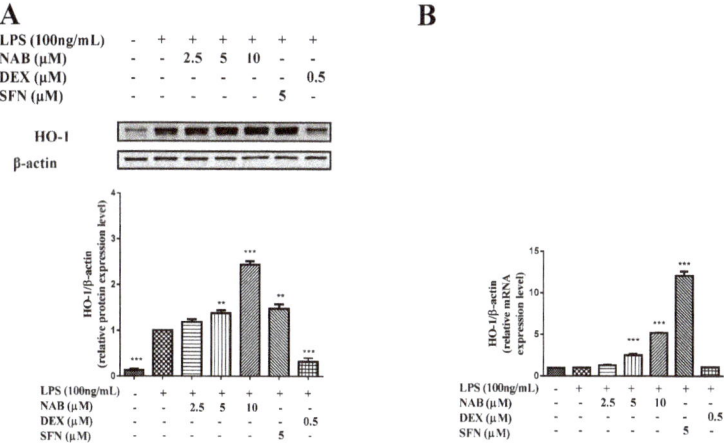

Figure 4. The effect of NAB on expression level of HO-1 in LPS-stimulated RAW264.7 cells. (**A**) Effect of NAB on HO-1 expression level in LPS-stimulated RAW264.7 cells. Cells were pretreated with NAB or positive control drug (dexamethasone, DEX) for 1 h and then stimulated with LPS (100 ng/mL) for 6 h. The total protein of the cells was prepared, and the expression level of HO-1 protein was measured by Western blotting. (**B**) Effect of NAB on the mRNA expression level in LPS-stimulated RAW264.7 cells. Cells were pretreated with NAB or positive control drug (dexamethasone, DEX, or sulforaphane, SFN) for 1 h and then stimulated with LPS (100 ng/mL) for 6 h. The total mRNA was prepared, and the expression level was evaluated by qRT-PCR. The density ratio of the LPS group (model control) was set to 1. Results are expressed as the mean ± SEM of three independent experiments. ** $P < 0.01$ and *** $P < 0.001$ vs. LPS-stimulated cells.

2.2.2. NAB Promoted Nrf2 Protein Translocation into the Nucleus in RAW264.7 Macrophages

As shown in Figure 5, the pretreatment of NAB promoted Nrf2 protein entering the nucleus in RAW264.7 cells, similar to the effect of SFN.

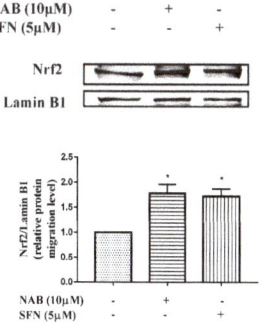

Figure 5. Effect of NAB on Nrf2 protein migration level in nucleoprotein of RAW264.7 macrophages. The RAW264.7 cells were treated with NAB or positive control drug (sulforaphane, SFN) for 6 h. The nuclear fraction was extracted, and the nuclear protein was measured by Western blotting. The density ratio of the CON group (normal control) was set to 1. Results are expressed as the mean ± SEM of three independent experiments. * $P < 0.05$ vs. normal cells.

2.2.3. NAB Suppressed the Production of TNF-α, IL-1β, and IL-6

The results show that the LPS stimulation of RAW264.7 cells increased the expression levels of TNF-α (Figure 6A), IL-1β (Figure 6C), and IL-6 (Figure 6E) in the culture medium. The mRNA expression levels of TNF-α (Figure 6B), IL-1β (Figure 6D), and IL-6 (Figure 6F) were induced by LPS as well. The treatment of NAB downregulated the expression levels of TNF-α (Figure 6A,B), IL-1β (Figure 6C,D), and IL-6 (Figure 6E,F). The positive control drug sulforaphane also significantly inhibited the expression level of these inflammatory mediators (Figure 6).

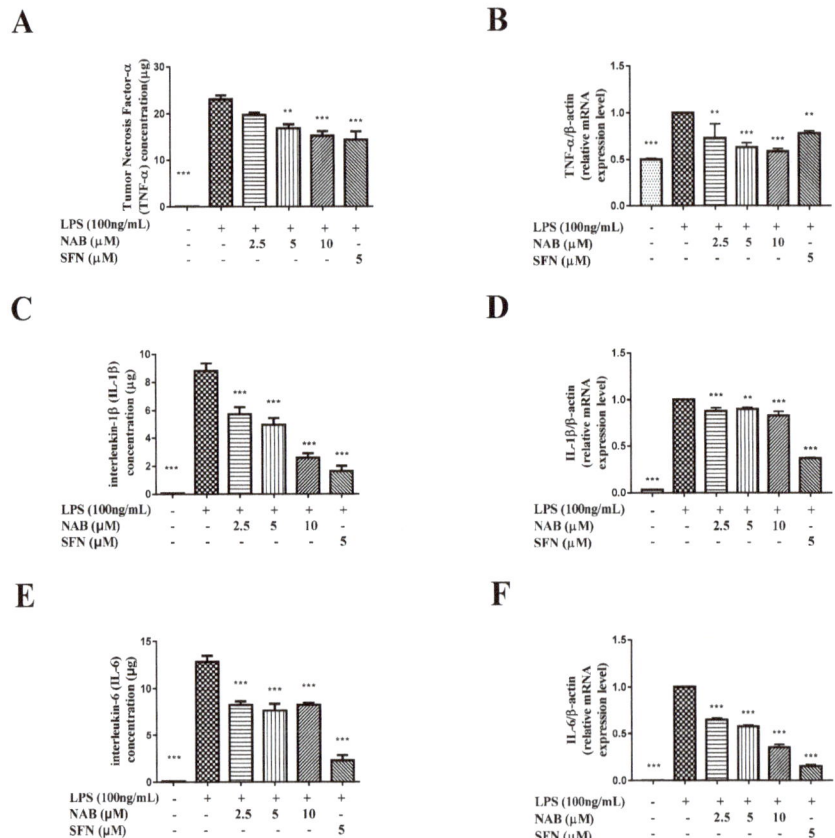

Figure 6. The effect of NAB on the production of TNF-α, IL-1β, and IL-6 in LPS-activated RAW264.7 cells. Effects of NAB on the expression level of TNF-α (**A,B**), IL-1β (**C,D**), and IL-6 (**E,F**) in LPS-stimulated RAW264.7 cells. Cells were pretreated with NAB or positive control drug (sulforaphane, SFN) for 1 h and then stimulated with LPS (100 ng/mL) for 18 h. Total mRNA was prepared, and the mRNA expression of TNF-α, IL-1β, and IL-6 was detected. Culture medium was collected, and ELISA was used to measure the expression level of TNF-α, IL-1β, and IL-6. In the qRT-PCR analysis, the density ratio of the LPS group (model control) was set to 1. In the ELISA analysis, the variances were compared with the LPS group. Results are expressed as mean ± SEM of three independent experiments. ** $P < 0.01$ and *** $P < 0.001$ vs. LPS-stimulated cells.

2.2.4. NAB Failed to Inhibit the Activation of the NF-κB and MAPK Pathways in LPS-Stimulated RAW264.7 Cells

As shown in Figure 7, the LPS stimulation of RAW264.7 cells increased the expression levels of phospho-p65 (p-p65), phospho-p38 (p-p38), and phospho-extracellular regulated protein kinase (p-ERK). However, NAB failed to inhibit the increased expression levels of p-p65 (Figure 7A), p-ERK (Figure 7B), and p-p38 (Figure 7C).

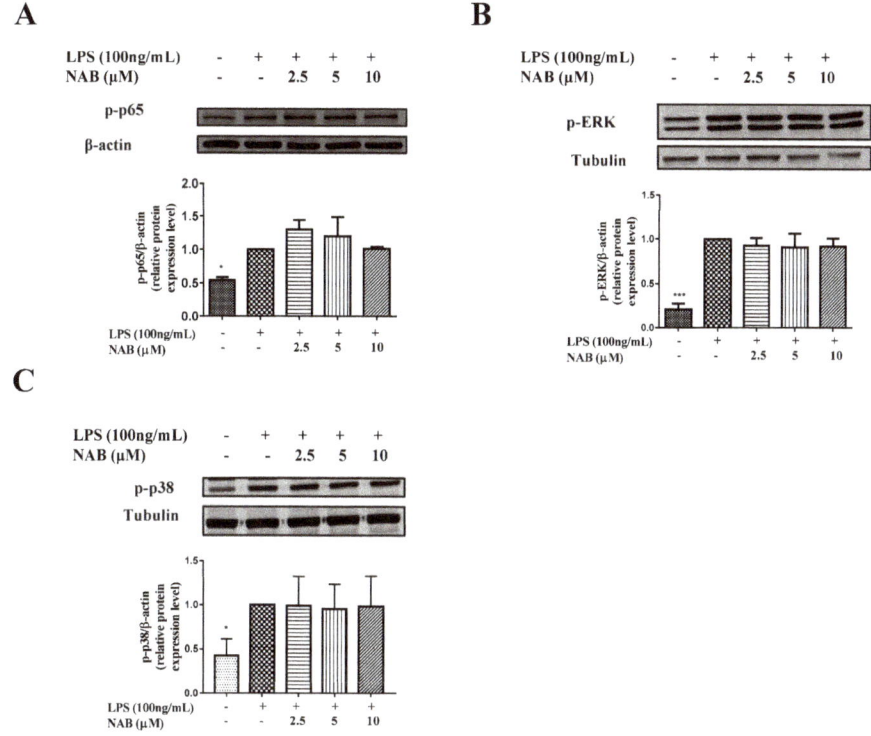

Figure 7. Effect of NAB on protein expression level of phospho-p65 (p-p65), phospho-extracellular regulated protein kinase (p-ERK), and phosphor-p38 (p-p38) in LPS-stimulated RAW264.7 cells. Cells were pretreated with NAB for 1 h and then stimulated with LPS (100 ng/mL) for 18 h. The total protein of the cells was collected, and the expression levels of p-p65 (**A**), p-ERK (**B**), and p-p38 (**C**) were analyzed with Western blotting. The density ratio of the LPS group (model control) was set to 1. Results are expressed as the mean ± SEM of three independent experiments. * $P < 0.05$ and *** $P < 0.001$ vs. LPS-stimulated cells.

3. Discussion

As described before, macrophages play an important role in inflammation as they are able to release different kinds of cytokines to ignite inflammatory reactions [9]. The LPS-stimulated RAW264.7 macrophages is a kind of classical inflammatory cell model widely used in evaluating the anti-inflammatory effect and mechanisms of many natural products derived from Chinese medicines [25]. Therefore, we chose the LPS-stimulated RAW264.7 cells as the cell model in this study. Dexamethasone (DEX) and sulforaphane (SFN) were chosen as the positive control drugs in this study. DEX is a classic anti-inflammatory drug that is widely used in the clinic [26]. It is a steroidal anti-inflammatory drug that has been widely used to treat rheumatoid arthritic knees [9], pneumonia [27], and bronchiolitis [11]. SFN is a kind of drug that has been confirmed as a Nrf2 activator. It is a natural isothiocyanate, and it has been proved that SFN could suppress LPS-induced inflammation in mouse peritoneal macrophages through activating the Nrf2 pathway and upregulating the HO-1 expression [28]. Moreover, SFN inhibited the expression of some inflammatory mediators, including TNF-α, IL-1β, and IL-6 [29], through activating the Nrf2 pathway. So, DEX was chosen as the positive control drug in the study to evaluate the anti-inflammatory activity of NAB, and SFN was chosen as the positive control in the study to evaluate the Nrf2 pathway-related mechanism of NAB.

In this study, we firstly evaluated the cytotoxicity of NAB and found that NAB had no significant cytotoxicity to LPS-stimulated RAW264.7 cells at the concentrations lower than 20 µM (Figure 2A,B). Thus, we selected the concentrations of NAB ranging from 2.5 µM to 10 µM to examine the anti-inflammatory activity of NAB in the LPS-stimulated RAW264.7 cells. Then, following evaluation of the effect of NAB on the production of NO and PGE$_2$ by the LPS-induced RAW264.7 cells, we examined the effect of NAB on the expression of iNOS and COX-2 by LPS-stimulated RAW264.7 macrophages, since iNOS and COX-2 are the enzymes responsible for the production of NO and PGE$_2$, respectively. After that, the expression level of HO-1 in LPS-stimulated RAW264.7 cells was detected with the treatment of NAB, because HO-1 is one of the regulating factors of the expression of iNOS. As the translocation of Nrf2 protein into the cell nucleus mediates the expression of HO-1, the migration level of Nrf2 protein in the RAW264.7 macrophages was evaluated. Moreover, as the macrophages release cytokines (e.g., TNF-α, IL-1β, and IL-6) [30] to promote and encourage the development and progression of inflammation in vivo, these inflammatory mediators were detected in this study.

NO and PGE$_2$ are two of the most important inflammatory mediators that participate in inflammatory processes. The inflammation and the exposure of tissue cells to bacterial products such as LPS, lipoteichoic acid (LTA), peptidoglycans, and bacterial DNA or whole bacteria will induce the high expression of iNOS and then enhance the production of NO. In these situations, the NO forms peroxynitrite, which acts as a cytotoxic molecule, resists invading microorganisms, and acts as a killer [31]. However, it has been reported that in aseptic inflammation, the iNOS expression and NO formation would also be induced in human macrophages; for example, in rheumatoid arthritis and osteoarthritis [32]. In these bacteria-free inflammatory processes, the synthesis of NO can be an important factor that helps maintain the inflammatory and osteolytic processes [13]. PGE$_2$ mediates the increasing of arterial dilation and microvascular permeability. This action will cause blood to flow into the inflamed tissue and thus causes redness and edema [33]. COX-2 belongs to the regulatory enzymes involved in the production of PGE$_2$, and it also regulates the synthesis of prostaglandin I$_2$ (PGI$_2$, also called as prostacyclin) and thromboxaneA$_2$ (TXA$_2$) [34]. It is known that TXA$_2$ is the major cyclooxygenase product in platelets. It is also a potent vasoconstrictor and can stimulate the aggregation of platelets in vitro. PGI$_2$ is produced and synthesized in vascular endothelial cells. It is a vasodilator and inhibitor of platelets [34]. It has been proven that the inhibition of COX-2 may break the balance between PGI$_2$ and TXA$_2$, leading to cardiovascular risks [35]. Fortunately, in this study, the results show that NAB only targets and inhibits NO and iNOS and does not affect the expression of COX-2 (Figure 2C,D and Figure 3). Thus, NAB may have low cardiovascular side effects compared with DEX. However, the results showed that the protein expression level of iNOS was inhibited by the concentration of 2.5 µM NAB, while the mRNA expression level was not; thus, it was considered that NAB may affect the translation process of iNOS from gene to protein.

TNF-α, IL-1β, and IL-6 belong to the inflammatory cytokines and are can also be involved in inflammatory processes [36]. In this research, all these inflammation cytokines and regulatory enzymes (iNOS and COX-2) were upregulated by the LPS stimulation (Figures 3 and 6). Then, the increases of these inflammatory mediators were significantly inhibited by NAB (Figure 6). More importantly, the inhibitory effect of NAB on the mRNA expression level of TNF-α is better than that of SFN, meaning that NAB has obvious anti-inflammatory activity in LPS-stimulated RAW264.7 macrophage cells.

Usually, the inflammatory processes are accompanied by the activation of the NF-κB pathway, which also promotes the expression of inflammatory mediators in macrophages [37]. Previous research has shown that the production of inflammatory cytokines is related to the LPS-induced activation of the NF-κB pathway [38]. The mitogen-activated protein kinases (MAPK) pathway also plays an critical role in inflammatory responses [39]. The activation of both NF-κB and MAPK signaling pathways is involved in the development of inflammation [25]. Therefore, under normal circumstances, inhibiting NF-κB and MAPK signaling pathways is considered as an effective way to combat inflammatory reaction. The activation of NF-κB resulted in the phosphorylation of nuclear factor of kappa light polypeptide gene enhancer in B-cells inhibitor, alpha (IκBα), IκB kinase-α (IKKα), and p65, leading to the transcription of inflammatory genes and the expression of inflammatory proteins [40]. The activation of the MAPK pathway results in the phosphorylation of p38, c-Jun N-terminal kinase (JNK), and ERK [41], which may promote proinflammatory cytokine production [42]. Some reports showed that the deactivation of NF-κB and MAPK pathways in RAW264.7 cells leads to the inhibition of LPS-induced NO, PGE_2, iNOS, COX-2, TNF-α, and IL-6 production [25,43]. Other studies have reported that the extracts of *N. chinensis* inhibited the p38 MAPK pathway to inhibit the expression of inflammatory mediators [44]. To study the anti-inflammatory mechanism of NAB, we first investigated the effect of NAB on the activation of the NF-κB and MAPK pathways in LPS-stimulated RAW264.7 cells. However, the results showed that NAB did not inhibit the activation of the NF-κB and MAPK pathways (Figure 7), so NAB may not act on the NF-κB and MAPK pathways to exert its anti-inflammatory effects.

The activation of the Nrf2 pathway is another possible way to prevent LPS-induced transcriptional upregulation of proinflammatory cytokines, including TNF-α, IL-1β, and IL-6 [45]. These inflammatory cytokines were decreased by the Nrf2-dependent antioxidant genes HO-1 and NQO-1. In Nrf2-knockout mice, the mRNA and protein levels of COX-2, iNOS, IL-6, and TNF-α increased [46] and the anti-inflammatory effect also disappeared [47]. Since the current result showed that NAB inhibited TNF-α, IL-1β, and IL-6 obviously (Figure 6), it was hypothesized that NAB may activate the Nrf2 pathway to exert its anti-inflammatory effect.

In this study, it was found that NAB inhibited the expression of the inflammatory protein iNOS (Figure 3A,C) and inflammatory cytokines including NO, TNF-α, and IL-6 (Figures 2C and 6), accompanied by the increase of antioxidant protein HO-1 (Figure 4). More importantly, the study found that NAB had no inhibitory effect on COX-2 (Figure 3B,D) and PGE_2 (Figure 2D), suggesting that NAB has potential to be developed as a selective iNOS/NO inhibitor, a kind of anti-inflammatory drug that helps to reduce airway inflammatory responses, such as the compound 1400W [48], and relieve the pain caused by mechanical damage, such as the compound AR-C102222 [49]. Further, since NAB did not affect the expressions of COX-2 and PGE_2, it is safer than NSAIDs, which inhibit PGE_2 to exert their anti-inflammatory effect through inhibiting COX-2 expression. At the same time, our study found that the inhibitory effect of NAB on NO is very similar to that of the positive control drug DEX, suggesting that NAB has great development value in future study.

Oxidative or nitrosative stress, cytokines, and other mediators may cause the cells to overproduce HO-1 to protect themselves [22,50]. The induction of HO-1 reduces the production of inflammatory mediators and modulates the inflammatory process [51]. HO-1 can be rapidly induced by various oxidative response-inducing agents, including LPS [22]. The current results also show that LPS increased the level of HO-1 slightly, but compared with the LPS group, NAB further increased the level of HO-1 protein dramatically (Figure 4). The NO production induced by LPS was inhibited by the high expression of HO-1 [52]. In this study, NAB reduced NO production while increasing HO-1 expression (Figure 4); the current results are consistent with the finding that the high expression of HO-1 can inhibit LPS-induced NO production [52].

Another factor that is related to the expression of HO-1 is the expression of interleukin (IL)-10. IL-10 induces the phosphorylation of Janus Kinase (Jak) 1 and the activation of signal transducer and activator of transcription (STAT)-1 and STAT-3 [53]. Also, IL-10 activates phosphatidylinositol-3 kinase (PI3K), which is involved in the proliferative effects of IL-10 [54]. It has been proven that IL-10 can induce the expression of HO-1 [55]. Also, it has been reported that the IL-10-induced activation of

STAT-3 and PI3K was associated with the expression of HO-1 [56]. Thus, further study will focus on the role of NAB in the expression of IL-10 and the associated production such as STAT-1 and PI3K.

Taken together, the results suggest that the activation of the Nrf2/HO-1 pathway is the potential mechanism by which NAB exerts its anti-inflammatory effects against LPS-activated inflammation (Figure 8).

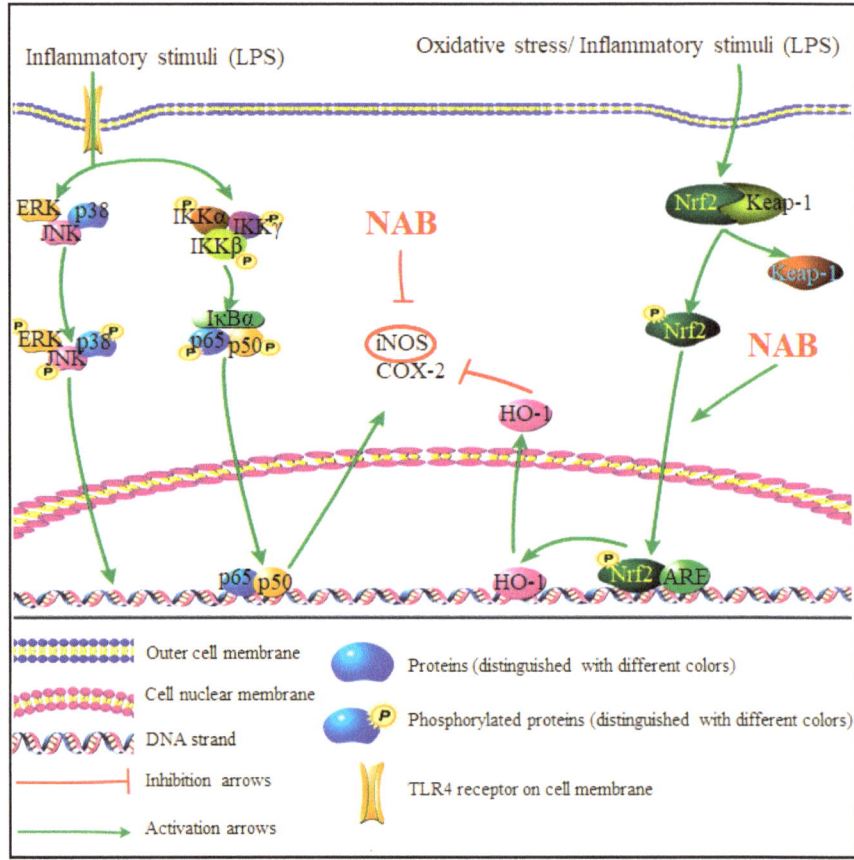

Figure 8. Proposed molecular mechanisms underlying the inhibitory effect of NAB on the LPS-activated RAW264.7 macrophages. NAB activates the Nrf2 pathway, leading to the high expression of HO-1, then contributing to the anti-inflammatory effects in LPS-activated RAW264.7 macrophages. Abbreviations in the figure: NAB, nardochinoid B; TLR4, Toll-like receptors; ERK, extracellular regulated protein kinase; JNK, c-Jun N-terminal kinase; HO-1, heme oxygenase (HO)-1; Nrf2, nuclear factor erythroid 2-related factor 2; Keap-1, Kelch-like ECH-associated protein-1; ARE, antioxidant response element; iNOS, inducible nitric oxide synthase; COX-2, cyclooxygenase-2; IKK$\alpha/\beta/\gamma$, IκB kinase $\alpha/\beta/\gamma$; IκBα, inhibitor of nuclear factor kappa-B kinase α.

4. Materials and Methods

4.1. Materials

Nardochinoid B (NAB) (Figure 1) (HPLC purity >98%) was provided by the Institute of Traditional Chinese Medicine and Natural Products, Jinan University (Guangzhou, China). Dimethyl sulfoxide (DMSO) (Sigma, Cat. No. D2625, St. Louis, MO, USA) was used to dissolve the NAB powder to give a stock solution of 30 mM concentration. Lipopolysaccharide (LPS), dexamethasone (DEX), and sulforaphane (SFN) were purchased from Sigma Chemical Co. (St. Louis, MO, USA). Antibodies to iNOS [57], COX-2 [58], heme oxygenase (HO)-1 [58], Nrf2 [18], p-p65 [18], p-p38 [18], and phospho-extracellular regulated protein kinases (p-ERK) [18] were obtained from Cell Signaling Technology (Boston, MA, USA). Antibodies to β-actin and laminin B1 [18] were from Santa Cruz Biotechnology (Santa Cruz, CA, USA). Antibody to α-tubulin [18] was from Sigma Chemical Co. (St. Louis, MO, USA). The secondary antibodies for Western blot were from Li-COR Biotechnology (Lincoln, NE, USA). ELISA kits for IL-1β, IL-6, and TNF-α was from eBioscience (eBioscience, Inc., San Diego, CA, USA). ELISA kit for PGE$_2$ was from Cayman Chemical (Cayman Chemical, Ann Arbor, MI, United States). The nitric oxide (NO) production level was measured by a Griess Reagent System kit, which was obtained from Promega Corporation (Madison, WI, USA).

4.2. Cell Culture

The immortalized mouse macrophage cell line RAW264.7 was obtained from the American Type Culture Collection (ATCC, Manassas, VA, USA). Dulbecco's modified Eagle's medium (DMEM) supplement with 10% heat-inactivated fetal bovine serum (FBS) (Gibco BRL Co, Grand Island, NY, USA), penicillin G (100 units/mL), streptomycin (100 mg/mL), and L-glutamine (2 mM) (Gibco BRL Co, Grand Island, NY, USA) was chosen to maintain the cells. The cells were incubated at 37 °C in a humidified atmosphere containing 5% CO$_2$ and 95% air.

4.3. Cell Viability Assay

The cells were seeded in 96-well plates at the density of 1.4×10^4 cells/well and were incubated for 24 h. After incubation, the cells were pretreated with different concentrations (1.25, 2.5, 5, 10, 20, and 40 µM) of NAB for 1 h. Then, the cells were stimulated with or without LPS (100 ng/mL) for 18 h. Cytotoxicity was analyzed by using MTT assay. MTT solution (5 g/L) was added to each well and incubated for 4 h at 37 °C. Then, 100 µL 10% sodium dodecyl sulfate (SDS)–HCl solution was added to the wells and incubated for another 18 h. The optical density was read at 570 nm (reference, 650 nm) using a microplate UV/VIS spectrophotometer (Tecan, Mannedorf, Switzerland). The control group, in which the cells were not treated with compounds and LPS, was set as 100% for its cell viability.

4.4. Determination of NO, PGE$_2$, TNF-α, IL-1β, and IL-6 Production

The cells were plated in 24-well plates at the density of 8×10^4 cells/well and were incubated for 24 h. Then, the cells were pretreated with different concentrations (2.5, 5, and 10 µM) of NAB and positive control drug (dexamethasone, DEX, or sulforaphane, SFN) for 1 h, respectively. LPS (100 ng/mL) was added to the culture medium and the cells were stimulated with LPS for another 18 h. After incubating the cells with drugs and LPS, the cells and the medium were collected and stored at −80 °C. NO production was measured as the nitrite concentration in the medium by the Griess reagent (Promega, Madison, WI, USA). The TNF-α, IL-1β, and IL-6 concentrations in the culture medium were measured by using the enzyme-linked immunosorbent assay (ELISA) kit (eBioscience, Inc., San Diego, CA, USA), and the PGE$_2$ concentration in the cell supernatant was detected by the ELISA kit from Cayman Chemical (Cayman Chemical, Ann Arbor, MI, United States).

4.5. Protein Preparation and Western Blot Analysis

The cells in 24-well plates were collected after being treated with drugs and LPS for 6 h (for HO-1 proteins) or 18 h (for other inflammation-related proteins). RIPA lysis buffer (Cell Signaling technology, Boston, MA, USA) was mixed with 1× protease inhibitor (Roche Applied Science, Mannheim, Germany) and the mixture was used to lyse the collected cells to extract total protein. For the measurement of Nrf2 protein, cells were treated with NAB (10 µM) and SFN (5 µM) for 6 h, and then the NE-PER Nuclear and Cytoplasmic Extraction Reagents (Thermo Scientific, Rockford, IL, USA) were used to extract the cytoplasmic and nuclear extracts. The protein concentration was determined with the Bio-Rad Protein

Assay (Bio-Rad, Hercules, CA, USA). Thirty micrograms of these protein samples was resolved by 6% (for Nrf2 measurement), 10% (for iNOS, COX-2, p-p65, p-ERK, and p-p38 measurements), and 12% (for HO-1 measurement) sodium dodecyl sulfate polyacrylamide gel electrophoresis (SDS-PAGE). After electrophoresis separation, the proteins were transferred from the gel onto nitrocellulose membrane (GE Healthcare Life Sciences, Buckinghamshire, UK). Then, the membrane was blocked with 5% skimmed milk and then incubated with the primary antibodies (iNOS, COX-2, HO-1, Nrf-2, p-ERK, p-p65, and p-p38) and mouse antibodies specific for β-actin (for iNOS, COX-2, HO-1, and p-p65 measurements), α-tubulin (for p-ERK and p-p38 measurements), and laminin B1 (for Nrf2 measurement) at 4 °C overnight. After that, the membrane was incubated with IRDye 800CW goat anti-mouse IgG (H + L) or IRDye 800CW goat anti-rabbit IgG (H + L) secondary antibodies (Li-COR, Lincoln, NE, USA) at room temperature for 1 h. The antigen–antibody complex bands were examined with an Odyssey CLxImager (Li-COR, Lincoln, NE, USA) and the protein expression level was quantified by using Odyssey v3.0 software (Li-COR, USA). The density ratios of iNOS, COX-2, HO-1, Nrf-2, p-ERK, p-p65, and p-p38 to β-actin, α-tubulin, or laminin B1 were calculated for evaluating the anti-inflammatory effect and underlying mechanism of NAB.

4.6. RNA Extraction and Quantitative Real-Time Polymerase Chain Reaction (qRT-PCR)

The cells in 24-well plates were collected after being treated by tested drugs and LPS for 6 h (for the HO-1 test) or 18 h (for iNOS, COX-2, TNF-α, IL-1β, and IL-6 tests). Total RNA was isolated from cells with the NucleoSpin RNA kit (Macherey-Nagel, Düren, Germany). The total RNA concentration for each sample was detected by using a NanoDrop spectrophotometer (Thermo Scientific, USA). One microgram of total RNA of each sample were used for reverse transcription into cDNA by using the reverse transcription Universal cDNA Master Kit (Roche Applied Science, Germany). Target RNA levels were determined by using ViiATM 7 real-time PCR, where 1 μL cDNA, 2 μL primers, 10 μL SYBER Green PCR Master Mix (Roche, Mannheim, Germany), and 7 μL PCR-grade water were used in the PCR reaction. The denaturation step of the PCR reactions was set to 95 °C for 10 min. Forty cycles were repeated at 95 °C for 15 s and 60 °C for 1 min. The $2^{-\Delta\Delta Ct}$ cycle threshold method was used to normalize the relative mRNA expression levels to the internal control. The primers used in this study are listed in Table 1.

Table 1. The primers used in this study.

Target Gene	Primer Sequences
β-actin_F	5'-CGGTTCCGATGCCCTGAGGCTCTT-3'
β-actin_R	5'-CGTCACACTTCATGATGGAATTGA-3'
iNOS_F	5'-CAGCACAGGAAATGTTTCAGC-3'
iNOS_R	5'-TAGCCAGCGTACCGGATGA-3'
COX-2_F	5'-TTTGGTCTGGTGCCTGGTC-3'
COX-2_R	5'-CTGCTGGTTTGGAATAGTTGCTC-3'
TNF-α_F	5'-TATGGCTCAGGGTCCAACTC-3'
TNF-α_R	5'-CTCCCTTTGCAGAACTCAGG-3'
IL-6_F	5'-GGTGACAACCACGGCCTTCCC-3'
IL-6_R	5'-AAGCCTCCGACTTGTGAAGTGGT-3'
HO-1_F	5'-CCCACCAAGTTCAAACAGCTC-3'
HO-1_R	5'-AGGAAGGCGGTCTTAGCCTC-3'
IL-1β_F	5'-TTGACGGACCCCAAAAGATG-3'
IL-1β_R	5'-AGAAGGTGCTCATGTCCTCA-3'

4.7. Data Analysis

All data are presented as the mean ± SEM of three independent experiments. The statistical analyses for these results were carried out with GraphPad Prism 7 (GraphPad Software, San Diego, CA, USA) by using one-way ANOVA followed by post-hoc analysis with Tukey's multiple comparison

5. Conclusions

From the above study, it has been proven that the compound NAB inhibited the activation of LPS-induced RAW264.7 cells. It is clear that NAB increased the expression of HO-1 to reduce NO production. Also, inflammatory mediators, including NO, TNF-α, IL-1β, and IL-6, were inhibited by the pretreatment of NAB. More importantly, the study found that NAB has no inhibitory effect on COX-2, suggesting that it may be safer than NSAIDs. At the same time, our study found that the inhibitory effect of NAB on NO is similar to that of the positive control drug DEX, suggesting that NAB has great potential for future drug development. In conclusion, NAB may be a potential HO-1 inducer for the treatment of inflammatory diseases.

As described previously, the results suggested that NAB exerted its anti-inflammatory effects against LPS-induced inflammation via activating the Nrf2/HO-1 pathway (Figure 8). Also, the potential unique anti-inflammatory mechanism of NAB provides a new therapeutic solution for oxidative damage- and inflammation-related diseases. Although more experiments are needed in vivo and in vitro to verify the effect and mechanism of NAB in future research, this study helps to provide a potential treatment mechanism of *Nardostachys chinensis* and evidence for the use of this recently discovered natural compound in the treatment of diseases related to inflammation and oxidative stress.

Author Contributions: Conceptualization, H.Z. and Z.-Q.L.; methodology, H.Z., Z.-Q.L., J.M., Y.X., P.L., J.-X.L., Y.D., and X.-S.Y.; formal analysis, Y.-D.Y. and H.Z.; investigation, Y.-D.Y., J.-F.L., C.-K.L., Y.Y., and X.-Y.S.; resources, Y.D. and X.-S.Y.; data curation, Y.-D.Y. and H.Z.; writing—original draft preparation, Y.-D.Y. and H.Z.; supervision, H.Z., Z.-Q.L., Y.D., and X.-S.Y.; funding acquisition, H.Z. and Z.-Q.L.

Funding: This research was supported by the Joint Research Fund for Overseas Chinese Scholars and Scholars in Hong Kong and Macao of the National Natural Science Fund of China (Project No.: 81628016) and the Macao Science and Technology Development Fund (Project No: 062/2017/A2, 0027/2017/AMJ).

Acknowledgments: The authors would like to thank the State Key Laboratory of Quality Research in Chinese Medicine (Macau University of Science and Technology) for their instrumental support to the study.

Conflicts of Interest: The authors declare no conflict of interest.

Abbreviations

Nardochinoid B, NAB; nonsteroidal anti-inflammatory drugs, NSAIDs; dexamethasone, DEX; sulforaphane, SFN; lipopolysaccharide, LPS; lipoteichoic acid, LTA; inducible nitric oxide synthase, iNOS; cyclooxygenases, COXs; cyclooxygenase-2, COX-2; heme oxygenase-1, HO-1; nuclear factor erythroid 2-related factor 2, Nrf2; phospho-p65, p-p65; phospho-p38, p-p38; phospho-extracellular regulated protein kinase, p-ERK; nuclear factor of kappa light polypeptide gene enhancer in B-cells inhibitor, alpha, IκBα; IκB kinase-α, IKKα; c-Jun N-terminal kinase, JNK; Janus Kinase, Jak; signal transducer and activator of transcription, STAT; phosphatidylinositol-3 kinase, PI3K; nitric oxide, NO; prostaglandin E_2, PGE_2; prostaglandin I_2, PGI_2; thromboxane A_2, TXA_2; interleukin-1β, IL-1β; interleukin-6, IL-6; tumor necrosis factor alpha, TNF-α; nuclear factor-κB, NF-κB; mitogen-activated protein kinase, MAPK; enzyme-linked immunosorbent assay, ELISA; quantitative real-time polymerase chain reaction, qRT-PCR.

References

1. Ashley, N.T.; Weil, Z.M.; Nelson, R.J. Inflammation: Mechanisms, costs, and natural variation. *Annu. Rev. Ecol. Evol. Syst.* **2012**, *43*, 385–406. [CrossRef]
2. Al-Duaij, A.; De Brito, F.; Sedgwick, A.; Scott, D.; Willoughby, D. Susceptibility of cartilage to damage by immunological inflammation. *Int. Arch. Allergy Immunol.* **1986**, *80*, 435–437. [CrossRef]
3. Rao, P.; Knaus, E.E. Evolution of nonsteroidal anti-inflammatory drugs (nsaids): Cyclooxygenase (cox) inhibition and beyond. *J. Pharm. Pharm. Sci.* **2008**, *11*, 81s–110s. [CrossRef] [PubMed]
4. Koeberle, A.; Werz, O. Inhibitors of the microsomal prostaglandin e2 synthase-1 as alternative to non steroidal anti-inflammatory drugs (nsaids)-a critical review. *Curr. Med. Chem.* **2009**, *16*, 4274–4296. [CrossRef] [PubMed]
5. Frangogiannis, N.G.; Smith, C.W.; Entman, M.L. The inflammatory response in myocardial infarction. *Cardiovasc. Res.* **2002**, *53*, 31–47. [CrossRef]

6. Chamorro, Á. Role of inflammation in stroke and atherothrombosis. *Cerebrovasc. Dis.* **2004**, *17*, 1–5. [CrossRef] [PubMed]
7. Dorfmüller, P.; Perros, F.; Balabanian, K.; Humbert, M. Inflammation in pulmonary arterial hypertension. *Eur. Respir. J.* **2003**, *22*, 358–363. [CrossRef]
8. Anker, S.D.; von Haehling, S. Inflammatory mediators in chronic heart failure: An overview. *Heart* **2004**, *90*, 464–470. [CrossRef]
9. Linde, A.; Mosier, D.; Blecha, F.; Melgarejo, T. Innate immunity and inflammation—New frontiers in comparative cardiovascular pathology. *Cardiovasc. Res.* **2007**, *73*, 26–36. [CrossRef]
10. Parameswaran, N.; Patial, S. Tumor necrosis factor-α signaling in macrophages. *Crit. Rev. Eukaryot. Gene Expr.* **2010**, *20*, 87–103. [CrossRef]
11. Marini, M.; Vittori, E.; Hollemborg, J.; Mattoli, S. Expression of the potent inflammatory cytokines, granulocyte-macrophage-colony-stimulating factor and interleukin-6 and interleukin-8, in bronchial epithelial cells of patients with asthma. *J. Allergy Clin. Immunol.* **1992**, *89*, 1001–1009. [CrossRef]
12. Humes, J.L.; Bonney, R.J.; Pelus, L.; Dahlgren, M.E.; Sadowski, S.J.; Kuehl, F.A.; Davies, P. Macrophages synthesise and release prostaglandins in response to inflammatory stimuli. *Nature* **1977**, *269*, 149–151. [CrossRef] [PubMed]
13. Moilanen, E.; Moilanen, T.; Knowles, R.; Charles, I.; Kadoya, Y.; Al-Saffar, N.; Revell, P.A.; Moncada, S. Nitric oxide synthase is expressed in human macrophages during foreign body inflammation. *Am. J. Pathol.* **1997**, *150*, 881–887. [PubMed]
14. Miller, B.E.; Krasney, P.A.; Gauvin, D.M.; Holbrook, K.B.; Koonz, D.J.; Abruzzese, R.V.; Miller, R.E.; Pagani, K.A.; Dolle, R.E.; Ator, M.A. Inhibition of mature il-1β production in murine macrophages and a murine model of inflammation by win 67694, an inhibitor of il-1β converting enzyme. *J. Immunol.* **1995**, *154*, 1331–1338. [PubMed]
15. Coussens, L.M.; Werb, Z. Inflammation and cancer. *Nature* **2002**, *420*, 860–867. [CrossRef]
16. Lu, C.-L.; Zhu, Y.-F.; Hu, M.-M.; Wang, D.-M.; Xu, X.-J.; Lu, C.-J.; Zhu, W. Optimization of astilbin extraction from the rhizome of smilax glabra, and evaluation of its anti-inflammatory effect and probable underlying mechanism in lipopolysaccharide-induced raw264. 7 macrophages. *Molecules* **2015**, *20*, 625–644. [CrossRef]
17. Hwang, J.S.; Lee, S.A.; Hong, S.S.; Han, X.H.; Lee, C.; Lee, D.; Lee, C.-K.; Hong, J.T.; Kim, Y.; Lee, M.K. Inhibitory constituents of nardostachys chinensis on nitric oxide production in raw 264.7 macrophages. *Bioorg. Med. Chem. Lett.* **2012**, *22*, 706–708. [CrossRef]
18. Luo, J.-F.; Shen, X.-Y.; Lio, C.K.; Dai, Y.; Cheng, C.-S.; Liu, J.-X.; Yao, Y.-D.; Yu, Y.; Xie, Y.; Luo, P. Activation of nrf2/ho-1 pathway by nardochinoid c inhibits inflammation and oxidative stress in lipopolysaccharide-stimulated macrophages. *Front. Pharmacol.* **2018**, *9*, 911. [CrossRef]
19. Shen, X.Y.; Yu, Y.; Chen, G.D.; Zhou, H.; Luo, J.F.; Zuo, Y.H.; Yao, X.S.; Dai, Y. Six new sesquiterpenoids from nardostachys chinensis batal. *Fitoterapia* **2017**, *119*, 75–82. [CrossRef]
20. Shen, X.-Y.; Qin, D.-P.; Zhou, H.; Luo, J.-F.; Yao, Y.-D.; Lio, C.-K.; Li, H.-B.; Dai, Y.; Yu, Y.; Yao, X.-S. Nardochinoids a–c, three dimeric sesquiterpenoids with specific fused-ring skeletons from nardostachys chinensis. *Org. Lett.* **2018**, *20*, 5813–5816. [CrossRef]
21. Kim, J.; Cha, Y.-N.; Surh, Y.-J. A protective role of nuclear factor-erythroid 2-related factor-2 (nrf2) in inflammatory disorders. *Mutat. Res./Fundam. Mol. Mech. Mutagenesis* **2010**, *690*, 12–23. [CrossRef] [PubMed]
22. Chung, S.W.; Liu, X.; Macias, A.A.; Baron, R.M.; Perrella, M.A. Heme oxygenase-1–derived carbon monoxide enhances the host defense response to microbial sepsis in mice. *J. Clin. Investig.* **2008**, *118*, 239–247. [CrossRef] [PubMed]
23. Gold, R.; Kappos, L.; Arnold, D.L.; Bar-Or, A.; Giovannoni, G.; Selmaj, K.; Tornatore, C.; Sweetser, M.T.; Yang, M.; Sheikh, S.I. Placebo-controlled phase 3 study of oral bg-12 for relapsing multiple sclerosis. *N. Engl. J. Med.* **2012**, *367*, 1098–1107. [CrossRef] [PubMed]
24. Deeks, E.D. Nivolumab: A review of its use in patients with malignant melanoma. *Drugs* **2014**, *74*, 1233–1239. [CrossRef]
25. Liu, J.; Tang, J.; Zuo, Y.; Yu, Y.; Luo, P.; Yao, X.; Dong, Y.; Wang, P.; Liu, L.; Zhou, H. Stauntoside b inhibits macrophage activation by inhibiting nf-κb and erk mapk signalling. *Pharmacol. Res.* **2016**, *111*, 303–315. [CrossRef]

26. Kim, M.-J.; Kim, S.-J.; Kim, S.S.; Lee, N.H.; Hyun, C.-G. Hypochoeris radicata attenuates lps-induced inflammation by suppressing p38, erk, and jnk phosphorylation in raw 264.7 macrophages. *EXCLI J.* **2014**, *13*, 123–136.
27. Meijvis, S.C.A.; Hardeman, H.; Remmelts, H.H.F.; Heijligenberg, R.; Rijkers, G.T.; van Velzen-Blad, H.; Voorn, G.P.; van de Garde, E.M.W.; Endeman, H.; Grutters, J.C.; et al. Dexamethasone and length of hospital stay in patients with community-acquired pneumonia: A randomised, double-blind, placebo-controlled trial. *Lancet* **2011**, *377*, 2023–2030. [CrossRef]
28. Lin, W.; Wu, R.T.; Wu, T.; Khor, T.O.; Wang, H.; Kong, A.N. Sulforaphane suppressed lps-induced inflammation in mouse peritoneal macrophages through nrf2 dependent pathway. *Biochem. Pharmacol.* **2008**, *76*, 967–973. [CrossRef] [PubMed]
29. Brandenburg, L.-O.; Kipp, M.; Lucius, R.; Pufe, T.; Wruck, C.J. Sulforaphane suppresses lps-induced inflammation in primary rat microglia. *Inflamm. Res.* **2010**, *59*, 443–450. [CrossRef]
30. Fujiwara, N.; Kobayashi, K. Macrophages in inflammation. *Curr. Drug Targets-Inflamm. Allergy* **2005**, *4*, 281–286. [CrossRef]
31. Hui-Yi, L.; Shing-Chuan, S.; Yen-Chou, C. Anti-inflammatory effect of heme oxygenase 1: Glycosylation and nitric oxide inhibition in macrophages. *J. Cell. Physiol.* **2005**, *202*, 579–590.
32. Mcinnes, I.B.; Leung, B.P.; Field, M.; Wei, X.Q.; Huang, F.P.; Sturrock, R.D.; Kinninmonth, A.; Weidner, J.; Mumford, R.; Liew, F.Y. Production of nitric oxide in the synovial membrane of rheumatoid and osteoarthritis patients. *J. Exp. Med.* **1996**, *184*, 1519. [CrossRef] [PubMed]
33. Ricciotti, E.; FitzGerald, G.A. Prostaglandins and inflammation. *Arterioscler. Thromb. Vasc. Biol.* **2011**, *31*, 986–1000. [CrossRef] [PubMed]
34. Heller, A.; Koch, T.; Schmeck, J.; van Ackern, K. Lipid mediators in inflammatory disorders. *Drugs* **1998**, *55*, 487–496. [CrossRef] [PubMed]
35. Fitzgerald, G.A.; Pedersen, A.K.; Patrono, C. Analysis of prostacyclin and thromboxane biosynthesis in cardiovascular disease. *Circulation* **1983**, *67*, 1174–1177. [CrossRef]
36. Bradley, J.R. Tnf-mediated inflammatory disease. *J. Pathol.* **2008**, *214*, 149–160. [CrossRef]
37. DiDonato, J.A.; Mercurio, F.; Karin, M. Nf-kappa b and the link between inflammation and cancer. *Immunol. Rev.* **2012**, *246*, 379–400. [CrossRef]
38. Ghosh, S.; Hayden, M.S. New regulators of nf-κb in inflammation. *Nat. Rev. Immunol.* **2008**, *8*, 837–848. [CrossRef]
39. Liu, Y.S.; Shepherd, E.G.; Nelin, L.D. Mapk phosphatases—Regulating the immune response. *Nat. Rev. Immunol.* **2007**, *7*, 202–212. [CrossRef]
40. Ghosh, S.; May, M.J.; Kopp, E.B. Nf-kappa b and rel proteins: Evolutionarily conserved mediators of immune responses. *Annu. Rev. Immunol.* **1998**, *16*, 225–260. [CrossRef]
41. Rao, K.M.K. Map kinase activation in macrophages. *J. Leukoc. Biol.* **2001**, *69*, 3–10. [PubMed]
42. Sun, L.D.; Wang, F.; Dai, F.; Wang, Y.H.; Lin, D.; Zhou, B. Development and mechanism investigation of a new piperlongumine derivative as a potent anti-inflammatory agent. *Biochem. Pharmacol.* **2015**, *95*, 156–169. [CrossRef] [PubMed]
43. Kim, J.-B.; Han, A.-R.; Park, E.-Y.; Kim, J.-Y.; Cho, W.; Lee, J.; Seo, E.-K.; Lee, K.-T. Inhibition of lps-induced inos, cox-2 and cytokines expression by poncirin through the nf-κb inactivation in raw 264.7 macrophage cells. *Biol. Pharm. Bull.* **2007**, *30*, 2345–2351. [CrossRef] [PubMed]
44. Shin, J.Y.; Bae, G.-S.; Choi, S.-B.; Jo, I.-J.; Kim, D.-G.; Lee, D.-S.; An, R.-B.; Oh, H.; Kim, Y.-C.; Shin, Y.K. Anti-inflammatory effect of desoxo-narchinol-a isolated from nardostachys jatamansi against lipopolysaccharide. *Int. Immunopharmacol.* **2015**, *29*, 730–738. [CrossRef] [PubMed]
45. Kobayashi, E.H.; Suzuki, T.; Funayama, R.; Nagashima, T.; Hayashi, M.; Sekine, H.; Tanaka, N.; Moriguchi, T.; Motohashi, H.; Nakayama, K. Nrf2 suppresses macrophage inflammatory response by blocking proinflammatory cytokine transcription. *Nat. Commun.* **2016**, *7*, 11624. [CrossRef] [PubMed]
46. Rojo, A.I.; Innamorato, N.G.; Martín-Moreno, A.M.; De Ceballos, M.L.; Yamamoto, M.; Cuadrado, A. Nrf2 regulates microglial dynamics and neuroinflammation in experimental parkinson's disease. *Glia* **2010**, *58*, 588–598. [CrossRef] [PubMed]
47. Thimmulappa, R.K.; Scollick, C.; Traore, K.; Yates, M.; Trush, M.A.; Liby, K.T.; Sporn, M.B.; Yamamoto, M.; Kensler, T.W.; Biswal, S. Nrf2-dependent protection from lps induced inflammatory response and mortality by cddo-imidazolide. *Biochem. Biophys. Res. Commun.* **2006**, *351*, 883–889. [CrossRef]

48. Koarai, A.; Ichinose, M.; Sugiura, H.; Yamagata, S.; Hattori, T.; Shirato, K. Allergic airway hyperresponsiveness and eosinophil infiltration is reduced by a selective inos inhibitor, 1400w, in mice. *Pulm. Pharmacol. Ther.* **2000**, *13*, 267–275. [CrossRef]
49. Labuda, C.J.; Koblish, M.; Tuthill, P.; Dolle, R.E.; Little, P.J. Antinociceptive activity of the selective inos inhibitor ar-c102222 in rodent models of inflammatory, neuropathic and post-operative pain. *Eur. J. Pain* **2012**, *10*, 505. [CrossRef]
50. Ryter, S.W.; Alam, J.; Choi, A.M. Heme oxygenase-1/carbon monoxide: From basic science to therapeutic applications. *Physiol. Rev.* **2006**, *86*, 583–650. [CrossRef]
51. Alcaraz, M.; Fernandez, P.; Guillen, M. Anti-inflammatory actions of the heme oxygenase-1 pathway. *Curr. Pharm. Des.* **2003**, *9*, 2541–2551. [CrossRef] [PubMed]
52. Lin, H.-Y.; Juan, S.-H.; Shen, S.-C.; Hsu, F.-L.; Chen, Y.-C. Inhibition of lipopolysaccharide-induced nitric oxide production by flavonoids in raw264. 7 macrophages involves heme oxygenase-1. *Biochem. Pharmacol.* **2003**, *66*, 1821–1832. [CrossRef]
53. Finbloom, D.S.; Winestock, K.D. Il-10 induces the tyrosine phosphorylation of tyk2 and jak1 and the differential assembly of stat1 alpha and stat3 complexes in human t cells and monocytes. *J. Immunol.* **1995**, *155*, 1079–1090. [PubMed]
54. Crawley, J.B.; Williams, L.M.; Mander, T.; Brennan, F.M.; Foxwell, B.M. Interleukin-10 stimulation of phosphatidylinositol 3-kinase and p70 s6 kinase is required for the proliferative but not the antiinflammatory effects of the cytokine. *J. Biol. Chem.* **1996**, *271*, 16357–16362. [CrossRef] [PubMed]
55. Lee, T.-S.; Chau, L.-Y. Heme oxygenase-1 mediates the anti-inflammatory effect of interleukin-10 in mice. *Nat. Med.* **2002**, *8*, 240–246. [CrossRef] [PubMed]
56. Ricchetti, G.A.; Williams, L.M.; Foxwell, B.M. Heme oxygenase 1 expression induced by il-10 requires stat-3 and phosphoinositol-3 kinase and is inhibited by lipopolysaccharide. *J. Leukoc. Biol.* **2004**, *76*, 719–726. [CrossRef]
57. Hwang, D.; Kang, M.-j.; Jo, M.J.; Seo, Y.B.; Park, N.G.; Kim, G.-D. Anti-inflammatory activity of β-thymosin peptide derived from pacific oyster (crassostrea gigas) on no and pge2 production by down-regulating nf-κb in lps-induced raw264. 7 macrophage cells. *Mar. Drugs* **2019**, *17*, 129. [CrossRef]
58. Choo, G.S.; Lim, D.P.; Kim, S.M.; Yoo, E.S.; Kim, S.H.; Kim, C.H.; Woo, J.S.; Kim, H.J.; Jung, J.Y. Anti-inflammatory effects of dendropanax morbifera in lipopolysaccharide-stimulated raw264. 7 macrophages and in an animal model of atopic dermatitis. *Mol. Med. Rep.* **2019**, *19*, 2087–2096.

Sample Availability: Samples of the compounds are available from the authors.

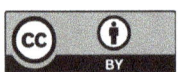

© 2019 by the authors. Licensee MDPI, Basel, Switzerland. This article is an open access article distributed under the terms and conditions of the Creative Commons Attribution (CC BY) license (http://creativecommons.org/licenses/by/4.0/).

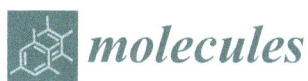

Article

Long-Lasting Anti-Inflammatory and Antinociceptive Effects of Acute Ammonium Glycyrrhizinate Administration: Pharmacological, Biochemical, and Docking Studies

Francesco Maione [1,†], Paola Minosi [2,†], Amalia Di Giannuario [2], Federica Raucci [1], Maria Giovanna Chini [3], Simona De Vita [3], Giuseppe Bifulco [3], Nicola Mascolo [1] and Stefano Pieretti [2,*]

1. Department of Pharmacy, School of Medicine and Surgery, University of Naples Federico II, Via Domenico Montesano 49, 80131 Naples, Italy
2. National Centre for Drug Research and Evaluation, Istituto Superiore di Sanità, Viale Regina Elena 299, 00161 Rome, Italy
3. Department of Pharmacy, University of Salerno, Via Giovanni Paolo II 132, 84084 Fisciano (SA), Italy
* Correspondence: stefano.pieretti@iss.it; Tel.: +39-0649902451
† These authors contributed equally to this work.

Academic Editors: Ericsson Coy-Barrera
Received: 21 May 2019; Accepted: 3 July 2019; Published: 4 July 2019

Abstract: The object of the study was to estimate the long-lasting effects induced by ammonium glycyrrhizinate (AG) after a single administration in mice using animal models of pain and inflammation together with biochemical and docking studies. A single intraperitoneal injection of AG was able to produce anti-inflammatory effects in zymosan-induced paw edema and peritonitis. Moreover, in several animal models of pain, such as the writhing test, the formalin test, and hyperalgesia induced by zymosan, AG administered 24 h before the tests was able to induce a strong antinociceptive effect. Molecular docking studies revealed that AG possesses higher affinity for microsomal prostaglandin E synthase type-2 compared to type-1, whereas it seems to locate better in the binding pocket of cyclooxygenase (COX)-2 compared to COX-1. These results demonstrated that AG induced anti-inflammatory and antinociceptive effects until 24–48 h after a single administration thanks to its ability to bind the COX/mPGEs pathway. Taken together, all these findings highlight the potential use of AG for clinical treatment of pain and/or inflammatory-related diseases.

Keywords: ammonium glycyrrhizinate; docking; long-lasting effect; nociception; inflammation

---

1. Introduction

The most prevalent medical issues strongly affecting people in terms of health and quality of life are acute and chronic pain [1]. Acute and chronic pain are different clinical entities. Acute pain resolves with healing of the underlying injury and it is usually nociceptive, whereas chronic pain is a pathophysiological state connected with the alteration of the peripheral and/or central nervous systems and it is commonly coupled with inflammation caused by tissue trauma, chemical stimuli, and infectious agents. A considerable number of studies have demonstrated that several mediators, including cytokines (Interleukin (IL) -1β, IL-6, IL-17, IL-10, tumor necrosis factor (TNF) -α), chemokines (chemokine (CXCL1), Motif Chemokine Ligand (CCL2), C-X-C chemokine receptor type 2 (CXCR2)), lipid mediators (prostaglandins and leukotrienes) and growth factors (nerve growth factor (NGF), and brain-derived neurotrophic factor (BDNF)), play an important role in inflammatory pain [2].

Two types of treatments can be used to treat inflammatory pain: nonsteroidal anti-inflammatory drugs (NSAIDs) and opioids. Very often there are several side effects, such as gastrointestinal lesions [3] and nephrotoxicity [4], in the case of treatment with NSAIDs, when they are used for a long time, and respiratory depression, tolerance, and physical dependence for opioids [5]. Thus, the identification of new potential targets to treat pain without inducing side effects is crucial.

Glycyrrhiza glabra L., commonly known as liquorice, is a perennial, herbaceous shrub, belonging to the family of Leguminosae. This plant is endemic to Mediterranean countries, such as Greece, Spain, and Southern Italy [6]. Liquorice root has been used since prehistoric times. It contains triterpenoid saponins (3–5%), mainly glycyrrhizin, a mix of calcium and potassium salts of 18β-glycyrrhizic acid (also known as glycyrrhizic or glycyrrhizinic acid and a glycoside of glycyrrhetinic acid) and flavonoids (1–1.5%) [7,8]. Responsible for the anti-inflammatory effect, owing an indirect strengthening of the glucocorticoid activity, are triterpenes [9]. Liquorice is a herb that people have used for thousands of years to treat a variety of ailments, such as dermatitis, psoriasis, and eczema, and shows comparable efficacy to that of corticosteroids [10–12]. In particular, the ammonium salt of glycyrrhizic acid (AG) has strong anti-inflammatory activity [13]. Furthermore it is clear that glycyrrhizin leads to a decrease in inflammatory events due to spinal cord injury (edema, tissue damage, apoptosis, inducible expression of nitric oxide synthase (iNOS)) and nuclear factor kappa-light-chain-enhancer of activated B cells (NFκB) activation, improving the recovery of limb function [14].

Antinociceptive effects were also reported for glycyrrhizic acid and derivatives. Disodium glycyrrhetinic acid hemiphthalate significantly suppressed acetic acid-induced writhing responses in mice, with a potency ~12 times higher than acetylsalicylic acid [15]. Glycyrrhizin in mice significantly inhibited the nociception induced by acetic acid and formalin, downregulating the expression levels of TNF-α, IL-6, iNOS, and COX-2 [16]. Recent evidence confirm the anti- inflammatory and antinociceptive effectiveness of glycyrrhizin and suggest that these effects depend upon the glycyrrhizin inhibition of microglial high-mobility group box 1 protein (HMGB1) [17].

The above-mentioned activities were observed in a short time range after administration of AG and AG derivates. Therefore, in the present study, we investigated the long-lasting anti-inflammatory and antinociceptive effects of AG after a single administration and we have explored its mechanism of action by biochemical and molecular docking studies.

2. Results

2.1. Edema Induced by Zymosan

In animals treated with vehicle (Hepes, 10 mL/kg, i.p.) 10 min before zymosan, we discovered a rise in paw volume that achieved the maximal value 3–4 h after the injection, followed by a slight reduction in the following 48 h (Figure 1). In this set of experiments, we noticed significant differences in the behavioral responses between treatments ($F_{2,33} = 16.30$, $p < 0.0001$) and in the time elapsed after zymosan administration ($F_{5,165} = 38.59$, $p < 0.0001$). The i.p. administration of AG at the dose of 50 mg/kg 10 min before zymosan generated a considerable reduction of paw edema induced by zymosan injection, from 1 to 3 h after zymosan injection (Figure 1). The i.p. administration of AG at the dose of 150 mg/kg induced a robust reduction of paw edema starting from 1 h and lasting for the full course of treatment (Figure 1).

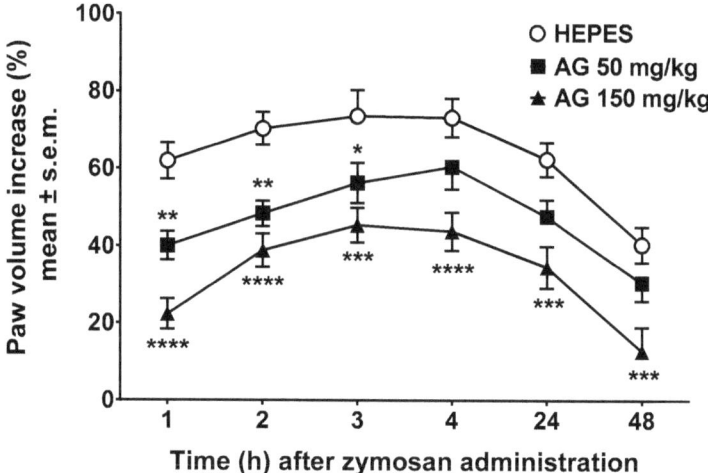

Figure 1. Zymosan-induced paw edema. Effects induced by vehicle (Hepes, 10 mL/kg, intraperitoneally (i.p.)) and ammonium glycyrrhizate (AG, 50 or 150 mg/kg, i.p.) administered 10 min before zymosan (2.5% w/v in saline, 20 µL/paw). * denotes $p < 0.05$, ** denotes $p < 0.01$, *** denotes $p < 0.001$ and **** denotes $p < 0.0001$ vs. Vehicle. $n = 12$.

2.2. Writhing Test

The antinociceptive effect of AG in acetic acid writhing test is shown in Figure 2. Statistical analysis revealed significant differences between treatments ($F_{2,24} = 17.69$, $p < 0.0001$). In this test, AG administered i.p. at the dose of 50 mg/kg reduced writhes induced by acetic acid. Severe inhibition of the number of writhes was discovered when AG was administered at the dose of 150 mg/kg.

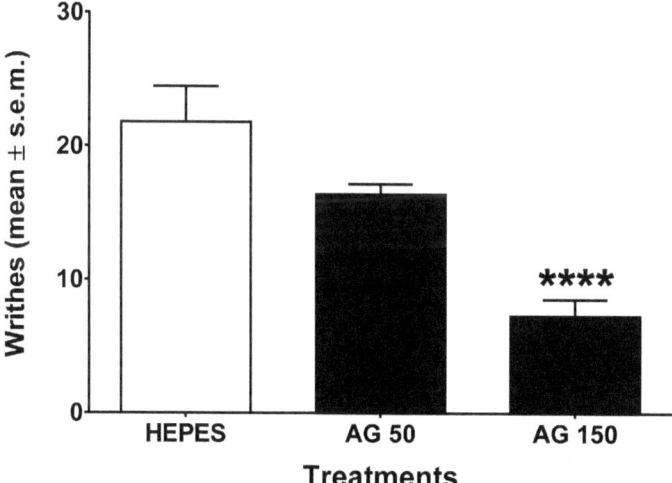

Figure 2. Writhing test. Effects induced by vehicle (Hepes, 10 mL/kg, intraperitoneally (i.p.)) and ammonium glycyrrhizate (AG, 50 or 150 mg/kg, i.p.) administered 24 h before acetic acid (0.6% v/v in salina, 10 mL/kg, i.p.). **** denotes $p < 0.0001$ vs. Vehicle. $n = 9$.

2.3. Formalin Test

Subcutaneous injection of formalin induced a nociceptive behavioural response that showed a biphasic trend. There was an early phase (from 0 to 10 min after formalin injection) produced by the direct stimulation of peripheral nociceptors, and a late prolonged phase (from 15 to 40 min) which reflected the response to inflammatory pain. The total time the animal spent licking or biting its paw during the early and late phase of formalin-induced nociception was recorded. The results obtained in these experiments are reported in Figure 3. The administration of AG at the dose of 50 or 150 mg/kg i.p. 24 h before formalin, did not modify the nociceptive response induced by aldehyde in the early phase of the test ($F_{2,27}$ = 2.903, $p > 0.05$). A considerable decrease of the formalin-induced licking and biting activity was instead observed in the late phase of the test ($F_{2,27}$ = 24.69, $p < 0.0001$). When the confront was restricted to two means, AG administered at the dose of 50 mg/kg induced a light but nonsignificant reduction of formalin-induced behaviour ($p > 0.05$) in the late phase. On the contrary, AG administered at the dose of 150 mg/kg strongly reduced the nociceptive behavior induced by formalin ($p < 0.0001$).

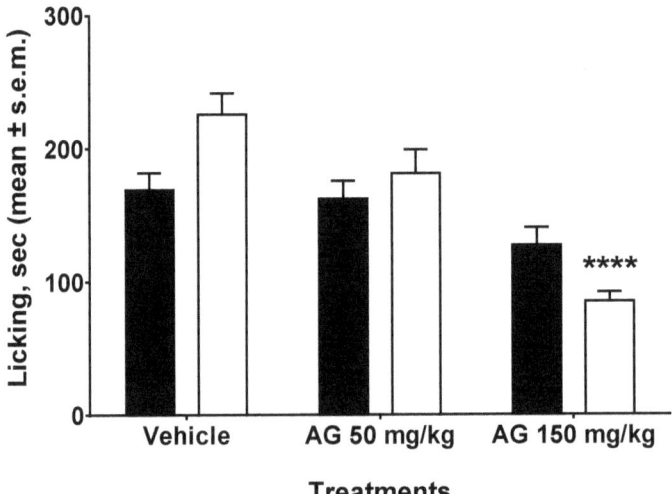

Figure 3. Formalin test. Effects induced by vehicle (Hepes, 10 mL/kg, i.p.) and ammonium glycyrrhizate (AG, 50 or 150 mg/kg, i.p.) administered 24 h before formalin (1% in saline, 20 µL/paw) in the formalin test. Black bars represent the early phase and the white bars represent the late phase of the formalin test. **** is for $p < 0.0001$ vs. Vehicle. $n = 10$.

2.4. Zymosan-Induced Hyperalgesia

This experimental pain model is characterized by the measurements of time-dependent hyperalgesia after zymosan administration. This measurement is equivalent to time-dependent reduction in the latency to respond to the thermal stimuli applied to the injected paw compared with the baseline measurements. In particular, 20 µL of zymosan A (2.5% *w/v* in saline) was administered s.c. into the dorsal surface of one hind paw.

In our experiments, treatments were given i.p. 10 min before the first measurement of the pain threshold, i.e., 1 h after zymosan administration. Figure 4 shows the results of these experiments. With the use of two-way ANOVA, we can notice that there are significant differences in treatments ($F_{2,27}$ = 6.901, $p < 0.01$) and in the time point when pain threshold was recorded ($F_{5,135}$ = 30.51, $p < 0.0001$). Tukey's multiple comparison test showed significant differences from 1 to 24 h after zymosan administration between animals treated with AG at the dose of 150 mg/kg, i.p. and those deal with vehicle. AG administered at low dose (50 mg/kg, i.p) induced a light but nonsignificant increase in pain threshold (Figure 4).

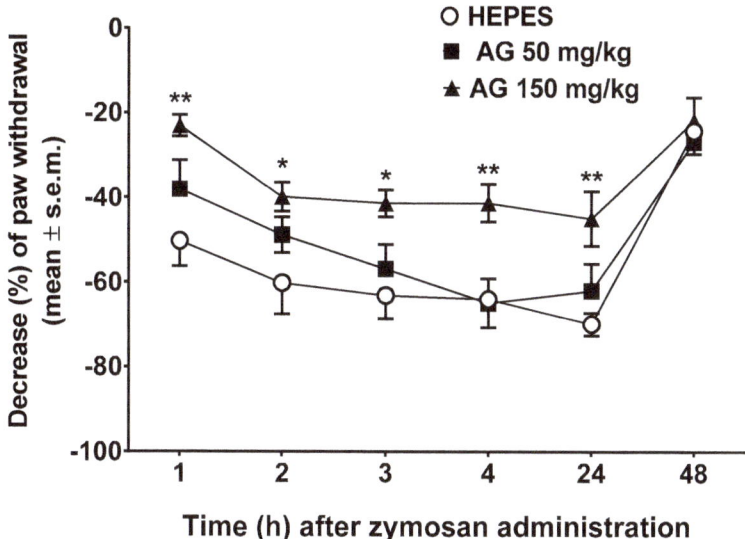

Figure 4. Zymosan-induced hyperalgesia. Effects induced by vehicle (Hepes, 10 mL/kg, intraperitoneally (i.p.)) and ammonium glycyrrhizate (AG, 50 or 150 mg/kg, i.p.) administered 10 min before zymosan (2.5% *w/v* in saline, 20 µL/paw). * denotes $p < 0.05$ and ** denotes $p < 0.01$ vs. Vehicle. $n = 10$.

2.5. Zymosan Peritonitis and Cytokines-Chemokines Protein Array

To investigate the molecular mechanisms behind the selective long-lasting anti-inflammatory and antinociceptive effects of AG, we firstly compared the recruitment of total inflammatory cells and the cytokines and chemokines profiles of collected inflammatory fluids obtained from mice receiving zymosan and zymosan plus AG at 4 and 24 h. As shown in Figure 5a, 4 h after zymosan (500 mg/kg) or zymosan + AG (150 mg/kg) injection, mice exhibited no significant difference in the number of recruited inflammatory leukocytes. In contrast, at 24 h, mice receiving AG (150 mg/kg) showed a marked decrease ($p < 0.01$) in the number of inflammatory infiltrates compared to zymosan-treated mice (Figure 5b). Administration of AG at 50 and 150 mg/kg did not show any significant effect, both at 4 and 24 h (data not shown). Contingently, as shown in Figure 6, zymosan administration at 4 h caused a massive production of cyto/chemokines (Figure 6a) that was not counterbalanced in AG-treated mice (Figure 6b), except for macrophage inflammatory proteins (MIP)-1α and keratinocyte chemoattractant (KC) production and with a less extent IL-6, SDF-1 and TNF-α (Figure 6c). Interestingly, comparison of the inflammatory profile of fluids from zymosan (Figure 7a) and zymosan + AG (Figure 7b) at 24 h revealed a striking difference in the semiquantitative levels of IL-6, IL-10, IL-1β, IP-10, KC, MCP-5, macrophage inflammatory proteins (MIP) 1-α, 1-β, 2, and TNF-α (Figure 7c,d).

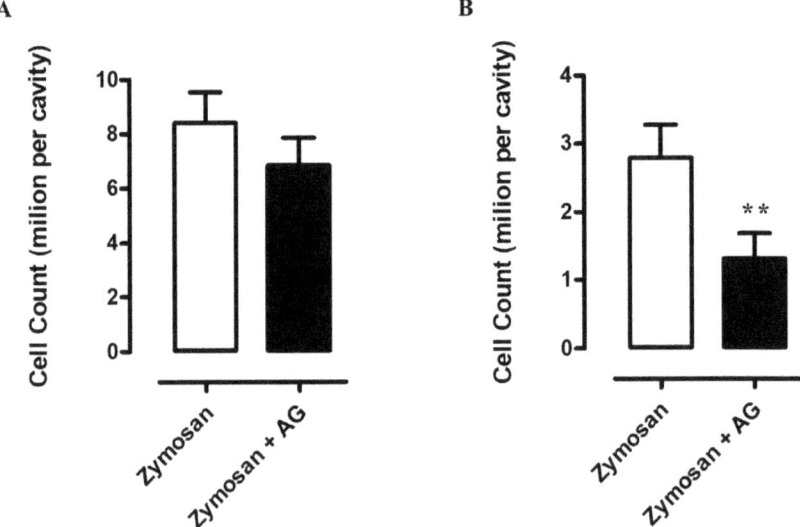

Figure 5. (**A**) Cell infiltration into mouse peritoneal cavity of mice that have received an intraperitoneal (i.p.) injection of zymosan (500 mg/kg) or zymosan + AG (150 mg/kg) at 4 and (**B**) 24 h. Bars represent group mean values ± Standard Error of the Mean (S.E.M) of three separate experiments with $n = 7$ mice. ** $p < 0.01$ vs. zymosan-treated mice.

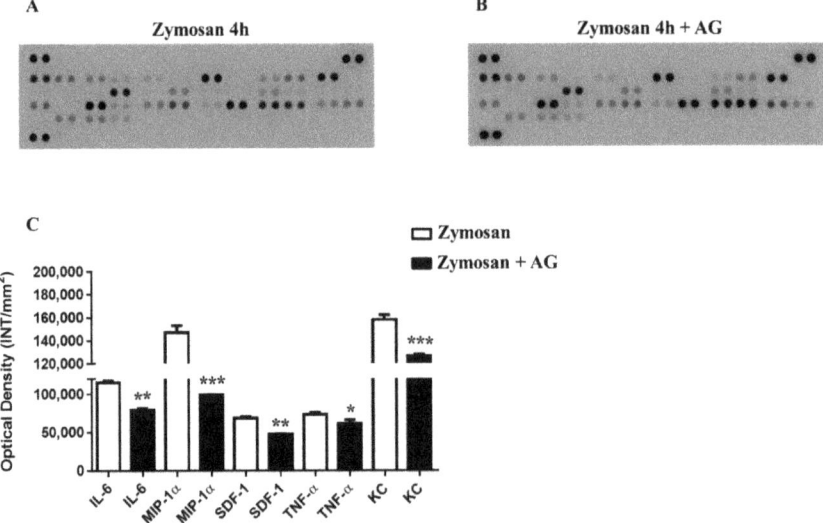

Figure 6. (**A**) Inflammatory fluids in zymosan and zymosan + AG-injected mice at 4 h. Inflammatory fluids obtained from peritoneal cavities were assayed using a proteome profiler cytokine array. Mean changes (± S.E.M) between zymosan (500 mg/kg) and (**B**) zymosan + AG-injected mice (150 mg/kg) of three separate experiments with $n = 7$ mice, (**C**) are expressed as increase in the optical density (INT/mm$_2$) between the two groups. * $p < 0.05$, ** $p < 0.01$ and *** $p < 0.001$ vs. zymosan-treated mice.

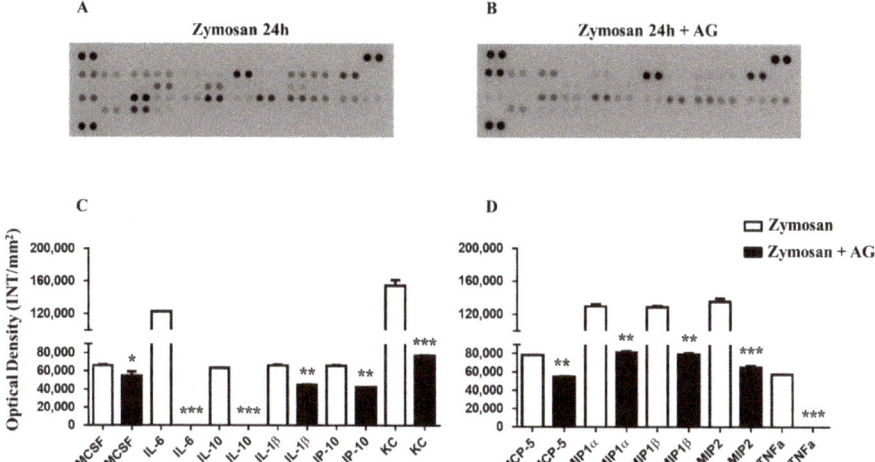

Figure 7. (**A**) Inflammatory fluids in zymosan and zymosan + AG-injected mice at 24 h. Inflammatory fluids obtained from peritoneal cavities were assayed using a proteome profiler cytokine array. (**B**) Mean changes (± S.E.M) between zymosan (500 mg/kg) and zymosan + AG-injected mice (150 mg/kg) of three separate experiments with n = 7 mice, (**C**, **D**) are expressed as increase in the optical density (INT/mm2) between the two groups. * p < 0.05, ** p < 0.01 and *** p < 0.001 vs. zymosan-treated mice.

2.6. Docking Experiments

The molecular docking studies were used to evaluate and to rationalize the anti-inflammatory activity of glycyrrhizic acid towards some key enzymes of the arachidonic acid cascade such as 5-lipoxygenase (5-LO), 5-lipoxygenase-activating protein (FLAP, Supporting Information), microsomal prostaglandin E synthase 1 and 2 (mPGES-1 and mPGES-2), and COX-1 and COX-2, responsible for leukotrienes (LTs) and prostaglandin (PG) biosynthesis, respectively. These enzymes are involved in the generation of inflammatory mediators and their role in the progression of inflammation is well-established; therefore, they were suitable targets for the study of the glycyrrhizic acid anti-inflammatory activity.

2.7. mPGES-1 and mPGES-2

Prostaglandin E_2 (PGE_2) is one of the key mediators of inflammation and it is synthesized by members of the prostaglandin E synthase (PGESs) family from the unstable prostaglandin H_2 (PGH_2). The most known and studied isoforms are mPGES-1 and mPGES-2; the first one is an inducible isoform, whereas mPGES-2 is constitutively expressed [18]. They differ also in tissue localization, with mPGES-1 mainly expressed in lung, kidney, and reproductive organs and mPGES-2 mainly expressed in heart and brain [18,19]. Key amino acids for the binding are: Arg38, Asp49, Arg52, His53, Arg70, Arg73, Asn74, Glu77, Arg110, Leu121, Arg122, Arg126, Ser127, Ile125, Thr129, and Tyr130 for mPGES-1 [20–23], and Cys110, His241, His244, Ser247, Arg292, and Arg296 for mPGES-2 [24]. Molecular docking experiments involving both microsomal prostaglandin E synthase proteins revealed that AG has a higher affinity for mPGES-2 than mPGES-1. In particular, in the case of mPGES-1, the only interaction shown is one H-bond between the OH group and Arg52 and His53 on chain B. Regarding mPGES-2, instead, the three polar groups of AG are all involved in H-bonds with the target. In more detail:

- The OH group interacts both with the side chain and the backbone of Thr109,
- The carbonyl group interacts with Ser247, and
- The carboxyl group forms an H-bond and a salt bridge with Arg296 (Figures 8 and 9).

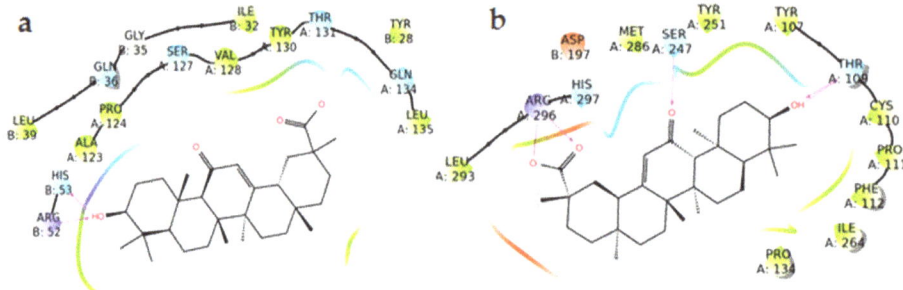

Figure 8. (**a**) 2D panels represent the interactions between AG with the microsomal prostaglandin E synthase 1 (mPGES-1) and 2 (mPGES-2) (**b**) binding sites. Positively charged residues are colored violet, negatively charged residues are colored red, polar residues are colored light blue, hydrophobic residues are colored green. Red-to-blue lines represent salt bridges and H-bonds (side chain) are reported as dotted pink arrows.

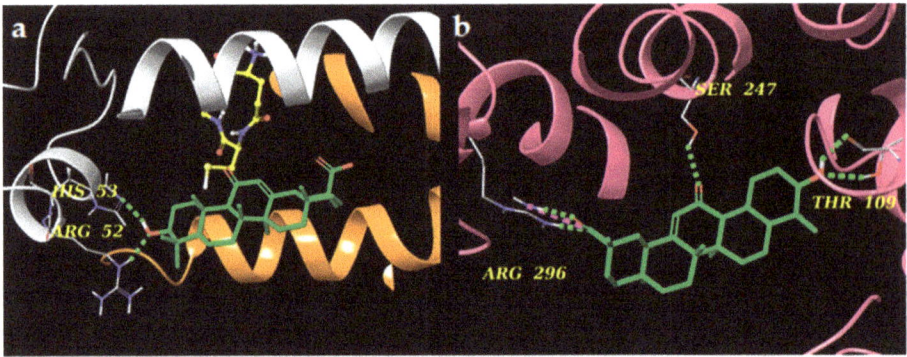

Figure 9. (**a**) 3D models of AG (colored by atom types: C green, O red, polar H white) in the binding site of microsomal prostaglandin E synthase 1 (mPGES-1) (panel a, chain A and chain B are reported in orange and white ribbons, respectively) and (**b**) microsomal prostaglandin E synthase 2 (mPGES-2) (chain A is reported in pink ribbons). Green dotted lines represent H-bonds and pink dotted lines represent salt bridges.

2.8. COX-1 and COX-2

Cyclooxygenases are the starting point in the production of eicosanoids, as they convert fatty acids into PGH_2. Like mPGESs, they are present in two main isoforms: COX-1, which is constitutively expressed, and COX-2, which is inducible [25,26]. COX-1 and COX-2 monomers consist of three different domains: the EGF domain, the membrane-binding domain, and the catalytic domain containing the catalytic triad Arg120, Tyr355, and Glu524. Among these, the catalytic domain represents the main target for NSAID and, particularly, Arg120, Tyr355, Tyr385, Ser530, and Arg513 are essential for the inhibitory activity [27]. The study of the interaction between AG and the two isoforms of COX required a flexible docking approach (induced fit) [28] to allow the entrance of the ligand into the catalytic site of the enzymes. AG seems to locate better in the binding pocket of COX-2 as it interacts with key amino acids such as Trp387 and Ser530 (H-bonds) and Arg120 (salt bridge). In the case of COX-1, on the other hand, AG forms H-bonds and a salt bridge with Arg120 that do not reach the inner part of the binding pocket (Figures 10 and 11). These data suggest a preference of glycyrrhetic acid (AG) for isoform 2 of COX.

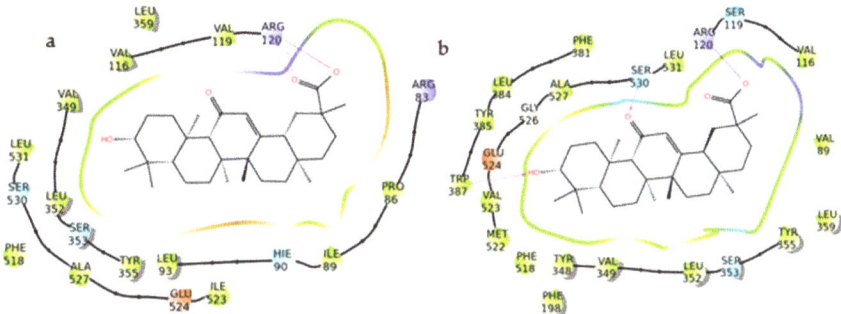

Figure 10. (**a**) 2D panels represent the interactions between AG with cyclooxygenase 1 (COX-1) and (**b**) cyclooxygenase 2 (COX-2) binding sites. Positively charged residues are colored violet, negatively charged residues are colored red, polar residues are colored light blue, hydrophobic residues are colored green. Red-to-blue lines represent salt bridges and H-bonds (side chain) are reported as dotted pink arrows. Neutral histidine with hydrogen on the δ nitrogen is shown as HIE.

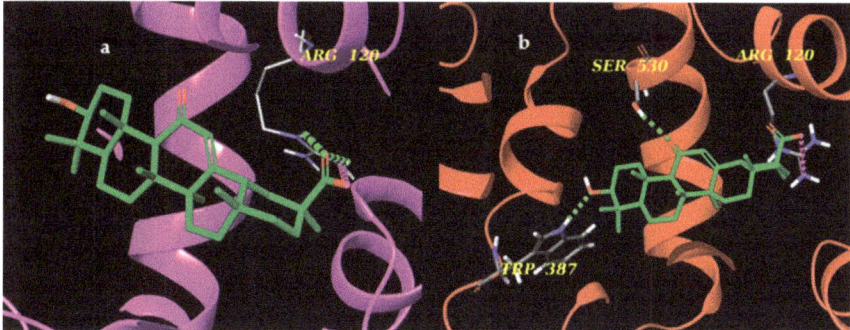

Figure 11. (**a**) 3D models of AG (colored by atom types: C green, O red, polar H white) in the binding site of cyclooxygenase 1 (COX-1) (purple ribbons) and (**b**) cyclooxygenase 2 (COX-2) (red ribbons). Green dotted lines represent H-bonds and pink dotted lines represent salt bridges.

2.9. 5-LO

The mammalian 5-lipoxygenase (5-LO) pathway produces potent mediators, such as leukotriene B4 (LTB4) and peptide leukotrienes (LTC4, LTD4 or LTE4), that have well-known functions and are involved in different pathologies and disorders [29–31]. To date, four different class of 5-LO direct inhibitors are classified: 1) iron-ligand inhibitors, 2) non-redox-active 5-LO inhibitors, which compete with arachidonic acid for binding to the enzyme 3) redox-active 5-LO inhibitors, interfering with the catalytic cycle of the enzyme, and 4) inhibitors that act with an unrecognized mechanism [30]. To computationally evaluate the binding of AG to 5-LO, a combined approach of rigid and flexible docking was used to predict its possible mechanism of action.

The human 5-LO structure (PDB ID: 3V99) [32] in complex with its substrate, arachidonic acid (AA), was used as the target for molecular docking studies [33]. The computational analysis highlighted two possible binding modes for the AG molecule (Figure 12), compatible with two different class of direct 5-LO inhibitors [30]. The results of the rigid docking approach are compatible with a non-redox type binding mode (Figure 12a), where AG was able to partially occupy the same binding site of AA and establishes hydrogen bonds with the side chain of Lys409 and with the backbone of Phe177. On the other hand, considering the induced fit molecular docking approach, the carboxylate group of AG was able to coordinate Fe^{2+} (Figure 12b) in a bidentate manner, and the OH group formed a hydrogen bond with the backbone of Arg666, behaving as an iron-ligand inhibitor.

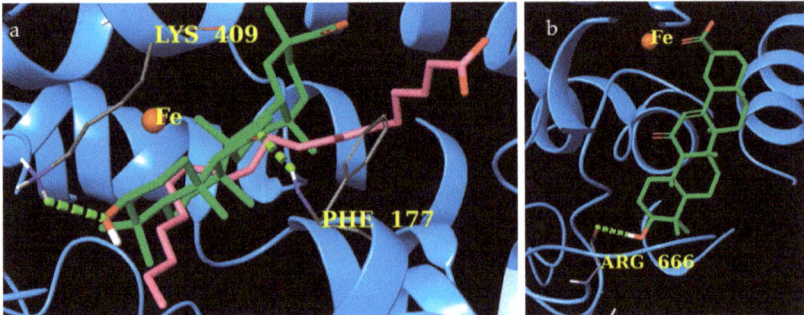

Figure 12. (**a**) Rigid docking and induced fit (**b**) of AG (colored by atom types: C green, O red, polar H white) in the binding site of 5-lipoxygenase (5-LO) (blue ribbons and Fe^{2+} as an orange sphere). Green dotted lines represent H-bonds, and original arachidonic acid (AA) molecule is in pink.

These computational data have suggested a probable binding between AG and 5-LO by one of the two proposed mechanisms, which could represent a novel finding regarding its biological activity profile, especially with respect to glycyrrhizin from *Glycyrrhiza glabra L.* as reported by Chandrasekaran et al. [34].

3. Discussion

Available therapy for the management of chronic and inflammatory pain is not fully adequate in most cases. Furthermore, the common treatments of inflammatory pain, NSAIDs and opioids, lead to severe toxicities, including gastrointestinal lesions and nephrotoxicity [4] in the case of NSAIDs and respiratory depression, tolerance, and physical dependence for opioids when they are used for a long time [35]. Thus, identification of new potential targets which may affect pain and inflammatory processes is becoming an urgent clinical and therapeutic need. In our present study, we investigated the possible long-lasting anti-inflammatory and antinociceptive effects of AG using pharmacological, biochemical, and in silico tools. Our experimental method demonstrated that AG caused significant long-lasting reduction of inflammation and nociception, revealing that effects are most likely due to the inhibition of different aspects and mediators of inflammation. Moreover, these effects were observed at AG doses which have already been demonstrated to be free of toxic effects [36].

Several investigators have reported that the anti-inflammatory mechanism of AG involves cytokines such as IFN-γ, TNF-α, IL-1β, IL-4, IL-5, IL-6, IL-8, IL-10, IL-12, and IL-17 [37–42], intercellular cell adhesion molecule 1 (ICAM-1) and P-selectin, enzymes such as iNOS, and transcription factors such as NF-kappaB, signal transducer and activator of transcription (STAT)-3 and STAT-6 [33].

The anti-inflammatory efficacy of AG was evaluated using zymosan-induced paw edema and peritonitis. Zymosan consists of insoluble polysaccharides from yeast cell wall that induces an inflammatory reaction [43]. In this context, zymosan-induced ear or paw edema are preliminary models for screening potential anti-inflammatory drugs, characterized by pronounced dose- and time-dependent edema with moderate to severe infiltration of neutrophils and, to a lesser extent, macrophages and lymphocytes [44]. Furthermore, zymosan-induced paw edema is COX-2-dependent since it is significantly reduced in COX-$2^{-/-}$ mice [45]. In this context, previous studies demonstrated that AG was able to reduce paw [15,16] or ear [16] edema formation and these effects were observed from 1 to 5 h after its administration [46]. After carrageenan injection in mouse paw, TNF-α, IL-6, iNOS, and COX-2 mRNA expressions increased and AG treatment (150 mg/kg, i.p.) markedly suppressed carrageenan's effects [16]. The results of our experiments demonstrated that AG had a significant long-lasting anti-inflammatory activity since AG reduced paw edema formation until 48 h after administration.

Accordingly, to better investigate the long-lasting anti-inflammatory effect of AG, we next aimed to assess its action using zymosan-induced peritonitis. Intraperitoneal injection of zymosan is a model of acute inflammation and has been widely used for the quantification of cell types and inflammation-related soluble factors [47]. It is well known that the use of zymosan as experimental model of inflammation results in a range of benefits: following the injection with zymosan, it is possible to collect a reasonable amount of exudate for the analysis of several inflammatory mediators; the normal inflammatory response of an immunocompetent individual is imitated by zymosan injection. Furthermore, injection into a serosal cavity instead of an artificially formed cavity, such as a sterile air pouch, means that leukocytes exit from the site of inflammation via their natural conduits to the draining lymph node [48,49]. This model is simple, accurate, and capable of being reproduced [47].

When administered in the mouse peritoneal cavity, zymosan-induced acute inflammation characterized by increased vascular permeability, leukocyte influx, and release of inflammatory mediators [50]. In mice receiving AG 24 h before zymosan, AG induced a high decrease in the number of inflammatory cells and a significant decrease in IL-6, IL-10, IL-1β, IP-10, KC, MCP-5, MIP1-α, MIP1-β, MIP2, and TNF-α release in inflammatory fluids from zymosan-treated animals. This scenario was partially evoked even at 4 h post-AG administration. At this time-point, AG was able to reduce the levels of IL-6, MIP-1α, SDF-1, TNF-α, and KC. No data have previously been reported, to our knowledge, on AG effects in a zymosan-peritonitis model. However, in a model of acute lung injury induced by intratracheal administration of lipopolysaccharide (LPS) from *Escherichia coli*, AG was able to reduce lung edema, total leukocyte number, and neutrophil percentage in the bronchoalveolar lavage fluid (BALF), and AG downregulated TNF-α level in the lung [51]. Further investigation using a similar model of lung inflammation indicated that AG was able to reduce the concentrations of pro-inflammatory cytokines IL-1β in BALF and AG suppressed the expression of COX-2 and iNOS in lung tissue [52]. All reported data confirm the anti-inflammatory effects of AG, and these AG-related anti-inflammatory effects were until present 24–48 h after a single AG administration.

The writhing test, formalin test, and zymosan-induced hyperalgesia test were performed 24 h after AG administration to evaluate the possible long-lasting antinociceptive property of AG. Several studies have already demonstrated that AG is able to induce antinociceptive effects in the writhing test [15,16], formalin test, and thermal hyperalgesia [16] and these effects were observed from 1 to 5 h after AG administration. Our data demonstrated for the first time that AG exerts long-lasting antinociceptive effects, since AG-induced antinociception was observed until 24–48 h after a single administration.

To better investigate its analgesic profile, we finally tested the AG pharmacological profile in an acetic acid-induced writhing test, a commonly used method for monitoring preliminary antinociceptive activity, since in this test both central and peripheral analgesics are detected [53]. The injection of acetic acid directly activates the visceral and somatic nociceptors that innervate the peritoneum and induces inflammation not only in subdiaphragmatic visceral organs, but also in the subcutaneous muscle walls [54]. Furthermore, the nociceptive activity of acetic acid in the writhing model may be due to the release of TNF-α, IL-1β, and IL-8 by resident peritoneal macrophages and mast cells [55]. Our results revealed that AG administered 24 h before the test significantly reduced the number of writhes, suggesting that AG possessed long-lasting antinociceptive effects. Because of the lack of drug specificity, caution is required in interpreting the results obtained in the writhing test [53], and other tests could be conducted to scientifically asses the obtained results.

The formalin test for nociception, which is mainly used with rats and mice, involves moderate and continuous pain generated by injured tissue. This test in mice is a well-founded and trustworthy model of nociception and is sensitive for various classes of analgesic drugs [56]. Plantar injections of formalin in the mouse induce a characteristic behaviour evoked in two temporal phases. The first phase is observed immediately after the formalin injection, followed by a quiescent period, and then a second phase appears, which lasts until the end of the period of observation. The first phase depends upon direct stimulation of nociceptors, whereas the second involves a period of sensitization during which inflammatory phenomena occurs, involving the release of pain mediators such as histamine, serotonin, prostaglandins, bradykinin, and cytokines. Opioid analgesics appear to be antinociceptive for both phases, whereas NSAIDs seem to suppress only the second phase [53]. In our research,

AG substantially diminished the second phase of the formalin test when administered 24 h before the test, thus confirming the results obtained in the writhing test.

Furthermore, in vivo tests of AG show the efficiency of the drug in terms of increase of nociceptive threshold after zymosan administration. Associated with paw edema, the injection of zymosan in the mouse paw produces a decrease of pain thresholds, which indicates a state of hyperalgesia [44,45]. In this pain model, a time-dependent hyperalgesia was noticed after zymosan administration and measured as a time-dependent reduction in the latency to respond to the thermal stimuli applied to the injected paw compared to the baseline measurements. We also have outstanding results in terms of the highest increase in pain threshold after AG administration. We observed that AG caused a significant reduction of zymosan-induced hyperalgesia until 48 h after administration.

It is well known that several components of liquorice can suppress COX-2 [57,58] and this seems to be true also for AG [16]. In addition to above-mentioned effects of AG on COX-2 [51,52], in skin tumor, AG significantly inhibited NF-κB, COX-2, prostaglandin E$_2$ (PGE$_2$), and nitric oxide (NO) levels [59]. Furthermore, in focal cerebral ischemic-reperfusion injury in mice, AG administered for seven days significantly improved neurofunction, decreased infarct size, and suppressed edema [60]. The neuroprotective effect of AG was associated with a significant reduction in IL-1, TNF-α, COX-2, iNOS, NF-κB, and GFAP levels [60]. Further recent studies showed that AG downregulates the expression of iNOS and COX-2 in the inflamed kidney [61] and skin [62], blocking NF-κB activation. In HaCaT cells, AG inhibited the UV-B-mediated increase in intracellular ROS and downregulated the release of IL-6, IL-1α, IL-1β, TNF-α, and PGE$_2$ [63]. In LPS-stimulated mouse endometrial epithelial cells, AG considerably repressed LPS-induced TNF-α, IL-1β, NO, and PGE$_2$ production, attenuated LPS-induced iNOS, COX-2, and TLR4 expression and NF-κB activation [64].

Our docking studies, for the first time, suggest that AG's effects on inflammation and nociception might also depend upon the interaction with mPGES-1/2, COX-1/2, and 5-LO. In fact, from the analysis of the results, it emerged that AG interacted with key amino acids of mPGES-2 and COX-2, highlighting a preferential binding with these two isoforms. AG seems to locate better in the binding pocket of COX-2 as it interacts with key amino acids like Trp387, Ser530 (H-bonds), and Arg120 (salt bridge). Moreover, by combined rigid and flexible molecular docking studies, two possible mechanisms of interaction between AG and 5-LO were proposed: non-redox competitive binding and Fe^{2+} complexation. Here, the binding energy calculated is lower compared to those obtained with the other proteins, namely mPGES-1 and 2, COX-1 and 2, (data not shown), but consistent with putative inhibitor activity. These data suggest that further experiments should be performed to evaluate the effects of AG's interaction with 5-LO.

4. Materials and Methods

4.1. Reagents

Ethylenediaminetetraacetate (EDTA), enhanced chemiluminescence detection kit (ECL), and glycyrrhizic acid ammonium salt from glycyrrhiza root (≥95%) were purchased from Sigma-Aldrich (Milan, Italy). The proteome profiler mouse cytokine array kit was from R&D System (Abingdon, UK). All the other reagents were from Carlo Erba (Milan, Italy), unless otherwise specified.

4.2. Animals and Ethical Statement

We used male CD-1 mice (Harlan, Italy) weighing 25 g in all of the experiments. Mice were housed in colony cages (seven mice per cage) under standard conditions of light, temperature, and relative humidity for at least one week before the start of experimental sessions. Food and water were available ad libitum.

All experiments were performed according to Legislative Decree 26/14, which implements the European Directive 2010/63/UE on laboratory animal protection in Italy, and were approved by the local ethics committee. Animal studies are reported in accordance with the ARRIVE (Animal Research:

Reporting of In Vivo Experiments) guidelines [65,66]. The research protocol was approved by the Service for Biotechnology and Animal Welfare of the Istituto Superiore di Sanità and authorized by the Italian Ministry of Health.

4.3. Edema Induced by Zymosan

Edema was induced with a subcutaneous injection of 2.5% *w/v* zymosan A in saline, in the dorsal surface of the right hind paw (20 μL/paw). Paw volume was measured three times before the injections and at 1, 2, 3, 4, 24, and 48 h thereafter by the use of hydroplethysmometer specially modified for small volumes (Ugo Basile, Italy). AG (50 or 150 mg/kg) and vehicle (Hepes, 10 mL/kg) were administered intraperitoneally (i.p.) 10 min before zymosan A. The increase in paw volume was evaluated as percentage difference between the paw volume at each time point and the basal paw volume [67].

4.4. Writhing Test

Mice were given an intraperitoneal injection of 0.6% *v/v* acetic acid in a volume of 10 mL/kg. Acetic acid induces a series of writhes, consisting in abdominal contraction and hind limb extension [68]. AG (50 or 150 mg/kg) and vehicle (Hepes, 10 mL/kg) were administered i.p. 24 h before acetic acid. After vehicle or AG administration, the number of writhes were recorded over a 20 min period beginning 5 min after acetic acid injection.

4.5. Formalin Test

Male mice were split into three groups of ten animals each: vehicle (10 mL/kg, i.p.), AG (50 mg/kg, i.p.) and AG (150 mg/kg, i.p.). One percent formalin in saline was injected into the right mouse hind paw, twenty-four hours after saline and AG i.p. administrations. Formalin aroused nociceptive behavioural responses, such as licking and/or biting the injected paw, which are considered indices of nociception [69]. The nociceptive response showed a biphasic trend: an early phase (from 0 to 10 min after formalin injection) produced by the direct stimulation of peripheral nociceptors, and a late prolonged phase (from 15 to 40 min) which reflected the response to inflammatory pain. The total time the animal spent licking or biting its paw during the early and late phase of formalin-induced nociception was recorded. During the test, the mouse was located in a Plexiglas observation cage (30 × 14 × 12 cm) 1 h before the formalin administration to allow it to acclimatize to its surroundings.

4.6. Zymosan-Induced Hyperalgesia

In these experiments, AG (50 or 150 mg/kg) and vehicle (Hepes, 10 mL/kg) were administered intraperitoneally (i.p.) 10 min before a subcutaneous injection (20 μL/paw) of zymosan A (2.5% *w/v* in saline) into the dorsal surface of the right hind paw. Then, hyperalgesia measurements were performed [70]. The plantar test (Ugo Basile, Italy) was used to measure the sensitivity to a noxious heat stimulus with the aim of assessing thermal hyperalgesia after zymosan-induced inflammation of the mouse hind paw. The animals are located in cages with a glass floor covered with transparent plastic boxes and allowed to habituate to their surroundings for at least 1 h in a temperature-controlled room (21 °C) for three consecutive days prior to testing. On the test day, the animals were acclimatized to their environment for at least 1 h before paw withdrawal latency (PWL) was measured. Care was taken to initiate the test when the animal was at rest, not walking, with its hind paw in contact with the glass floor of the test apparatus. A radiant heat source was constantly directed at the mouse footpad until paw withdrawal, foot drumming, licking, or any other aversive action was observed. A timer started automatically when the heat source was activated, and a photocell stopped the timer when the mouse withdrew its hind paw. The heat source on the plantar apparatus was set to an intensity of 30 and a cut-off time of 15 s was used to avoid tissue damage. Animals were first tested to determine their baseline PWL; after zymosan injection, the PWL (seconds) of each animal in response to the plantar test was determined again at 1, 2, 3, 4, 5, 24, and 48 h.

4.7. Zymosan Peritonitis

Zymosan peritonitis was induced as previously reported [71,72]. Mice were injected intraperitoneally with 500 mg/kg of zymosan. Animals were killed by CO_2 exposure, peritoneal cavities washed with 3 mL of PBS containing 3 mM EDTA, at different time points. Aliquots of the lavage fluids were then stained with Turk's solution (0.01% crystal violet in 3% acetic acid) and differential counts performed using a Neubauer haemocytometer counting chamber (Thermo Fisher Scientific, Rome, Italy) and a light microscope. Lavage fluids were collected and used to measure the relative expression levels of ~40 cytokines and chemokines using the Mouse Cytokine Array Panel A from R&D System.

4.8. Cytokines and Chemokines Protein Array

Equal volumes (1.5 mL) of the peritoneal inflammatory fluids obtained at different time points (4 and 24 h) after the treatment with zymosan (500 mg/kg) or zymosan plus AG (150 mg/kg) were incubated with the precoated proteome profiler array membranes according to the manufacturer's instructions. Dot plots were detected by using ECL detection kit and ImageQuant 400 GE Healthcare (GE Healthcare Europe GmbH, Milan, Italy) and successively quantified as optical density (INT/mm_2) using GS 800 imaging densitometer software (Bio-Rad Laboratories, Milan, Italy) as previously described [73].

4.9. Molecular Docking Input Files Preparation

The crystal structure of mPGES1 in complex with inhibitors (5TL9) [74], mPGES-2 in complex with indomethacin (1Z9H) [24], COX-1 in complex with mofezolac (5WBE) [25], COX-2 in complex with meclofenamic acid (5IKQ) [38], and 5-lipoxygenase (3V99) [32] were used as molecular targets for the docking studies. All the protein 3D structures were produced using the Schrödinger Protein Preparation Wizard workflow [75]. First, all missing hydrogen atoms were added, bond orders were properly assigned, partial charges calculated, water molecules were eliminated, and protein termini were capped. Glycyrrhizic acid was built with Maestro's Build Panel (Maestro version 10.2, 2015), processed with LigPrep (LigPrep version 3.4, 2015) and, finally, minimized with the OPLS 2005 force field [76].

4.10. Docking Experiments

The cocrystallized inhibitors were used to generate the grid necessary for the molecular docking experiments, using the following coordinates: 10.75 (x), 15.07 (y), 28.45 (z) for mPGES-1; −21.10 (x), 54.51 (y), 11.75 (z) for mPGES-2; 19.34 (x), 2.67 (y), 31.22 (z) for COX-1; 24.25 (x), 3.52 (y), 33.07 (z) for COX-2; 9.21 (x), −82.00 (y), −32.69 (z) for 5-LO. The boundaries of the inner box were extended of 10 Å for COX-1 and mPGES1 and 13 Å for mPGES-2 and COX-2 in the three directions of space. Regarding 5-LO, in both calculations, the centre of the grid was set close to Asn544 and, in the rigid docking approach, the outer box boundaries were set at 40 Å from it. For the in silico docking experiments, the software Glide [77–79] was used. In the rigid docking approach, in a preliminary phase, in standard precision (SP) mode, 10,000 ligand poses were kept, and the best 800 poses were selected for energy minimization. Once the minimization was completed, only one output structure was saved for each ligand. After this phase, a post-docking optimization of the obtained molecules was carried out, setting the rejection cut-off at 0.5 kcal/mol and a maximum of ten poses per ligand were kept. The poses generated in the initial phase, were submitted to a second optimizations phase in extra precision glide (XP) mode. In this last phase, the post-docking optimization of the docking poses was performed accounting for a maximum of ten poses with the same parameters for the selection of initial poses and rejection cut off used during the SP docking experiments. The induced fit docking was carried out using the same settings of the rigid docking XP mode, but allowing a certain degree of flexibility to amino acids of the catalytic pocket. The first step consists in docking the ligand in the binding site with Glide [77–79]; then, the protein side chains are re-oriented with Prime [80,81] with the aim of better accommodating the molecule. At the last stage, a second rigid docking inside the new cavity is carried out.

4.11. Data Analysis and Statistics

The results achieved are given as the mean ± SEM. Statistical analysis was carried out by using one-way ANOVA followed by Dunnett's post-test when comparing more than two groups. In certain cases, one sample *t*-test was used to evaluate significance against the hypothetical zero value. Statistical analysis was conducted by using GraphPad Prism 6.0 software (San Diego, CA, USA). Data were considered statistically significant when a value of $p < 0.05$ was achieved. The data and statistical analysis comply with the recommendations on experimental design and analysis [82].

5. Conclusions

Results of the present study indicated that AG possesses long-lasting anti-inflammatory and antinociceptive effects as observed 24–48 h after the administration. Our data also suggest that its anti-inflammatory and antinociceptive effects might be attributed to the inhibition of the levels of different pro-inflammatory cytokines and chemokines. Taken together, all these findings indicate that AG is a long-acting therapeutic agent for the treatment of painful conditions and inflammatory-related diseases.

Supplementary Materials: The following are available online. Molecular docking studies between AG and FLAP and spectral data.

Author Contributions: S.P. designed the study and wrote the manuscript. F.M., P.M., F.R., M.G.C. and S.D.V. performed the experiments. A.D.G., G.B., N.M. and S.P. edited and revised the manuscript. All Authors gave final approval to the publication.

Funding: This work was in part supported by Ministero dell'Università e della Ricerca (MIUR) PRIN 2017 (2017A95NCJ/2017A95NCJ_002) "Stolen molecules – Stealing natural products from the depot and reselling them as new drug candidates".

Conflicts of Interest: The authors declare no competing conflict of interests.

References

1. Rahavard, B.B.; Candido, K.D.; Knezevic, N.N. Different pain responses to chronic and acute pain in various ethnic/racial groups. *Pain Manag.* **2017**, *7*, 427–453. [CrossRef] [PubMed]
2. Baral, P.; Udit, S.; Chiu, I.M. Pain and immunity: Implication for host defence. *Nat. Rev. Immunol.* **2019**, *15*, 1. [CrossRef] [PubMed]
3. Sinha, M.; Gautam, L.; Shukla, P.K.; Kaur, P.; Sharma, S.; Singh, T.P. Current perspectives in NSAID-induced gastropathy. *Mediat. Inflamm.* **2013**, *2013*, 258209. [CrossRef]
4. Musu, M.; Finco, G.; Antonucci, R.; Polati, E.; Sanna, D.; Evangelista, M.; Ribuffo, D.; Schweiger, V.; Fanos, V. Acute nephrotoxicity of NSAID from the foetus to the adult. *Eur. Rev. Med. Pharmacol. Sci.* **2011**, *15*, 1461–1472. [PubMed]
5. Benyamin, R.; Trescot, A.M.; Datta, S.; Buenaventura, R.; Adlaka, R.; Sehgal, N.; Glaser, S.E.; Vallejo, R. Opioid complications and side effects. *Pain Physician* **2008**, *11*, S105–S120. [PubMed]
6. Statti, G.A.; Tundis, R.; Sacchetti, G.; Muzzoli, M.; Bianchi, A.; Menichini, F. Variability in the content of active constituents and biological activity of *Glycyrrhiza glabra*. *Fitoterapia* **2004**, *75*, 371–374. [CrossRef]
7. Fu, Y.; Hsieh, T.C.; Guo, J.; Kunicki, J.; Lee, M.Y.; Darzynkiewicz, Z.; Wu, J.M. Licochalcone-A, a novel flavonoid isolated from licorice root (*Glycyrrhiza glabra*), causes G2 and late-G1 arrests in androgen-independent PC-3 prostate cancer cells. *Biochem. Biophys. Res. Commun.* **2004**, *322*, 263–270. [CrossRef]
8. Ignesti, G.; Maleci, L.; Medica, A.; Pirisino, R. *Piante Medicinali. Botanica,Chimica,Farmacologia,Tossicologia*; Pitagora Editrice: Bologna, Italy, 1999.
9. Chen, M.F.; Shimada, F.; Kato, H.; Yano, S.; Kanaoka, M. Effect of oral administration of glycyrrhizin on the pharmacokinetics of prednisolone. *Endocrinol. Jpn.* **1991**, *38*, 167–174. [CrossRef]
10. Herold, A.; Cremer, L.; Calugaru, A.; Tamas, V.; Ionescu, F.; Manea, S.; Szegli, G. Hydroalcoholic plant extracts with antiinflammatory activity. *Roum. Arch. Microbiol. Immunol.* **2003**, *62*, 117–129.

11. Fukai, T.; Satoh, K.; Nomura, T.; Sakagami, H. Preliminary evaluation of antinephritis and radical scavenging activities of glabridin from *Glycyrrhiza glabra*. *Fitoterapia* **2003**, *74*, 624–629. [CrossRef]
12. Morteza-Semnani, K.; Saeedi, M.; Shahnavaz, B. Comparison of antioxidant activity of extract from roots of licorice (*Glycyrrhiza glabra* L.) to commercial antioxidants in 2% hydroquinone cream. *J. Cosmet. Sci.* **2003**, *54*, 551–558. [PubMed]
13. Paolino, D.; Lucania, G.; Mardente, D.; Alhaique, F.; Fresta, M. Ethosomes for skin delivery of ammonium glycyrrhizinate: In vitro percutaneous permeation through human skin and in vivo anti-inflammatory activity on human volunteers. *J. Control. Release* **2005**, *106*, 99–110. [CrossRef] [PubMed]
14. Genovese, T.; Menegazzi, M.; Mazzon, E.; Crisafulli, C.; Di Paola, R.; Dal Bosco, M.; Zou, Z.; Suzuki, H.; Cuzzocrea, S. Glycyrrhizin reduces secondary inflammatory process after spinal cord compression injury in mice. *Shock* **2009**, *31*, 367–375. [CrossRef] [PubMed]
15. Khaksa, G.; Zolfaghari, M.E.; Dehpour, A.R.; Samadian, T. Anti-inflammatory and anti-nociceptive activity of disodium glycyrrhetinic acid hemiphthalate. *Planta Med.* **1996**, *62*, 326–328. [CrossRef] [PubMed]
16. Wang, H.L.; Li, Y.X.; Niu, Y.T.; Zheng, J.; Wu, J.; Shi, G.J.; Ma, L.; Niu, Y.; Sun, T.; Yu, J.Q. Observing Anti-inflammatory and Anti-nociceptive Activities of Glycyrrhizin Through Regulating COX_2 and Pro-inflammatory Cytokines Expressions in Mice. *Inflammation* **2015**, *38*, 2269–2278. [CrossRef] [PubMed]
17. Sun, X.; Zeng, H.; Wang, Q.; Yu, Q.; Wu, J.; Feng, Y.; Deng, P.; Zhang, H. Glycyrrhizin ameliorates inflammatory pain by inhibiting microglial activation-mediated inflammatory response via blockage of the HMGB1-TLR4-NF-kB pathway. *Exp. Cell. Res.* **2018**, *369*, 112–119. [CrossRef] [PubMed]
18. Koeberle, A.; Werz, O. Perspective of microsomal prostaglandin E_2 synthase-1 as drug target in inflammation-related disorders. *Biochem. Pharmacol.* **2015**, *98*, 1–15. [CrossRef]
19. Park, J.Y.; Pillinger, M.H.; Abramson, S.B. Prostaglandin E_2 synthesis and secretion: The role of PGE_2 synthases. *Clin. Immunol.* **2006**, *119*, 229–240. [CrossRef]
20. Iranshahi, M.; Chini, M.G.; Masullo, M.; Sahebkar, A.; Javidnia, A.; Chitsazian Yazdi, M.; Pergola, C.; Koeberle, A.; Werz, O.; Pizza, C.; et al. Can Small Chemical Modifications of Natural Pan-inhibitors Modulate the Biological Selectivity? The Case of Curcumin Prenylated Derivatives Acting as HDAC or mPGES-1 Inhibitors. *J. Nat. Prod.* **2015**, *78*, 2867–2879. [CrossRef]
21. Ding, K.; Zhou, Z.; Hou, S.; Yuan, Y.; Zhou, S.; Zheng, X.; Chen, J.; Loftin, C.; Zheng, F.; Zhan, C.G. Structure-based discovery of mPGES-$_1$ inhibitors suitable for preclinical testing in wild-type mice as a new generation of anti-inflammatory drugs. *Sci. Rep.* **2018**, *8*, 5205. [CrossRef]
22. Luz, J.G.; Antonysamy, S.; Kuklish, S.L.; Condon, B.; Lee, M.R.; Allison, D.; Yu, X.P.; Chandrasekhar, S.; Backer, R.; Zhang, A.; et al. Crystal Structures of mPGES-$_1$ Inhibitor Complexes Form a Basis for the Rational Design of Potent Analgesic and Anti-Inflammatory Therapeutics. *J. Med. Chem.* **2015**, *58*, 4727–4737. [CrossRef] [PubMed]
23. Lauro, G.; Tortorella, P.; Bertamino, A.; Ostacolo, C.; Koeberle, A.; Fischer, K.; Bruno, I.; Terracciano, S.; Gomez-Monterrey, I.M.; Tauro, M.; et al. Structure-Based Design of Microsomal Prostaglandin E_2 Synthase-$_1$ (mPGES-$_1$) Inhibitors using a Virtual Fragment Growing Optimization Scheme. *Chem. Med. Chem.* **2016**, *11*, 612–619. [CrossRef] [PubMed]
24. Yamada, T.; Komoto, J.; Watanabe, K.; Ohmiya, Y.; Takusagawa, F. Crystal structure and possible catalytic mechanism of microsomal prostaglandin E synthase type 2 (mPGES-$_2$). *J. Mol. Boil.* **2005**, *348*, 1163–1176. [CrossRef] [PubMed]
25. Cingolani, G.; Panella, A.; Perrone, M.G.; Vitale, P.; Di Mauro, G.; Fortuna, C.G.; Armen, R.S.; Ferorelli, S.; Smith, W.L.; Scilimati, A. Structural basis for selective inhibition of Cyclooxygenase-1 (COX-1) by diarylisoxazoles mofezolac and 3-(5-chlorofuran-2-yl)-5-methyl-4-phenylisoxazole (P6). *Eur. J. Med. Chem.* **2017**, *138*, 661–668. [CrossRef] [PubMed]
26. Orlando, B.J.; Malkowski, M.G. Substrate-selective inhibition of cyclooxygeanse-2 by fenamic acid derivatives is dependent on peroxide tone. *J. Biol. Chem.* **2016**, *291*, 15069–15081. [CrossRef] [PubMed]
27. Blobaum, A.L.; Marnett, L.J. Structural and Functional Basis of Cyclooxygenase Inhibition. *J. Med. Chem.* **2007**, *50*, 1425–1441. [CrossRef] [PubMed]
28. Sherman, W.; Day, T.; Jacobson, M.P.; Friesner, R.A.; Farid, R. Novel procedure for modeling ligand/receptor induced fit effects. *J. Med. Chem.* **2006**, *49*, 534–553. [CrossRef]
29. Pergola, C.; Werz, O. 5-Lipoxygenase inhibitors: A review of recent developments and patents. *Expert Opin. Ther. Pat.* **2010**, *20*, 355–375. [CrossRef]

30. Werz, O. Inhibition of 5-Lipoxygenase Product Synthesis by Natural Compounds of Plant Origin. *Planta Med.* **2007**, *73*, 1331–1357. [CrossRef]
31. Rådmark, O.; Samuelsson, B. Regulation of the activity of 5-lipoxygenase, a key enzyme in leukotriene biosynthesis. *Biochem. Biophys. Res. Commun.* **2010**, *396*, 105–110. [CrossRef]
32. Gilbert, N.C.; Rui, Z.; Neau, D.B.; Waight, M.T.; Bartlett, S.G.; Boeglin, W.E.; Brash, A.R.; Newcomer, M.E. Conversion of human 5-lipoxygenase to a 15-lipoxygenase by a point mutation to mimic phosphorylation at Serine-663. *FASEB J.* **2012**, *26*, 3222–3229. [CrossRef] [PubMed]
33. Tsolaki, E.; Eleftheriou, P.; Kartsev, V.; Geronikaki, A.; Saxena, K.A. Application of Docking Analysis in the Prediction and Biological Evaluation of the Lipoxygenase Inhibitory Action of Thiazolyl Derivatives of Mycophenolic Acid. *Molecules.* **2018**, *23*, 1621. [CrossRef] [PubMed]
34. Chandrasekaran, C.V.; Deepak, H.B.; Thiyagarajan, P.; Kathiresan, S.; Sangli, G.K.; Deepak, M.; Agarwal, A. Dual inhibitory effect of *Glycyrrhiza glabra* (GutGard™) on COX and LOX products. *Phytomedicine* **2011**, *18*, 278–284. [CrossRef] [PubMed]
35. Stamenkovic, D.M.; Laycock, H.; Karanikolas, M.; Ladjevic, N.G.; Neskovic, V.; Bantel, C. Chronic Pain and Chronic Opioid Use After Intensive Care Discharge—Is It Time to Change Practice? *Front. Pharmacol.* **2019**, *10*, 23. [CrossRef]
36. Cosmetic Ingredient Review Expert Panel. Final report on the safety assessment of Glycyrrhetinic Acid, Potassium Glycyrrhetinate, Disodium Succinoyl Glycyrrhetinate, Glyceryl Glycyrrhetinate, Glycyrrhetinyl Stearate, Stearyl Glycyrrhetinate, Glycyrrhizic Acid, Ammonium Glycyrrhizate, Dipotassium Glycyrrhizate, Disodium Glycyrrhizate, Trisodium Glycyrrhizate, Methyl Glycyrrhizate, and Potassium Glycyrrhizinate. Cosmetic Ingredient Review Expert Panel. *Int. J. Toxicol.* **2007**, *26*, 79–112.
37. Menegazzi, M.; Di Paola, R.; Mazzon, E.; Genovese, T.; Crisafulli, C.; Dal Bosco, M.; Zou, Z.; Suzuki, H.; Cuzzocrea, S. Glycyrrhizin attenuates the development of carrageenan-induced lung injury in mice. *Pharmacol. Res.* **2008**, *58*, 22–31. [CrossRef]
38. Sun, Y.; Cai, T.T.; Shen, Y.; Zhou, X.B.; Chen, T.; Xu, Q. Si-Ni-San a traditional Chinese prescription, and its active ingredient glycyrrhizin ameliorate experimental colitis through regulating cytokine balance. *Int. Immunopharmacol.* **2009**, *9*, 1437–1443. [CrossRef]
39. Feng, C.; Wang, H.; Yao, C.; Zhang, J.; Tian, Z. Diammonium glycyrrhizinate, a component of traditional Chinese medicine Gan-Cao, prevents murine T-cell-mediated fulminant hepatitis in IL-10- and IL-6-dependent manners. *Int. Immunopharmacol.* **2007**, *7*, 1292–1298. [CrossRef]
40. Yoshida, T.; Abe, K.; Ikeda, T.; Matsushita, T.; Wake, K.; Sato, T.; Sato, T.; Inoue, H. Inhibitory effect of glycyrrhizin on lipopolysaccharide and d-galactosamine-induced mouse liver injury. *Eur. J. Pharmacol.* **2007**, *576*, 136–142. [CrossRef]
41. Ram, A.; Mabalirajan, U.; Das, M.; Bhattacharya, I.; Dinda, A.K.; Gangal, S.V.; Ghosh, B. Glycyrrhizin alleviates experimental allergic asthma in mice. *Int. Immunopharmacol.* **2006**, *6*, 1468–1477. [CrossRef]
42. Matsui, S.; Sonoda, Y.; Sekiya, T.; Aizu-Yokota, E.; Kasahara, T. Glycyrrhizin derivative inhibits eotaxin 1 production via STAT6 in human lung fibroblasts. *Int. Immunopharmacol.* **2006**, *6*, 369–375. [CrossRef] [PubMed]
43. Calhoun, W.; Chang, J.; Carlson, R.P. Effect of selected antiinflammatory agents and other drugs on zymosan, arachidonic acid, PAF and carrageenan induced paw edema in the mouse. *Agents Actions* **1987**, *21*, 306–309. [CrossRef] [PubMed]
44. Suo, J.; Linke, B.; Meyer dos Santos, S.; Pierre, S.; Stegner, D.; Zhang, D.D.; Denis, C.V.; Geisslinger, G.; Nieswandt, B.; Scholich, K. Neutrophils mediate edema formation but not mechanical allodynia during zymosan-induced inflammation. *J. Leukoc. Biol.* **2014**, *96*, 133–142. [CrossRef] [PubMed]
45. Jain, N.K.; Ishikawa, T.O.; Spigelman, I.; Herschman, H.R. COX-$_2$ expression and function in the hyperalgesic response to paw inflammation in mice. *Prostaglandins Leukot. Essent. Fatty Acids* **2008**, *79*, 183–190. [CrossRef] [PubMed]
46. Mariancecci, C.; Rinaldi, F.; Di Marzio, L.; Mastriota, M.; Pieretti, S.; Celia, C.; Paolino, D.; Iannone, M.; Fresta, M.; Carafa, M. Ammonium glycyrrhizinate-loaded niosomes as a potential nanotherapeutic system for anti-inflammatory activity in murine models. *Int. J. Nanomed.* **2014**, *9*, 635–651. [CrossRef]
47. Cash, J.L.; White, G.E.; Greaves, D.R. Chapter 17. Zymosan-induced peritonitis as a simple experimental system for the study of inflammation. *Methods Enzymol.* **2009**, *461*, 379–396. [CrossRef] [PubMed]

48. Bellingan, G.J.; Caldwell, H.; Howie, S.E.; Dransfield, I.; Haslett, C. In vivo fate of the inflammatory macrophage during the resolution of inflammation: Inflammatory macrophages do not die locally, but emigrate to the draining lymph nodes. *J. Immunol.* **1996**, *157*, 2577–2585.
49. Schwab, J.M.; Chiang, N.; Arita, M.; Serhan, C.N. Resolvin E1 and protectin D1 activate inflammation-resolution programmes. *Nature* **2007**, *447*, 869–874. [CrossRef]
50. Leite, J.A.; Alves, A.K.; Galvão, J.G.; Teixeira, M.P.; Cavalcante-Silva, L.H.; Scavone, C.; Morrot, A.; Rumjanek, V.M.; Rodrigues-Mascarenhas, S. Ouabain Modulates Zymosan-Induced Peritonitis in Mice. *Mediat. Inflamm.* **2015**, *2015*, 265798. [CrossRef]
51. Shi, J.R.; Mao, L.G.; Jiang, R.A.; Qian, Y.; Tang, H.F.; Chen, J.Q. Monoammonium glycyrrhizinate inhibited the inflammation of LPS-induced acute lung injury in mice. *Int. Immunopharmacol.* **2010**, *10*, 1235–1241. [CrossRef]
52. Ni, Y.F.; Kuai, J.K.; Lu, Z.F.; Yang, G.D.; Fu, H.Y.; Wang, J.; Tian, F.; Yan, X.L.; Zhao, Y.C.; Wang, Y.J.; et al. Glycyrrhizin treatment is associated with attenuation of lipopolysaccharide-induced acute lung injury by inhibiting cyclooxygenase-2 and inducible nitric oxide synthase expression. *J. Surg. Res.* **2011**, *165*, e29–e35. [CrossRef] [PubMed]
53. Le Bars, D.; Gozariu, M.; Cadden, S.W. Animal models of nociception. *Pharmacol. Rev.* **2001**, *53*, 597–652. [PubMed]
54. Satyanarayana, P.S.; Jain, N.K.; Singh, A.; Kulkarni, S.K. Isobolographic analysis of interaction between cyclooxygenase inhibitors and tramadol in acetic acid-induced writhing in mice. *Prog. Neuropsychopharmacol. Biol. Psychiatry* **2004**, *28*, 641–649. [CrossRef] [PubMed]
55. Ribeiro, R.A.; Vale, M.L.; Thomazzi, S.M.; Paschoalato, A.B.; Poole, S.; Ferreira, S.H.; Cunha, F.Q. Involvement of resident macrophages and mast cells in the writhing nociceptive response induced by zymosan and acetic acid in mice. *Eur. J. Pharmacol.* **2000**, *387*, 111–118. [CrossRef]
56. Hunskaar, S.; Hole, K. The formalin test in mice: Dissociation between inflammatory and non-inflammatory pain. *Pain* **1987**, *30*, 103–114. [CrossRef]
57. Lau, G.T.; Ye, L.; Leung, L.K. The licorice flavonoid isoliquiritigenin suppresses phorbol ester-induced cyclooxygenase-2 expression in the non-tumorigenic MCF-10A breast cell line. *Planta Med.* **2010**, *76*, 780–785. [CrossRef]
58. Song, N.R.; Kim, J.E.; Park, J.S.; Kim, J.R.; Kang, H.; Lee, E.; Kang, Y.G.; Son, J.E.; Seo, S.G.; Heo, Y.S.; et al. Licochalcone A, a polyphenol present in licorice, suppresses UV-induced COX-2 expression by targeting PI3K, MEK1, and B-Raf. *Int. J. Mol. Sci.* **2015**, *16*, 4453–4470. [CrossRef]
59. Cherng, J.M.; Tsai, K.D.; Yu, Y.W.; Lin, J.C. Molecular mechanisms underlying chemopreventive activities of glycyrrhizic acid against UVB-radiation-induced carcinogenesis in SKH-1 hairless mouse epidermis. *Radiat. Res.* **2011**, *176*, 177–186. [CrossRef]
60. Hou, S.Z.; Li, Y.; Zhu, X.L.; Wang, Z.Y.; Wang, X.; Xu, Y. Ameliorative effects of diammonium glycyrrhizinate on inflammation in focal cerebral ischemic-reperfusion injury. *Brain Res.* **2012**, *1447*, 20–27. [CrossRef]
61. Zhao, H.; Zhao, M.; Wang, Y.; Li, F.; Zhang, Z. Glycyrrhizic Acid Attenuates Sepsis-Induced Acute Kidney Injury by Inhibiting NF-κB Signaling Pathway. *Evid. Based Complement. Alternat. Med.* **2016**, *2016*, 8219287. [CrossRef]
62. Liu, W.; Huang, S.; Li, Y.; Li, Y.; Li, D.; Wu, P.; Wang, Q.; Zheng, X.; Zhang, K. Glycyrrhizic acid from licorice down-regulates inflammatory responses via blocking MAPK and PI3K/Akt-dependent NF-κB signalling pathways in TPA-induced skin inflammation. *MedChemComm* **2018**, *9*, 1502–1510. [CrossRef] [PubMed]
63. Afnan, Q.; Kaiser, P.J.; Rafiq, R.A.; Nazir, L.A.; Bhushan, S.; Bhardwaj, S.C.; Sandhir, R.; Tasduq, S.A. Glycyrrhizic acid prevents ultraviolet-B-induced photodamage: A role for mitogen-activated protein kinases, nuclear factor kappa B and mitochondrial apoptotic pathway. *Exp. Dermatol.* **2016**, *25*, 440–446. [CrossRef] [PubMed]
64. Wang, X.R.; Hao, H.G.; Chu, L. Glycyrrhizin inhibits LPS-induced inflammatory mediator production in endometrial epithelial cells. *Microb. Pathog.* **2017**, *109*, 110–113. [CrossRef] [PubMed]
65. Kilkenny, C.; Browne, W.; Cuthill, I.C.; Emerson, M.; Altman, D.G. Animal research: Reporting in vivo experiments: The ARRIVE guidelines. *Br. J. Pharmacol.* **2010**, *160*, 1577–1579. [CrossRef] [PubMed]
66. McGrath, J.C.; Lilley, E. Implementing guidelines on reporting research using animals (ARRIVE etc.): New requirements for publication in BJP. *Br. J. Pharmacol.* **2015**, *172*, 3189–3193. [CrossRef] [PubMed]

67. Colucci, M.; Maione, F.; Bonito, M.C.; Piscopo, A.; Di Giannuario, A.; Pieretti, S. New insights of dimethyl sulphoxide effects (DMSO) on experimental in vivo models of nociception and inflammation. *Pharmacol. Res.* **2008**, *57*, 419–425. [CrossRef] [PubMed]
68. Pieretti, S.; Dal Piaz, V.; Matucci, R.; Giovannoni, M.P.; Galli, A. Antinociceptive activity of a 3(2H)-pyridazinone derivative in mice. *Life Sci.* **1999**, *65*, 1381–1394. [CrossRef]
69. Tjølsen, A.; Berge, O.G.; Hunskaar, S.; Rosland, J.H.; Hole, K. The formalin test: An evaluation of the method. *Pain* **1992**, *51*, 5–17. [CrossRef]
70. Niederberger, E.; Schmidtko, A.; Gao, W.; Kühlein, H.; Ehnert, C.; Geisslinger, G. Impaired acute and inflammatory nociception in mice lacking the p50 subunit of NF-kappaB. *Eur. J. Pharmacol.* **2007**, *559*, 55–60. [CrossRef]
71. Chatterjee, B.E.; Yona, S.; Rosignoli, G.; Young, R.E.; Nourshargh, S.; Flower, R.J.; Perretti, M. Annexin 1-deficient neutrophils exhibit enhanced transmigration in vivo and increased responsiveness in vitro. *J. Leukoc. Biol.* **2005**, *78*, 639–646. [CrossRef]
72. Damazo, A.S.; Yona, S.; Flower, R.J.; Perretti, M.; Oliani, S.M. Spatial and temporal profiles for anti-inflammatory gene expression in leukocytes during a resolving model of peritonitis. *J. Immunol.* **2006**, *176*, 4410–4418. [CrossRef] [PubMed]
73. Maione, F.; Piccolo, M.; De Vita, S.; Chini, M.G.; Cristiano, C.; De Caro, C.; Lippiello, P.; Miniaci, M.C.; Santamaria, R.; Irace, C.; et al. Down regulation of pro-inflammatory pathways by tanshinone IIA and cryptotanshinone in a non-genetic mouse model of Alzheimer's disease. *Pharmacol. Res.* **2018**, *129*, 482–490. [CrossRef] [PubMed]
74. Partridge, K.M.; Antonysamy, S.; Bhattachar, S.N.; Chandrasekhar, S.; Fisher, M.J.; Fretland, A.; Gooding, K.; Harvey, A.; Hughes, N.E.; Kuklish, S.L.; et al. Discovery and characterization of [(cyclopentyl) ethyl] benzoic acid inhibitors of microsomal prostaglandin E synthase-1. *Bioorg. Med. Chem. Lett.* **2017**, *27*, 1478–1483. [CrossRef] [PubMed]
75. Sastry, G.M.; Adzhigirey, M.; Day, T.; Annabhimoju, R.; Sherman, W. Protein and ligand preparation: Parameters, protocols, and influence on virtual screening enrichments. *J. Comput. Aided Mol. Des.* **2013**, *27*, 221–234. [CrossRef] [PubMed]
76. D'Ambola, M.; Fiengo, L.; Chini, M.G.; Cotugno, R.; Bader, A.; Bifulco, G.; Braca, A.; De Tommasi, N.; Dal Piaz, F. Fusicoccane Diterpenes from Hypoestes forsskaolii as Heat Shock Protein 90 (Hsp90) Modulators. *J. Nat. Prod.* **2019**, *82*, 539–549. [CrossRef] [PubMed]
77. Friesner, R.A.; Murphy, R.B.; Repasky, M.P.; Frye, L.L.; Greenwood, J.R.; Halgren, T.A.; Sanschagrin, P.C.; Mainz, D.T. Extra Precision Glide: Docking and Scoring Incorporating a Model of Hydrophobic Enclosure for Protein-Ligand Complexes. *J. Med. Chem.* **2006**, *49*, 6177–6196. [CrossRef] [PubMed]
78. Halgren, T.A.; Murphy, R.B.; Friesner, R.A.; Beard, H.S.; Frye, L.L.; Pollard, W.T.; Banks, J.L. Glide: A New Approach for Rapid, Accurate Docking and Scoring. 2. Enrichment Factors in Database Screening. *J. Med. Chem.* **2004**, *47*, 1750–1759. [CrossRef]
79. Friesner, R.A.; Banks, J.L.; Murphy, R.B.; Halgren, T.A.; Klicic, J.J.; Mainz, D.T.; Repasky, M.P.; Knoll, E.H.; Shaw, D.E.; Shelley, M.; et al. Glide: A New Approach for Rapid, Accurate Docking and Scoring. 1. Method and Assessment of Docking Accuracy. *J. Med. Chem.* **2004**, *47*, 1739–1749. [CrossRef]
80. Jacobson, M.P.; Pincus, D.L.; Rapp, C.S.; Day, T.J.F.; Honig, B.; Shaw, D.E.; Friesner, R.A. A hierarchical approach to all-atom protein loop prediction. *Proteins Struct. Funct. Bioinf.* **2004**, *55*, 351–367. [CrossRef]
81. Jacobson, M.P.; Friesner, R.A.; Xiang, Z.; Honig, B. On the Role of the Crystal Environment in Determining Protein Side-chain Conformations. *J. Mol. Biol.* **2002**, *320*, 597–608. [CrossRef]
82. Curtis, M.J.; Bond, R.A.; Spina, D.; Ahluwalia, A.; Alexander, S.P.A.; Giembycz, M.A.; Gilchrist, A.; Hoyer, D.; Insel, P.A.; Izzo, A.A.; et al. Experimental design and analysis and their reporting: New guidance for publication in BJP. *Br. J. Pharmacol.* **2015**, *172*, 3461–3471. [CrossRef] [PubMed]

Sample Availability: Not available.

© 2019 by the authors. Licensee MDPI, Basel, Switzerland. This article is an open access article distributed under the terms and conditions of the Creative Commons Attribution (CC BY) license (http://creativecommons.org/licenses/by/4.0/).

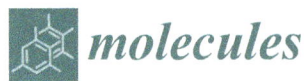

Article

Mechanism Investigation of *Tagetes patula* L. against Chronic Nonbacterial Prostatitis by Metabolomics and Network Pharmacology

Xueying Liu [1], Xiaoku Ran [1], Muhammad Riaz [1,2], Haixue Kuang [3,*], Deqiang Dou [1,*] and Decheng Cai [4]

1. College of Pharmacy, Liaoning University of Traditional Chinese Medicine, Dalian 116600, China; liuxueying0806@126.com (X.L.); xkran@163.com (X.R.); pharmariaz@outlook.com (M.R.)
2. Department of Pharmacy, Shaheed Benazir Bhutto Sheringal Dir Upper, Khyber Pakhtoon Khwa 18000, Pakistan
3. College of Pharmacy, Heilongjiang University of Chinese Medicine, Harbin 150040, China
4. Dalian Wuzhou Holy Herb Scientific and Techonological Co. Ltd, Dalian 116600, China; caidecheng1@126.com
* Correspondence: hxkuang@hotmail.com (H.K.); deqiangdou@126.com (D.D.); Tel.: +86-451-82193001 (H.K.); +86-411-87586014 (D.D.); Fax: +86-451-82110803 (H.K.); +86-411-85890128 (D.D.)

Academic Editor: Francesco Maione
Received: 21 May 2019; Accepted: 17 June 2019; Published: 18 June 2019

Abstract: The major objective of this study was to investigate the anti-chronic nonbacterial prostatitis (CNP) mechanism of *T. patula* by metabolomics and network pharmacology. The study demonstrated that the flavonoids and polysaccharides of *T. patula* could alleviate prostatitis by improving the level of DHT, reducing the secretion of PSA and TNF-α. Besides, both could enhance Na^+/K^+-ATPase activity, decrease the O_2 consumption, CO_2 production, heat production, energy expenditure of rats and promote respiratory exchange ratio of rats. Up to 28 potential biomarkers and 8 key metabolic pathways related to the treatment of CNP were elucidated by the metabolomics analysis, including phenylalanine metabolism, taurine and hypotaurine metabolism, tryptophan metabolism etc. Network pharmacology prediction also reflected the potential mechanism was associated with tryptophan metabolism and energy pathway. Generally, the potential anti-CNP mechanism of flavonoids and polysaccharides of *T. patula* might be through reducing the expression of inflammation factors, adjusting the level of hormone and regulating the amino acid metabolism, energy metabolism and glucose and lipid metabolism.

Keywords: *Tagetes patula* L.; chronic nonbacterial prostatitis; metabolomics; energy metabolism; network pharmacology

1. Introduction

Prostatitis is a common urinary system disease that endangers the health of adult males. Chronic nonbacterial prostatitis (CNP), as the most common type of prostatitis, is difficult to cure and easily recurs though there are several methods for treatment. *T. patula* is a perennial herb belonging to the family of Asteraceae, commonly known as French marigold, and it is also a traditional drug in Argentina, where it is used for the diuretic agent associated with prostatitis treatments [1,2]. We had illustrated that flavonoids were the main components of *T. patula* (Supplementary Materials Figure S1), and previous study had investigated that flavonoids and polysaccharides of *T. patula* were the effective constituents against CNP and their efficacy might be associated with hormone and the inflammatory mediators [3]. The emergence of metabolomics provided a new strategy to investigate the action mechanisms of *T. patula* anti-CNP. As a newly developed strategy, network pharmacology focused on searching for the relationships of active ingredients and their potential targets, which might be associated with pharmacological mechanisms in metabolomics. Therefore, this research aimed at deeply investigating the pharmacological mechanism of active constituents of *T. patula* against CNP through metabolomics and network pharmacology.

2. Results

2.1. The Levels of Physiological Indexes

Compared with the Sham-operated group (SOG), the levels of prostate-specific antigen (PSA) and tumor necrosis factor-α (TNF-α) in the chronic nonbacterial prostatitis model group (MOG) were a significant increase ($p < 0.05$, $p < 0.001$), and the levels of dihydrotestosterone (DHT) in MOG decreased obviously ($p < 0.01$). Serum DHT level was significantly higher in the polysaccharide treatment group (POL) and flavonoids treatment group (FLA) than in MOG ($p < 0.001$, $p < 0.0001$). Comparing with MOG, the serum PSA level in *Pule'an* tablet treatment group (TCM); Water decoction treatment group (WAD), POL and FLA all showed decreasing trends, and the content of TNF-α in levofloxacin treatment group (LEH), TCM, WAD, EOC and FLA also showed decreasing trends (Figure 1). The histological results of the prostate were shown in Supplementary Materials Figure S4: Histological analysis of prostate.

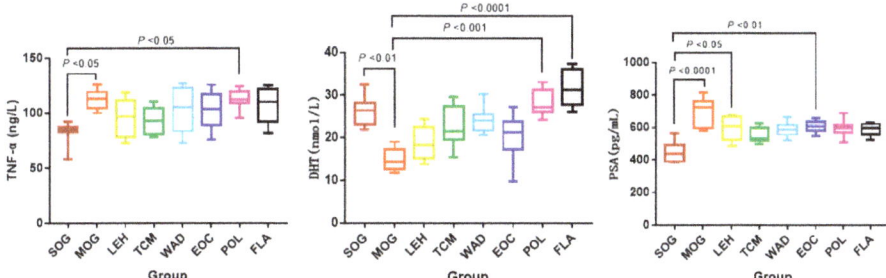

Figure 1. The concentrations of tumor necrosis factor-α (TNF-α), dihydrotestosterone (DHT) and prostate-specific antigen (PSA). Notes: Sham-operated group (SOG), Chronic nonbacterial prostatitis model group (MOG), Water decoction treatment group (WAD), Essential oil treatment group (EOC), Polysaccharide treatment group (POL), Flavonoids treatment group (FLA), *Pule'an* tablet treatment group (TCM), Levofloxacin treatment group (LEH).

2.2. The Activity of Na^+/K^+-ATPase

Comparing with SOG, Na^+/K^+-ATPase activity in MOG prostate was significantly reduced ($p < 0.01$). And comparing with MOG, water decoction and all the components of *T. patula* could enhance the Na^+/K^+-ATPase activity of prostate, in which POL and FLA were significantly increased extremely ($p < 0.001$) and WAD and EOC was increased significantly ($p < 0.05$, $p < 0.01$). Comparing with SOG, Na^+/K^+-ATPase activity of livers in MOG, LEH, TCM, WAD and EOC were substantially decreased ($p < 0.001$, $p < 0.01$, $p < 0.05$, $p < 0.001$, $p < 0.0001$). Na^+/K^+-ATPase activity of liver in FLA was significantly stronger than in MOG ($p < 0.05$) (Figure 2).

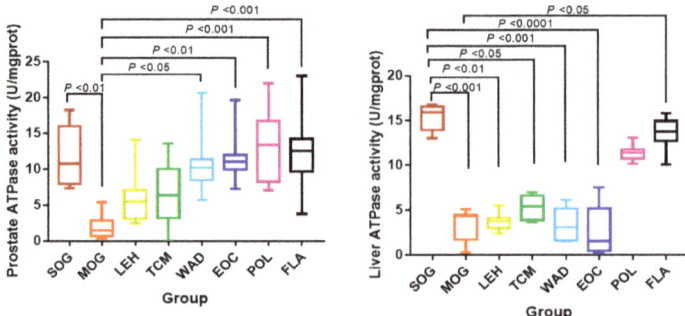

Figure 2. The activities of Na$^+$/K$^+$-ATPase in prostate and liver tissues. Notes: Sham-operated group (SOG), Chronic nonbacterial prostatitis model group (MOG), Water decoction treatment group (WAD), Essential oil treatment group (EOC), Polysaccharide treatment group (POL), Flavonoids treatment group (FLA), *Pule'an* tablet treatment group (TCM), Levofloxacin treatment group (LEH).

2.3. Results of Energy Metabolic Parameters

Based on actual animal weight calculations, comparing with SOG, the O$_2$ consumption (VO$_2$), CO$_2$ production (VCO$_2$), heat production (H) and energy expenditure (EE) in MOG and other treatment groups all show increasing trends no matter when the time was. However, energy metabolism parameters of WAD, POL and FLA all showed a decline at a certain degree. Respiratory exchange ratio (RER) of MOG and other treatment groups showed downtrends in comparison with SOG. From Figure 3, a difference between the model rats and sham rats in terms of energy metabolism can be seen.

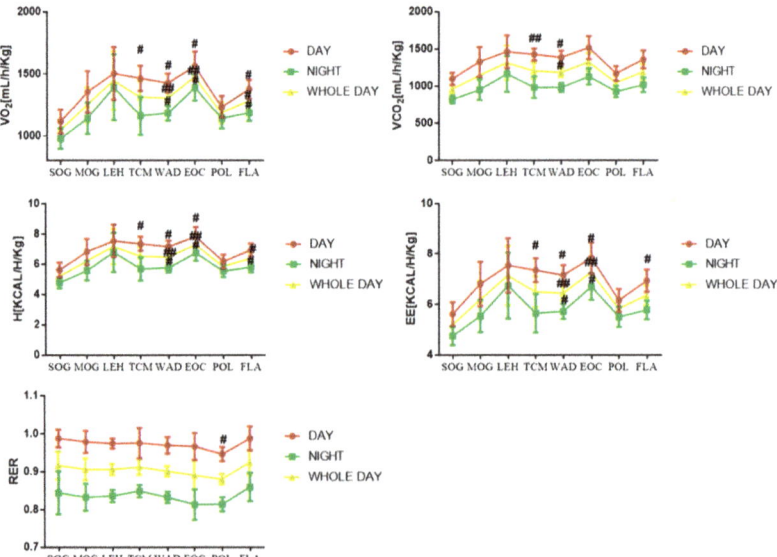

Figure 3. Changes of VO$_2$, VCO$_2$, H, EE and RER in rats during the day, night and the whole day. Notes: $^\#$ $p < 0.05$, $^{\#\#}$ $p < 0.01$ compared with SOG. Sham-operated group (SOG), Chronic nonbacterial prostatitis model group (MOG), Water decoction treatment group (WAD), Essential oil treatment group (EOC), Polysaccharide treatment group (POL), Flavonoids treatment group (FLA), *Pule'an* tablet treatment group (TCM), Levofloxacin treatment group (LEH), O$_2$ consumption (VO$_2$), CO$_2$ production (VCO$_2$), Heat production (H), Energy expenditure (EE), Respiratory exchange ratio (RER).

2.4. LC-MS Analysis of Metabolic Profiling

Using the super-high performance liquid chromatography-mass spectrum in series (UPLC-MS) conditions described in the methods, the representative total ion current (TIC) chromatograms of urine samples of different groups which harvested by UPLC/electrospray ionization quadrupole-time of flight (ESI-Q-TOF)/MS analysis were presented in Supplementary Materials Figure S2: TIC chromatograms on positive ion mode and Figure S3: TIC chromatograms on negative ion mode. The contours of these spectra differed between 3–5 min and 8–10 min in positive and negative TIC. The PCA and PLS-DA results displayed as score plots showed the scatter of the samples, which indicated similar metabolomics compositions when clustered together and compositional difference metabolomes when dispersed. Overall view of all PCA score plots, SOG and MOG were significantly divided into two classes, indicating that the model of CNP was successfully reproduced. As a supervised pattern recognition method, PLS-DA could better reflect the difference of distinct groups. The corresponding PLS-DA score plots also indicated that MOG is clearly separated from SOG, which implied that the metabolic characteristics of the various small molecules are obviously different. The 3D of PLS-DA score plot shows that SOG, MOG, POL and FLA were separated clearly, and the POL and FLA group was closer to SOG than MOG, which suggested that polysaccharides and flavonoids could reverse the pathological process of CNP (Figure 4).

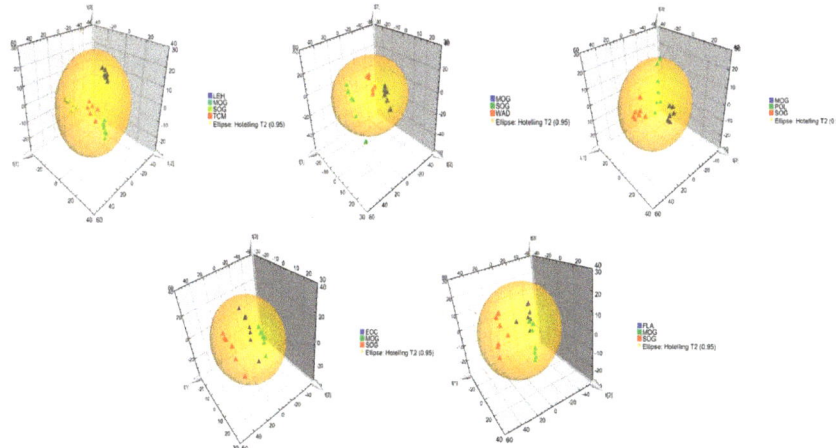

Figure 4. 3D PLS-DA score plot in positive ion mode. Notes: Sham-operated group (SOG), Chronic nonbacterial prostatitis model group (MOG), Water decoction treatment group (WAD), Essential oil treatment group (EOC), Polysaccharide treatment group (POL), Flavonoids treatment group (FLA), *Pule'an* tablet treatment group (TCM), Levofloxacin treatment group (LEH).

2.5. Identification of Metabolite Candidates

All collected samples were analyzed. Targeted and non-targeted metabolite candidates were identified as above described methods. Targeted metabolomics identified a total of 13 metabolites and non-targeted metabolomics provided 94 metabolites. A total of 28 metabolite candidates were designated by comprehensively comparative analysis of VIP and *P* values with significant differences (Table 1).

Table 1. Differential Metabolite Pathway Analysis Results.

Compound ID	Metabolite	Molecular Formula	Mode	Ret. Time	M/Z	Trend
HMDB0000158	Δ L-tyrosine	$C_9H_{11}NO_3$	ESI -	1.3987	180.0632	-
HMDB0006236	Phenylacetaldehyde	C_8H_8O	ESI +	1.5029	121.0663	-
HMDB0000205	Phenylpyruvic acid	$C_9H_8O_3$	ESI -	3.5141	163.0386	-
HMDB0000159	Δ L-phenylalanine	$C_9H_{11}NO_2$	ESI +	2.1193	120.0800	-
HMDB0003426	Pantetheine	$C_{11}H_{22}N_2O_4S$	ESI +	2.5712	279.1378	-
HMDB0000574	L-Cysteine	$C_3H_7NO_2S$	ESI +	4.8468	122.0283	-
HMDB0000210	Pantothenic Acid	$C_9H_{17}NO_5$	ESI -	2.3662	218.1016	-
HMDB0000300	Uracil	$C_7H_{10}N_2OS$	ESI +	1.5955	113.0465	+
HMDB0000929	Tryptophan	$C_{11}H_{12}N_2O_2$	ESI +	2.9052	205.1002	+
HMDB0000259	Serotonin	$C_{10}H_{12}N_2O$	ESI +	1.8983	177.1051	-
HMDB0000684	L-Kynurenine	$C_{10}H_{12}N_2O_3$	ESI +	2.3458	191.0838	-
HMDB0000734	Indoleacrylic acid	$C_{11}H_9NO_2$	ESI -	6.86	186.0561	+
HMDB0000978	4-(2-Aminophenyl)-2,4-dioxobutanoic acid	$C_{10}H_9NO_4$	ESI +	3.434	208.0615	-
HMDB0000197	3-Indoleacetic Acid	$C_{10}H_9NO_2$	ESI -	6.1042	174.0572	-
HMDB0001644	D-Xylulose	$C_5H_{10}O_5$	ESI -	1.6288	151.0607	-
HMDB0000127	D-Glucuronic acid	$C_6H_{10}O_7$	ESI -	3.6827	193.0474	+
HMDB0000177	Δ L-histidine	$C_6H_9N_3O_2$	ESI +	0.6353	156.0459	-
HMDB0062781	2-oxoglutarate	$C_5H_6O_5$	ESI -	0.8023	145.0105	+
HMDB0000156	Δ L-Malic acid	$C_4H_6O_5$	ESI -	0.7309	133.0072	+
HMDB0000094	Δ Citrate	$C_6H_8O_7$	ESI +	0.9318	193.0375	+
HMDB0000068	Epinephrine	$C_6H_7N_5O$	ESI +	2.3582	184.0994	-
HMDB0000073	Δ Dopamine	$C_8H_{11}NO_2$	ESI +	0.8783	154.0985	+
HMDB0002052	Maleylacetoacetic acid	$C_8H_8O_6$	ESI +	2.8867	201.042	-
HMDB0000251	Δ Taurine	$C_2H_7NO_3S$	ESI -	0.6159	124.0016	-
HMDB0000167	Δ L-threonine	$C_4H_9NO_3$	ESI +	0.7366	120.0690	+
HMDB0000123	Δ Glycine	$C_2H_5NO_2$	ESI +	4.2937	76.0406	-
HMDB0000289	Uric acid	$C_5H_4N_4O_3$	ESI +	1.0763	169.0381	-
HMDB0000034	Adenine	$C_6H_7N_5$	ESI +	0.9096	136.0654	-

Notes: Δ represents target metabolomics differential metabolites, and the rest are untargeted metabolomics differential metabolites. - indicates that MOG has a decreasing trend compared with SOG, + indicates that MOG showed an upward trend compared with SOG.

2.6. Pathway Analysis

To gain insight into the metabolic mechanism of CNP, metabolic pathways of the significantly altered metabolites were analyzed by using the pathway analysis module within the Masslynx V4.1 Workstations. Related pathways of biomarkers were identified by searching Kyoto Encyclopedia of Genes and Genomes (KEGG) and Human Metabolome Database (HMDB) PATHWAY Database. We identified a total of 31 metabolic pathways which were related to the metabolite candidates (Table 2). However, only 8 distinct metabolic pathways were significantly altered in the urine samples as compared with the model group ($p < 0.05$, impact > 0.1). The predominant hits were pathways involved in phenylalanine, tyrosine and tryptophan biosynthesis, phenylalanine metabolism, taurine and hypotaurine metabolism, tryptophan metabolism, tyrosine metabolism, glyoxylate and dicarboxylate metabolism, glycine, serine and threonine metabolism and citrate cycle (TCA cycle) (Figure 5). Results indicated that these pathways showed the marked perturbations over the formation of CNP and could contribute to the development of CNP.

Table 2. Metabolyst Approach Analysis Results Based on KEGG.

No.	Pathway Name	Match Status	P	Impact
1	Δ Phenylalanine, tyrosine and tryptophan biosynthesis	3/4	2.52×10^{-5}	1
2	Δ Phenylalanine metabolism	4/9	1.29×10^{-5}	0.77778
3	Δ Taurine and hypotaurine metabolism	2/8	0.0093149	0.42857
4	Ascorbate and aldarate metabolism	1/9	0.16098	0.4
5	Δ Tryptophan metabolism	5/41	8.37×10^{-4}	0.35955
6	Δ Tyrosine metabolism	4/42	0.0074067	0.32959
7	Δ Glyoxylate and dicarboxylate metabolism	2/16	0.036307	0.2963
8	Δ Glycine, serine and threonine metabolism	3/32	0.021783	0.29197
9	Histidine metabolism	1/15	0.25411	0.24194

Table 2. Cont.

No.	Pathway Name	Match Status	P	Impact
10	∆ Citrate cycle (TCA cycle)	3/20	0.0058413	0.16675
11	Cysteine and methionine metabolism	1/28	0.42297	0.12829
12	Pantothenate and CoA biosynthesis	4/15	1.29×10^{-4}	0.08163
13	Alanine, aspartate and glutamate metabolism	1/24	0.37538	0.06329
14	Primary bile acid biosynthesis	2/46	0.22107	0.05952
15	Pyrimidine metabolism	1/41	0.5547	0.04182
16	Purine metabolism	2/68	0.38017	0.02549
17	Glutathione metabolism	2/26	0.087435	0.00955
18	Ubiquinone and other terpenoid-quinone biosynthesis	1/3	0.056709	0
19	Thiamine metabolism	1/7	0.12752	0
20	Starch and sucrose metabolism	1/23	0.36291	0
21	Pyruvate metabolism	1/22	0.35019	0
22	Porphyrin and chlorophyll metabolism	1/27	0.41141	0
23	Pentose and glucuronate interconversions	2/14	0.028192	0
24	Nitrogen metabolism	2/9	0.011835	0
25	Methane metabolism	1/9	0.16098	0
26	Inositol phosphate metabolism	1/26	0.39963	0
27	D-glutamine and D-glutamate metabolism	1/5	0.09278	0
28	Cyanoamino acid metabolism	1/6	0.11031	0
29	Butanoate metabolism	1/20	0.32403	0
30	beta-Alanine metabolism	1/19	0.31057	0
31	Aminoacyl-tRNA biosynthesis	7/67	1.72×10^{-4}	0

Notes: ∆ represents pathway satisfied with the condition of both $p < 0.05$ and impact > 0.1

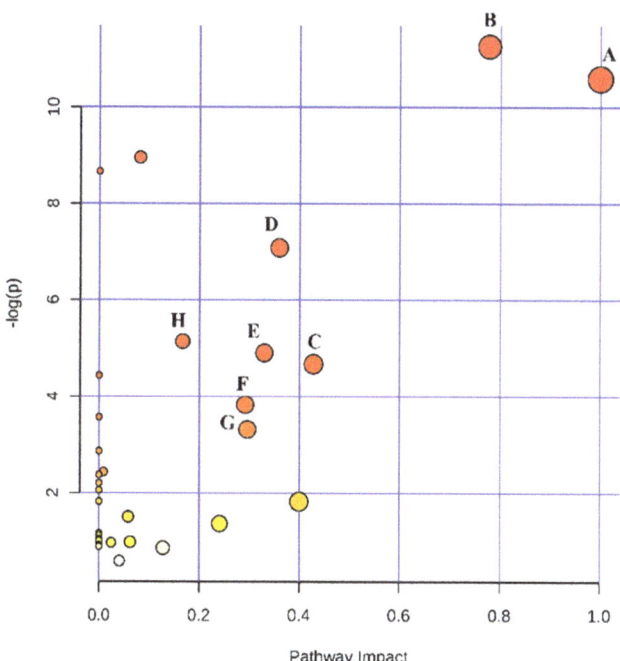

Figure 5. Summary of pathway analysis. Notes: A. Phenylalanine, tyrosine and tryptophan biosynthesis; B. Phenylalanine metabolism; C. Taurine and hypotaurine metabolism; D. Tryptophan metabolism; E. Tyrosine metabolism; F. Glyoxylate and dicarboxylate metabolism; G. Glycine, serine and threonine metabolism; H. Citrate cycle (TCA cycle).

2.7. Network Pharmacology

Figure 6 illustrates the interaction between the active compounds in *T. patula* and a potential target for prostatitis disease. In total, this network comprised 19 nodes (8 active compounds, 1 disease and 10 potential drug targets) and 25 edges. From Figure 6, we found that various compounds could hit multiple potential targets, while some could only hit less potential biomarkers. Compounds that can hit multiple potential targets were thought to be major active compounds in anti-prostatitis. Functional analysis by gene enrichment function of FunRich software indicated that up to 50% merge genes were associated with energy pathway and metabolism (Figure 7). And the results of enriched pathways showed that caffeine metabolism, omega-hydroxylase P450 pathway, ERBB signaling pathway, epoxygenase P450 pathway and tryptophan metabolism had more richfactor (Figure 8). The number of genes in RichFactor, P value, and enrichment pathways is a measure of KEGG enrichment. The larger the RichFactor, the greater the degree of enrichment is. The value of p value is [0,1], and the closer to 0, the more significant the enrichment is. Potential targets of active compounds and relevant target genes of prostatitis were shown in Supplementary Materials Table S1: Potential targets of active compounds. and Table S2: Relevant target genes of prostatitis. Information of merging gene was displayed in Supplementary Materials Table S3: The information of merging gene. Details of enriched pathways are summarized in the Supplementary Materials Table S4: Details of enriched pathways.

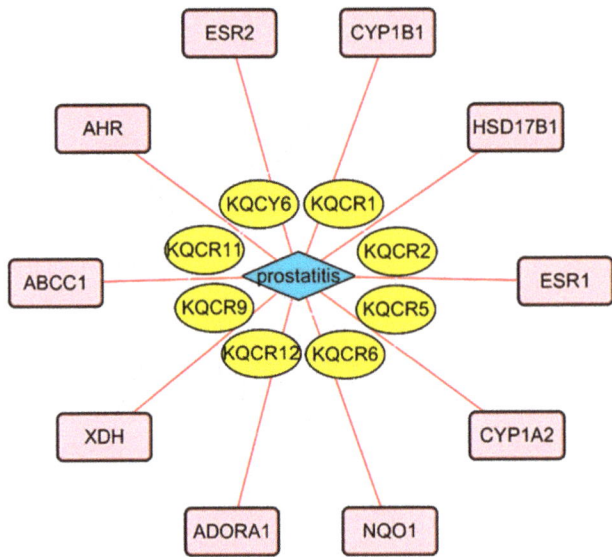

Figure 6. *T. patula* active compounds-target-prostatitis disease interaction.

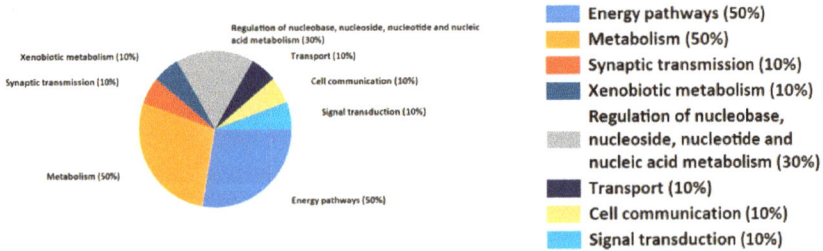

Figure 7. Biological process for merge gene.

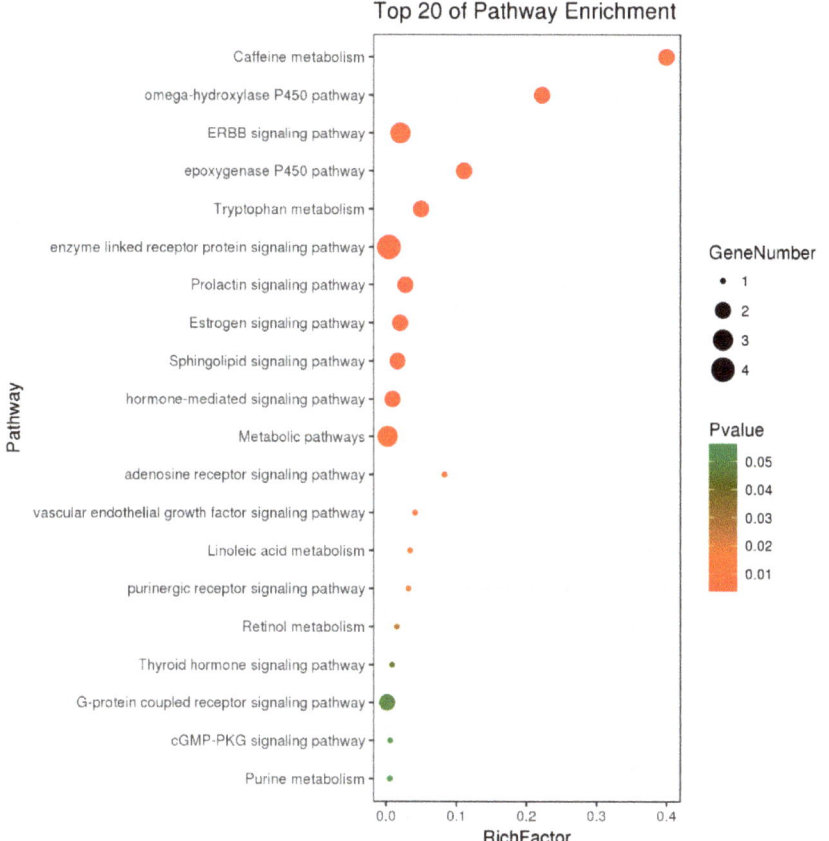

Figure 8. Pathway enrichment analysis of network pharmacology.

3. Discussion

As is well known, the main manifestations of prostatitis exhibited a pain in the pelvic region and dysfunction of urination. The main manifestations of pain exhibited anxiety, tachypnea, hypertension, hyperhidrosis and etc. It is interesting to note that the increasing of VO_2 and VCO_2 in this study might be caused by tachypnea, so as to promote the degree of H and EE and decrease RER. However, the flavonoids constituent and polysaccharides constituent of *T. patula* could reverse those. In addition, the increasing of Na^+/K^+-ATPase's activities in prostate and liver also reflected that the flavonoids and polysaccharides of *T. patula* could regulate energy metabolism.

Urine samples were analyzed by UPLC/ESI-TOF-MS and multivariate statistical analysis. The results showed that the area of dynamic metabolic profiles after polysaccharide and flavonoids treatment was close to the sham-operated group, demonstrating that polysaccharide and flavonoids of *T. patula* had therapeutic efficacy. Metabonomics analysis discovered that phenylalanine, tyrosine and tryptophan biosynthesis and phenylalanine metabolism in the rat prostatitis model showed abnormal metabolism. Compared with SOG, the levels of l-tyrosine, phenylacetaldehyde, phenylpyruvic acid, l-phenylalanine, pantetheine, l-cysteine, pantothenic acid, serotonin, l-kynurenine, 4-(2-Aminophenyl)-2,4-dioxobutanoic acid, 3-indoleacetic acid, d-xylulose, l-histidine, epinephrine, maleylacetoacetic acid, taurine, glycine, uric acid and adenine in the urine of model rats were reduced to varying degrees, and the contents of uracil, tryptophan, indoleacrylic acid, d-glucuronic acid, 2-oxoglutarate, l-malic acid, citrate, dopamine and l-threonine in the urine of model rats were increased to different degrees.

After the treatment of polysaccharide and flavonoids of *T. patula*, the concentration of L-tyrosine, L-phenylalanine, panteheine, L-cysteine, pantothenic acid, 4-(2-Aminophenyl)-2,4-dioxobutanoic acid, 3-indoleacetic acid, L-histidine, maleylacetoacetic acid, taurine, glycine, uric acid, adenine, tryptophan, indoleacrylic acid, D-glucuronic acid, 2-oxoglutarate, L-malic acid, citrate and L-threonine in urine were adjusted backwards to normal in certain degrees.

These above differential metabolite identification results referred the pathway related to phenylalanine, tyrosine and tryptophan biosynthesis, phenylalanine metabolism, pantothenate and CoA biosynthesis, tryptophan metabolism, pentose and glucuronate interconversions, aminoacyl-tRNA biosynthesis and taurine and hypotaurine metabolism. These disturbed metabolic pathways can be partially reversed by the polysaccharides and the total flavonoids of *T. patula*, in other words, they may help in repairing these metabolites.

Network pharmacology results also reflect the potential mechanism of active compounds in *T. patula* anti-prostatitis. The analysis results showed that the compounds in *T. patula* acts on multiple targets to anti-prostatitis. By integrating the metabolomics pathway and the target pathways predicted by network pharmacology, we found that they are similar, which could explain the accuracy of the predicted target. Research indicated that prostatitis is associated closely with hormone and inflammatory level. Uric acid has the antioxidant capacity and can prevent the emergence of an inflammatory environment [4–7]. Generally, the androgen of prostatitis patients is lower than healthy people. Amino acids are not merely the constituent units of proteins, but also can participate in hormone biosynthesis [8,9]. L-phenylalanine is the precursor of the tyrosine and catecholamines, while tyrosine is closely linked to the formation of certain hormones and neurotransmitters such as dopamine and epinephrine [10]. Phenylpyruvic acid and phenylacetaldehyde both are the intermediate or catabolic byproduct of phenylalanine metabolism [7]. Dopamine is a precursor to adrenaline and norepinephrine, which are synthesized by tyrosine [11]. Epinephrine is linked to the regulation of body temperature, which is derived from the phenylalanine and tyrosine [11]. L-threonine is oxidized by threonine dehydrogenase to form glycine [12]. Glycine is transformed into serine by the action of serine hydroxymethyltransferase, and serine further forms cysteine [13]. Cysteine is dehydrogenated to form cystine, which in turn can be hydrogenated to cysteine. Cystine is a structural component of many tissues and hormones. Besides, cysteine is also extremely important for energy metabolism which could be oxidatived to deaminate pyruvate and synthesize taurine [9]. Taurine has a wide range of physiological and pharmacological effects and is important in order to regulating the body's glucose and lipid metabolism. Pantothenic acid, vitamin B5, is a water-soluble vitamin required for life support which can form coenzyme A (CoA). CoA is mainly engaged in the breakdown of carbohydrates, fatty acid oxidation, amino acid decomposition, pyruvate degradation, and the tricarboxylic acid cycle. Pantothenic acid is critical to the metabolism and synthesis of carbohydrates, proteins, and fats and can also inhibit the metabolism of taurine [14]. Secretory epithelial cells of human and other animal prostate have unique citrate-related metabolic pathways regulated by testosterone and prolactin. This specialized hormone metabolic regulation is in charge of the production and secretion of a particularly high level of citric acid. Testosterone and prolactin are also engaged in the regulation of the gene of key regulatory enzymes of citrate production in prostate cells [15]. As the intermediate of the TCA cycle, malic acid and citric acid paticipate the metabolic pathways related to prostate [16]. Conclusively, TCA cycle is the hub of sugar, fat, and amino acid metabolism and most intermediates in the tricarboxylic acid cycle can be precisely or indirectly converted to various amino acids. Therefore, there are closely relationships among amino acid metabolism and energy metabolism (Figure 9). Besides, the results of Na^+/K^+-ATPase's activities and respiratory research also verified energy variety in the procession of CNP. Studies have demonstrated that the flavonoids such as curcumin could inhibit TNF-α to exert anti-inflammatory effects [17]. The flavonoids in *T. patula* can also reduce the increasing of TNF-α levels caused by CNP. Here we supposed that the flavonoids could decrease the secretion of TNF-α and other inflammatory cytokines, which might associate with the structure of flavonoids. The structure of flavonoids usually contains phenolic hydroxyl and ketone carbonyl, which have antioxidant effects in the study of the structure-activity relationship [18]. We just found the flavonoids are the effective fraction against CNP and we still need to investigate the specific compound and its potential mechanisms in further study.

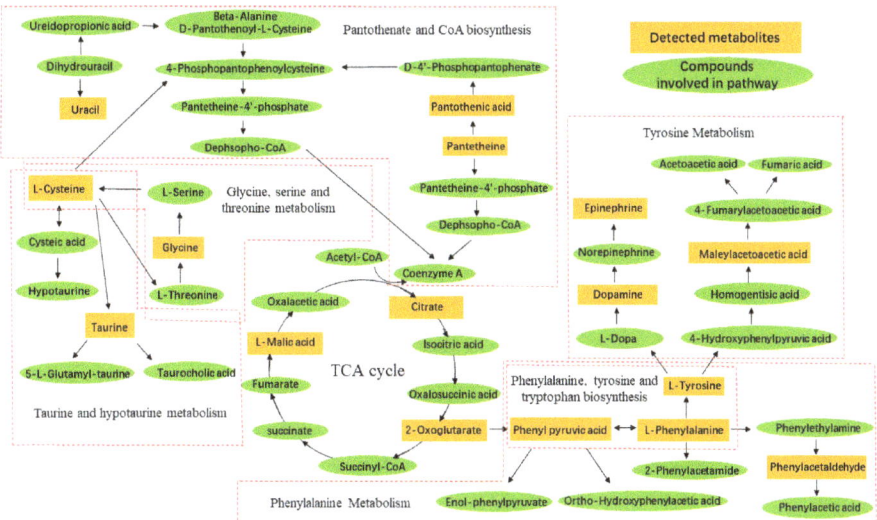

Figure 9. Related metabolic pathway.

In conclusion, the potential anti-CNP mechanism of flavonoids and polysaccharides of *T. patula* might be through reducing the expression of inflammation factors, adjusting the levels of hormone and regulating the amino acid metabolism, energy metabolism and glucose and lipid metabolism.

4. Materials and Methods

4.1. Materials and Reagents

T. patula was provided by Dalian Wuzhou Holy Herb Scientific and Technological Co. Ltd. (Dalian, China) and identified by Prof. Bing Wang in the Liaoning University of Traditional Chinese Medicine, the voucher specimens (No. 20160911) were deposited in the specimen herbarium, Liaoning University of Traditional Chinese Medicine. Acetonitrile, methanol and formic acid (HPLC grade) were acquired from Merck (Darmstadt, Germany). Milli-Q water purification system (Millipore, Bedford, MA, USA) was used for the purification of water and the preparation of samples and mobile phase. Estradiol benzoate was purchased from the Ningbo Second Hormone Factory (Ningbo, China). Levofloxacin hydrochloride was acquired from the Cisen Pharmaceutical Co., Ltd. (Jining, China). DHT and PSA ELISA kits were purchased from Shanghai Qiaodu Biotechnology Co. Ltd. (Shanghai, China). TNF-α ELISA kit, Na^+/K^+-ATPase assay kit and Total protein quantitative assay kit were all purchased from the Nanjing Jiancheng Biotechnology Co. Ltd. (Nanjing, China). 2-ketoglutaric acid, pyruvic acid, succinic acid, disodium fumarate, malic acid, stearic acid, 3-hydroxytyramine hydrochloride and mixed amino acid standards were purchased from Sigma (St. Louis., MO, USA). Betaine, allantoin, inosine, taurine, creatinine, L-carnitine, creatine, urea and citric acid were recruited from Aladdin (Shanghai, China). Sodium lactate, doxifluridine, D-(+)-pantothenic acid calcium salt and 6-hydroxypurine were purchased from the National Institutes for Food and Drug Control (Beijing, China). All the other chemicals employed in the experiments were commercial products of analytical grade. The preparation methods of each constituents are as follows, *T. patula* was extracted with distilled water and boiling to obtain water decoction. *T. patula* was extracted with distilled water and boiling to get the essential oil components with essential oil extractor. The resulting decoction was filtered. The residual was continued to extract with distilled water, and then, filtered. The filtrates and essential oil were collected respectively. The collected filtrates were concentrated, then adding alcohol to the concentrated solution to meet 70% alcohol for two times to provide the precipitate and supernatant constituents, respectively. The precipitate equal to POL and supernatant equal to FLA. The concrete preparation methods and administration solutions of different constituents of *T. patula* were obtained according to the reference [3].

4.2. Animals

Adult male SPF level Sprague-Dawley rats (weighing approximately 180–200 g) were offered by the Liaoning Changsheng Biotechnology Co. Ltd, Liaoning, China (License Key: SCXK (Liao) 20150001) and maintained under controlled condition (20 ± 2 °C, 40 ± 10% relative humidity and 12 hours light/dark cycle) with free access to standard food and water. Animal research was approved by the Animal Ethical and Welfare Committee of Liaoning University of Traditional Chinese Medicine and the experimental protocols were conducted according to the Guide for Care and Use of Laboratory Animals of Liaoning University of Traditional Chinese Medicine (131/2010).

After one week of acclimatization, the CNP model was induced by estradiol subcutaneously in castrated male rats according to the methods which established as Robinette described [19]. After the model was performed, the rats were randomly divided into 8 groups with 8 animals for each and intragastrically administrated with corresponding drugs for 9 days. SOG, MOG, WAD (1.8 g/kg/day), EOC (5.4 mg/kg/day), POL (254.3 mg/kg/day), FLA (207.5 mg/kg/day), TCM (540 mg/kg/day) and LEH (45 mg/kg/day) were intragastrically administrated with the corresponding drugs. And SOG and MOG were intragastrically administrated with 0.5% CMC-Na. The preparation methods of constituents of *T. patula* and the concentration of drugs for intragastrically administration was equated with the dose of human daily taking according to the reference [3].

4.3. Determination Eenergy Metabolic Parameters

After drugs administered on the 8th day 8:00 am, the rats in different groups were individually placed in the respiratory chambers of TSE phenoMaster/LabMaster (TSE phenoMaster/LabMaster, Bad Homburg, Germany) to monitor 24 h respiratory parameters in an isolated environment which temperature was controlled at 20 ± 2 °C. VO_2, VCO_2, H, EE and RER were measured by using the indirect calorimetry system.

4.4. Collection and Preparation of Biosamples

Urine samples were collected by metabolism cages at ambient temperature on the 9th of drug administration and centrifuged at 13,000 rpm at 4 °C for 10 min and stored frozen at −80 °C for metabolomic analysis.

4.5. Physiological Indexes

All rats were anesthetized after 24 h of the ending of the intragastric administration. Blood was drawn from the abdominal aorta. The serum was prepared and stored at −80 °C before estimation. Prostate and liver tissues were collected and stored at −80 °C. The left lateral lobe part of prostate were fixed in 4% paraformaldehyde solution for histological evaluation. Homogenate was obtained according to the ratio of tissue of right lateral lobe of prostate or liver and saline 1:9. The supernatant was harvested by centrifugation for 10 min at 3000 rpm. The levels of DHT and PSA in serum and TNF-α in prostate homogenate and Na^+/K^+-ATPase activity in prostate and liver homogenate were measured with correspondent measurement kit.

4.6. Metabolic Profiling Chromatography

Chromatography was performed using a Waters ACQUITYTM ultra performance liquid chromatography system (Waters Corporation, Milford, CT, USA) controlled with Masslynx (V4.1, Waters Corporation, Milford, CT, USA). An aliquot of 4 μL of the sample solution was injected onto an ACQUITY UPLC HSS T3 column (50 mm × 2.1 mm, 1.7 μm, Waters Corp, Milford, CT, USA) at 40 °C with a flow rate of 0.60 mL/min. The mobile phases were composed of 0.1% formic acid in acetonitrile (solvent A) and 0.1% formic acid in water (solvent B), the gradient was used as Supplementary Materials Table S5: Gradient elution program. The eluant was introduced to the mass spectrometer (Waters Corporation, Milford, CT, USA) directly and analyzed with positive/negative electrospray ion source (ESI). The quality control (QC) sample was used to optimize the condition of UPLC-MS, as it contained most information on whole urine samples. After every 10 samples injected, a pooled sample as the QC sample followed by a blank was injected in order to secure the stability and repeatability of the UPLC-MS systems.

4.7. Mass Spectrometry

Metabolic was analyzed and identified by Micromass Q-TOF micro^{TM} mass spectrometry and the optimal conditions of analysis were as follows. In positive ion mode, the capillary voltage was 3.0 kV, the sampling cone voltage was 45 V, desolvation gas temperature was 400 °C, desolvation gas flow was 800 L/h, the cone gas flow was 50 L/h. The data acquisition rate was set to 1 sec/scan with a 0.2 second interscan delay and the mass range was set at m/z 50–1200 using extended dynamic range. For accurate and repeatable mass acquisition, a lock-mass of leucine-enkephalin at a concentration of 50 fmol/μL was used via a lock spray interface at a flow rate of 60 μL/min monitoring for positive ion mode ([M + H] = 556.2771) and negative ion mode ([M − H] = 554.2615) to ensure accuracy during the MS analysis.

4.8. Data Processing

Testing and matching original peak through Markerlynx (SCN803) modules in Masslynx V4.1 workstation, and the peak intensity was normalized and denoised to extract data matrix consisting of metabolite retention time, m/z and corresponding peak intensities. Software specific parameter settings are shown in Supplementary Materials Table S6: Markerlynx Software parameter settings.

4.9. Multivariate Data Analysis

Data preprocessed analysis by using the extended statistics module in Masslynx V4.1 Workstations for compound statistics. All the data containing the retention time, peak intensity and exact mass were imported in the Masslynx V4.1 Workstations for multiple statistical analyses. Both principal component analysis (PCA) and partial least square discriminant analysis (PLS-DA) often could be taken, because of their ability to deal with highly multivariate, noisy, collinear and possibly incomplete data. PCA, unsupervised pattern recognition method, used to discern the presence of inherent similarities in spectral profiles initially. In the PCA plot, the longer distance the two samples' scores are, the greater the difference between them.

4.10. Biomarkers Identification

The retention time, precise molecular mass and m/z data for the structural identification of biomarkers were issued by the UPLC-MS analysis platform of the Masslynx V4.1 Workstations. The variable importance in projection value (VIP value) was obtained by PLS-DA, and the metabolites with VIP > 1 were selected to measure the significance of each metabolite in separating model from controls by one-way ANOVA with SPSS 17.0. Metabolites with VIP >1 and $p < 0.05$ were identified as differential metabolites and compound validation to verify the accuracy and eliminate unreliable differential metabolites.

Targeted Metabolomics: potential markers were identified by matching the retention time and *m/z* of these differential metabolites with the theoretical *m/z* based on the elemental composition of the standard products through the Molecular Weight Calculator module in Masslynx.

Non-targeted metabolomics: as a result of the relevant information on compounds structure types, elemental composition, and other information in urine samples were unknown, the identification of differential metabolites in this study mainly included the following methods. (1) Determination of differential metabolites $[M + H]^+$ or $[M - H]^-$ ions, through the molecular ion peak to find the possible elemental composition of the metabolite; (2) Analysis of elemental composition by MS and MS/MS spectra to find the fragment ion peaks of metabolites, according to the structure which metabolites might exist and meet the fragmentation peaks of mass spectrometry characteristics to infer the possible structures of the different metabolites and verified by an online database such as the MS/MS Spectrum Match module in the METLIN database (http://metlin.scripps.edu/). (3) Some of the metabolites did not split into debris due to the complexity of urine samples, the structure of metabolites were reverse analyzed of metabolically related networks and inferred through the possible mechanisms of prostatitis and according to the metabolic correlation networks which were identified by targeted metabolomics databases such as KEGG (http://www.genome.jp/kegg/), HMDB (http://www.hmdb.org/).

4.11. Metabolic Pathway Analysis

Metabolic pathways were obtained by analyzing and enriching differential metabolites that had been screened by MetaboAnalyst 3.0. Potential markers identified were compared with the accurate mass charge ratio in some databases, including HMDB, KEGG and Metlin database to discover related pathways. Pathway impact-alter was used to determine the statistical significance of the pathways.

4.12. Statistical Analysis

The PCA was used to uncover undiscovered trends in the treated groups. Statistically significant differences in mean values were tested by using one-way ANOVA, and $p < 0.05$ was considered statistically significant. Prior to multivariate analysis, the resultant data matrices from the two analytical techniques were mean-centered and pareto-scaled.

4.13. Network Pharmacology Predict Pathway

In the early stages, our laboratory was separated and identified the compound in *T. patula* and found that flavonoids is the main active component. Here, to certify the result of metabolism, the network-pharmacology was operating to illustrate the predictive action mechanism. The information of the active compound in *T. patula* was shown in Supplementary Materials Table S7: Structures of active compounds. Prediction of pathways that may be related to *T. patula* anti-prostatitis by screening out the common target genes of *T. patula* active compounds and prostatitis.

Potential targets of active compounds were predicted by SwissTargetPrediction server (http://www.swisstargetprediction.ch/) and stinted homo sapiens as organism. According to the CTD (https://ctdbase.org/) and Genecard (https://www.genecards.org/) databases to find relevant target genes of prostatitis, due to the large number of related genes and the complexed network, so selected gene with relevance score >30 to predict. The network was constructed using Cytoscape 3.7.1 software [20] to obtain the active compounds of *T. patula*—target map and prostatitis disease—target map. The common targets gene of *T. patula* active compounds and prostatitis was screened out by the merge function of Cytoscape, and the *T. patula* active compounds–target–prostatitis disease network map was constructed. Then the analysis of gene function was performed on the merge gene utilizing FunRich software [21,22]. The DAVID database (https://david.ncifcrf.gov/tools.jsp) was combined with KOPAS 3.0 (http://kobas.cbi.pku.edu.cn/anno_iden.php) to enrich the KEGG and GO pathways in the gene pathway. After the pathway enrichment, the broad pathways were excluded and the pathway information was obtained. Then Omicshare cloud platform (http://www.omicshare.com/forum/) was used to map the enriched pathways.

Supplementary Materials: The following are available online at http://www.mdpi.com/1420-3049/24/12/2266/s1, Figure S1: HPLC fingerprint of water decoction (a), supernatant (b) and essential oil (c) fractions of *T. patula.*, Figure S2: TIC chromatograms on positive ion mode, Figure S3: TIC chromatograms on negative ion mode, Figure S4 Histological analysis of prostate, Table S1: Potential targets of active compounds, Table S2: Relevant target genes of prostatitis, Table S3: The information of merging gene, Table S4: Details of enriched pathways, Table S5: Gradient elution program, Table S6: Markerlynx Software parameter settings, Table S7: Structures of active compounds.

Author Contributions: X.L. and D.D. planned and designed the experiment. X.L., X.R., M.R., H.K., D.D. and D.C. conducted the experiments, X.L. analyze the data, and prepared the figures. X.L. and D.D. wrote the paper. All authors agreed to the final version of this manuscript.

Funding: This research was funded by Liaoning Province Distinguished Professor Support Program, China.

Acknowledgments: This work received the support of Liaoning Province Distinguished Professor Support Program, China. Besides, we would like to express our gratitude to Heilongjiang University of Chinese Medicine to supply UPLC-MS equipment to us.

Conflicts of Interest: The authors declared no conflict of interest.

Abbreviations

CNP	Chronic nonbacterial prostatitis
PSA	prostate-specific antigen
TNF-α	tumor necrosis factor-α
DHT	dihydrotestosterone
SOG	Sham-operated group
MOG	Chronic nonbacterial prostatitis model group
WAD	Water decoction treatment group
EOC	Essential oil treatment group
POL	Polysaccharide treatment group
FLA	Flavonoids treatment group
TCM	Pule'an tablet treatment group
LEH	Levofloxacin treatment group
VO_2	O_2 consumption
VCO_2	CO_2 production
H	Heat production
EE	Energy expenditure
RER	Respiratory exchange ratio
ESI	electrospray ion source
QC	The quality control
PCA	principal component analysis
PLS-DA	partial least square discriminant analysis

References

1. Bano, H.; Ahmed, S.W.; Azhar, I.; Ali, M.S.; Alam, N. Chemical constituents of *Tagetes patula* L. *Pak. J. Pharm. Sci.* **2002**, *15*, 1–12. [PubMed]
2. Kasahara, Y.; Yasukawa, K.; Kitanaka, S.; Khan, M.T.; Evans, F.J. Effect of methanol extract from flower petals of *Tagetes patula* L. on acute and chronic inflammation model. *Phytotherapy Res. Ptr.* **2002**, *16*, 217–222. [CrossRef] [PubMed]
3. Liu, X.; Ran, X.; Dou, D.; Cai, D. Effectiveness of *Tagetes patula* against chronic nonbacterial prostatitis in rat model. *Bangl. J. Pharmacol.* **2017**, *12*, 376–383. [CrossRef]
4. Malik, R.; Aneni, E.C.; Shahrayar, S.; Freitas, W.M.; Ali, S.S.; Veledar, E.; Latif, M.A.; Aziz, M.; Ahmed, R.; Khan, S.A. Elevated serum uric acid is associated with vascular inflammation but not coronary artery calcification in the healthy octogenarians: The Brazilian study on healthy aging. *Aging Clin. Exper. Res.* **2016**, *28*, 359–362. [CrossRef] [PubMed]
5. Alemzadeh, R.; Kichler, J. Uric Acid-Induced Inflammation Is Mediated by the Parathyroid Hormone: 25-Hydroxyvitamin D Ratio in Obese Adolescents. *Metab. Syndrome Related Dis.* **2016**, *14*, 167. [CrossRef] [PubMed]

6. Sumner, S.J.; Fennell, T.R. Review of the metabolic fate of styrene. *Crit. Rev. Toxicol.* **1994**, *24* (Suppl. 1), S11–S33. [CrossRef] [PubMed]
7. Tang, A.; Wang, Q. Phenylalanine metabolic disorders and diseases. *J. Clin. Med. Pathol.* **2001**, *6*, 451–453.
8. Jin, G. *Biochemistry*; Shanghai Science and Technology Press: Shanghai, China, 2006; pp. 156–158.
9. Liu, J.; Xu, C.; Ying, L.; Zang, S.; Zhuang, Z.; Lv, H.; Yang, W.; Luo, Y.; Ma, X.; Wang, L. Relationship of serum uric acid level with non-alcoholic fatty liver disease and its inflammation progression in nonobese adults. *Hepatol. Res. Off. J. Japan Soc. Hepatol.* **2016**, *47*, E104. [CrossRef] [PubMed]
10. Zhou, H.; Zhang, T. Research progress of tyrosine pharmacology. *Chin. Pharmacol. Bull.* **1993**, 251–253.
11. Yin, D.; Qi, Z. Biosynthesis and metabolism of catecholamines. *Adv. Physiol. Sci.* **1965**, 58–67. [CrossRef]
12. Boehm, G.; Cervantes, H.; Georgi, G.; Jelinek, J.; Sawatzki, G.; Wermuth, B.; Colombo, J.P. Effect of increasing dietary threonine intakes on amino acid metabolism of the central nervous system and peripheral tissues in growing rats. *Pediatr. Res.* **1998**, *44*, 900–906. [CrossRef] [PubMed]
13. Li, X.; Zhu, X.; Chen, Q. Protective effect of glycine in cardiovascular diseases. *Adv. Biochem. Biophy.* **2015**, 810–816. [CrossRef]
14. Jie, N. Vitamin B5. *Chinese Health Food* **2013**, 12–14.
15. Costello, L.C.; Franklin, R.B. Testosterone and Prolactin Regulation of Metabolic Genes and Citrate Metabolism of Prostate Epithelial Cells. *Horm. Metab. Res.* **2002**, *34*, 417–424. [CrossRef] [PubMed]
16. Liu, J.; Xu, C.; Ying, L.; Zang, S.; Zhuang, Z.; Lv, H.; Yang, W.; Luo, Y.; Ma, X.; Wang, L. Research and Application on L-Malic Acid. *China Food Addict.* **2003**, 52–56.
17. Veronika, F.; Janez, K.; Urban, B. Inverse Molecular Docking as a Novel Approach to Study Anticarcinogenic and Anti-Neuroinflammatory Effects of Curcumin. *Molecules* **2018**, *23*, 3351. [CrossRef]
18. Sun, Q.; Wang, X.; Liu, J.; Cheng, C.; Jiang, T. Study on structure-antioxidation relationship of plant flavonoids. *Food Sci.* **2006**, *26*, 69–73. [CrossRef]
19. Robinette, C.L. Sex-hormone-induced inflammation and fibromuscular proliferation in the rat lateral prostate. *Prostate* **1988**, *12*, 271. [CrossRef] [PubMed]
20. Shannon, P.; Markiel, A.; Ozier, O.; Baliga, N.S.; Wang, J.T.; Ramage, D.; Amin, N.; Schwikowski, B.; Ideker, T. Cytoscape: A software environment for integrated models of biomolecular interaction networks. *Genome Res.* **2013**, *11*, 2498–2504. [CrossRef]
21. Pathan, M.; Keerthikumar, S.; Chisanga, D.; Alessandro, R.; Ang, C.S.; Askenase, P.; Batagov, A.O.; Benito-Martin, A.; Camussi, G.; Clayton, A.; et al. A novel community driven software for functional enrichment analysis of extracellular vesicles data. *J. Extracell. Vesicles* **2017**, *1*, 1321455. [CrossRef]
22. Pathan, M.; Keerthikumar, S.; Ang, C.S.; Gangoda, L.; Quek, C.M.J.; Williamson, N.J.; Mouradov, D.; Sieber, O.M.; Simpson, R.J.; Salim, A.; et al. FunRich: a standalone tool for functional enrichment analysis. *Proteomics* **2015**, *15*, 2597–2601. [CrossRef] [PubMed]

Sample Availability: Not available.

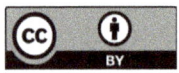

© 2019 by the authors. Licensee MDPI, Basel, Switzerland. This article is an open access article distributed under the terms and conditions of the Creative Commons Attribution (CC BY) license (http://creativecommons.org/licenses/by/4.0/).

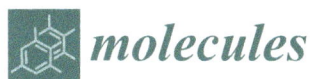

Article

Inhibitory Effects on NO Production and DPPH Radicals and NBT Superoxide Activities of Diarylheptanoid Isolated from Enzymatically Hydrolyzed Ehthanolic Extract of *Alnus sibirica*

Hye Soo Wang, Yoon Jeong Hwang, Jun Yin and Min Won Lee *

Laboratory of Pharmacognosy and Natural Product based Medicine, College of Pharmacy, Chung-Ang University, Seoul 06974, Korea; envi2308@hanmail.net (H.S.W.); g_intention@naver.com (Y.J.H.); yinjun89@naver.com (J.Y.)
* Correspondence: mwlee@cau.ac.kr; Tel.: +82-2-820-5602

Academic Editor: Ericsson Coy-Barrera
Received: 16 April 2019; Accepted: 17 May 2019; Published: 20 May 2019

Abstract: *Alnus sibirica* (AS) is geographically distributed in Korea, Japan, Northeast China, and Russia. Various anti-oxidant, anti-inflammation, anti-atopic dermatitis and anti-cancer biological effects of AS have been reported. Enzymatic hydrolysis decomposes the sugar bond attached to glycoside into aglycone which, generally, has a superior biological activity, compared to glycoside. Enzymatic hydrolysis of the extract (EAS) from AS was processed and the isolated compounds were investigated—hirsutanonol (**1**), hirsutenone (**2**), rubranol (**3**), and muricarpon B (**4**). The structures of these compounds were elucidated, and the biological activities were assessed. The ability of EAS and the compounds (**1**–**4**) to scavenge 2,2-diphenyl-1-picrylhydrazyl (DPPH) radicals and Nitroblue tetrazolium (NBT) superoxide, and to inhibit NO production was evaluated in vitro. EAS showed more potent antioxidant and anti-inflammatory activity than AS. All investigated compounds showed excellent antioxidant and anti-inflammatory activities.

Keywords: *Alnus sibirica*; oregonin; hirsutanonol; enzymatic hydrolysis; antioxidant; anti-inflammatory

1. Introduction

Alnus sibirica (AS), belonging to the family *Betulaceae*, is geographically distributed in Korea, Japan, China, and Russia [1]. The Korean Plant Names Index (KPNI), reports that fifteen *Alnus* species are native to Korea. The *Alnus* species are well-known in traditional Korean medicine, such as anti-cancer drugs, cathartics, hemostatics, and skin tonics. AS is used in cough lozenges and as a herbal decoction to treat alcoholism [1]. Previous studies on the chemical constituents of the *Alnus* species have led to the isolation of various diarylheptanoids [2–5], flavonoids [6,7], triterpenoids [8,9], and tannins [10,11]. AS is also reported to have anti-oxidant, anti-inflammatory [12], anti-atopic dermatitis [13], anti-adipogenic [14], and cytotoxic [15] properties.

Enzymatic modifications are used to transform compounds isolated from natural sources [16–18]. Enzymes are used in various industrial applications where specific catalysts are required. For instance, amylases are used for splitting polysaccharides and proteins in malt, in the brewing industry, and for producing sugars from starch, in food processing industries [11,19]. Aglycones—glycosides in which the sugar molecules have been replaced by hydrogen atoms after enzymatic hydrolysis by intestinal or colonic microflora—are more easily absorbed from the small intestine than glycosides [20,21]. Glycosidation enhances water solubility but reduces chemical reactivity. Therefore, glycosidases play a major role in biological processes and are important in the biological, biomedical, and industrial fields [22].

From our previous study, 17 compounds from fermented AS (FAS) were isolated and evaluated for their antioxidant, anti-inflammatory, and anti-atopic dermatitis activities, in vitro and in vivo, including the quantitative analysis of its components [23–25]. The present paper describes the evaluation of antioxidant and anti-inflammatory effects on the enzymatic hydrolysis (EAS). Through this study, diverse but expected chemical and biological changes, such as increased bioavailability or biological activities, were observed, after the glycosides were converted to aglycones.

2. Results and Discussion

2.1. Enzymatic Hydrolysis

Extracts from *A. sibirica* processed by enzymatic hydrolysis (EAS) was prepared by using Fungamyl Super AX (Novozymes, Bagsvaerd, Denmark). The differences between EAS and AS were observed by thin layer chromatography (TLC). (TLC results data not shown, reaction pathway shows in Figure 1)

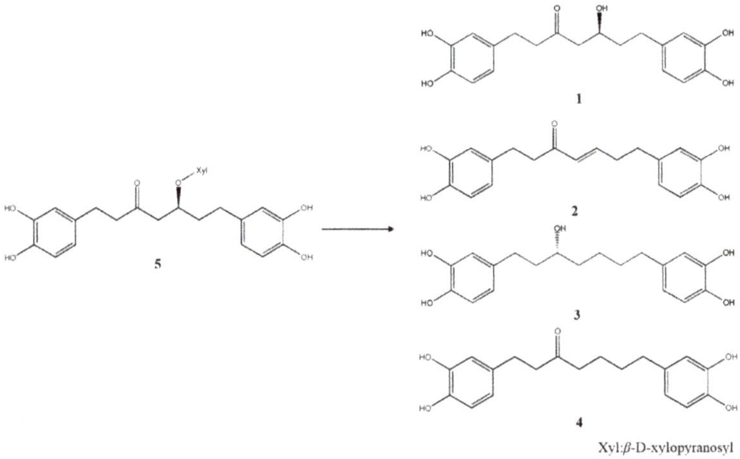

Figure 1. Chemical structure of **1–5** and the hydrolysis reaction pathway

2.2. Isolation and Structural Identification

The chromatographic isolation of EAS yielded four diarylheptanoids (**1–4**). Compound **1** was in the form of an amorphous brown oil. A navy-blue spot was observed after spraying the TLC strip with FeCl$_3$ solution. A dark-blue/deep-violet spot was also observed after spraying with 10% H$_2$SO$_4$ solution and heating. The ^{1}H-NMR (600 MHz, DMSO-d_6 + D$_2$O) spectrum of **1** showed two aromatic AMX-spin systems indicated by the ortho-meta coupled aromatic signals [δ 6.37–6.36 (2H in total, m, H-6′,6′′)], a meta-ortho coupled aromatic signal [δ 6.59–6.52 (4H in total, m, H-2′, 2′′, 5′, 5′′)], one hydroxyl-bearing methine [δ 3.36–3.32 (1H in total, m, H-5)], and five methylenes [δ 2.67–2.30 (8H in total, m, H-1,2,4,7) and 1.56–1.45 (2H in total, m, H-6)]. (Supplementary Materials Table S1) Thus, **1** was identified as hirsutanonol, 1,7-bis-(3,4-dihydroxyphenyl)-5-hydroxyheptane-3-one, after comparison of this spectrum with the reported spectral data for hirsutanonol [26].

Compound **2** was in the form of an amorphous brown oil. A navy-blue spot was observed after spraying the TLC strip with FeCl$_3$ solution. A dark-blue/deep-violet spot was also observed after spraying with 10% H$_2$SO$_4$ solution and heating. The ^{1}H-NMR (300 MHz, Acetone-d_6 + D$_2$O) spectrum of **2** showed two aromatic AMX-spin systems indicated by ortho-meta coupled aromatic signals [δ 6.94–6.90 (2H in total, m, H-6′, 6′′)], a meta-ortho coupled aromatic signal [δ 7.19–7.11 (4H in total, m, H-2′, 2′′, 5′, 5′′)], an alkene [δ 7.37 (1H, dt, J = 13.2, 6.6 Hz, H-5) and 6.57 (1H, d, J = 13.2 Hz, H-4)], and four methylenes [δ 3.25–2.89 (8H in total, m, H-1, 2, 6, 7)]. (Supplementary Materials Table S2)

Thus, **2** was identified as hirsutenone, 1,7-bis-(3,4-dihydroxyphenyl)-4-hepten-3-one, after comparison of this spectrum with the reported spectral data for hirsutenone [26].

Compound **3** was in the form of a dark-yellow oil. A dark-green spot was observed on the TLC strip after spraying with $FeCl_3$ solution. A violet spot was also observed after spraying with anisaldehyde-H_2SO_4 solution and heating. The ^{1}H-NMR (300 MHz, Acetone-d_6 + D_2O) spectrum of **3** showed two aromatic AMX-spin systems indicated by an ortho-meta-coupled aromatic signal [δ 6.71–6.66 (4H in total, m, H-2′, 2″, 5′, 5″), 6.51 (1H, dd, J = 6.3, 2.1 Hz, H-6′), and 6.45 (1H, dd, J = 6.3, 2.1 Hz, H-6″)] and six methylenes [δ 3.57–3.51 (1H in total, m, H-5), 2.68–2.42 (4H in total, m, H-1, 7), 1.69–1.42 (8H in total, m, H-2, 3, 4, 6)]. (Supplementary Materials Table S3) Thus, compound **3** was identified as rubranol, 1,7-bis-(3,4-dihydroxyphenyl)-5-hydroxyheptane, after comparison of this spectrum with the reported spectral data for rubranol [27].

Compound **4** was in the form of an amorphous brown oil. A navy-blue spot was observed after spraying the TLC strip with $FeCl_3$ solution. A dark-green spot was also observed after spraying with 10% H_2SO_4 solution and heating. The ^{1}H-NMR (600 MHz, Acetone-d_6 + D_2O) spectrum of **5** showed two aromatic AMX-spin systems indicated by a meta-ortho-coupled aromatic signal [δ 6.68 (1H, d, J = 7.2 Hz, H-5′), 6.67 (1H, d, J = 7.2 Hz, H-5″), 6.66 (1H, d, J = 2.1 Hz, H-2′), 6.64 (1H, d, J = 2.1 Hz, H-2″)], ortho-meta-coupled aromatic signals [δ 6.45 (1H, dd, J = 7.2, 2.1 Hz, H-6′), 6.44 (1H, dd, J = 7.2, 2.1 Hz, H-6″)], and six methylenes [2.67–2.61 (4H in total, m, H-1, 2), 2.42 (2H, t, J = 7.2 Hz, H-4), 2.40 (2H, t, J = 7.2 Hz, H-7), 1.49 (4H, m, H-5, 6)]. The ^{13}C-NMR (150 MHz, Acetone-d_6 + D_2O) spectrum of **4** also showed the presence of an aromatic AMX-spin system indicated by hydroxyl-bearing aromatic carbon signals [δ 144.8, 144.7, 143.1, and 142.9 ppm (C-3′, 3″, 4′ and 4″)] in a region downfield from the signals [δ 119.3, 119.2, 115.3, 115.2, 115.1, and 114.0 ppm (C-2′, 2″, 5′, 5″, 6′ and 6″)]. In the upfield region, a ketone group was observed at δ 210.4 (C-3). (Supplementary Materials Table S4) Thus, **4** was identified as muricarpon B, 1,7-bis(3,4-dihydroxyphenyl)-3-heptanone, after comparison of this spectrum with the reported spectral data for muricarpon B [28].

2.3. Biological Activities

The 2,2-diphenyl-1-picrylhydrazyl (DPPH) radical scavenging activities of AS, EAS, and the four compounds were assessed. According to the results (Table 1), EAS (IC_{50} = 16.68 ± 0.37 µg/mL) showed superior DPPH radical scavenging activity to that of AS (IC_{50} = 21.80 ± 0.55 µg/mL). Compounds **1** (IC_{50} = 26.02 ± 0.57 µM), **2** (IC_{50} = 19.39 ± 0.32 µM), **3** (IC_{50} = 23.30 ± 1.00 µM), and **4** (IC_{50} = 38.70 ± 0.71 µM) showed potent DPPH radical scavenging activities, compared with the positive control, L-ascorbic acid.

Table 1. IC_{50} values of *Alnus sibirica* (AS), enzymatic hydrolysis (EAS), and the isolated compounds for the 2,2-diphenyl-1-picrylhydrazyl (DPPH) radical scavenging activity.

Samples	IC_{50} (µg/mL)	Compounds	IC_{50} (µM)
AS	21.80 ± 0.55 [c]	1	26.02 ± 0.57 [a]
EAS	16.68 ± 0.37 [b]	2	19.39 ± 0.32 [a]
Ascorbic acid	11.18 ± 0.60 [a]	3	23.30 ± 1.00 [a]
		4	38.70 ± 0.71 [c]
		Ascorbic acid	44.67 ± 1.75 [b,c]

Values are presented as mean ± SD (n = 3). Values bearing different superscripts (a–c) in same columns are significantly different ($p < 0.05$).

The Nitroblue tetrazolium (NBT) superoxide scavenging activities of AS, EAS, and the four compounds were assessed. According to the results (Table 2), EAS (IC_{50} = 3.12 ± 0.75 µg/mL) showed a more potent NBT superoxide scavenging activity compared to that of AS (IC_{50} = 4.59 ± 0.68 µg/mL). According to the results (Table 2), compounds **1** (IC_{50} = 19.03 ± 8.79 µM), **2** (IC_{50} = 16.68 ± 6.74 µM), **3** (IC_{50} = 11.62 ± 7.86 µM), and **4** (IC_{50} = 12.65 ± 11.05 µM) showed good NBT superoxide scavenging activities, compared with those of the positive control, allopurinol.

Table 2. IC$_{50}$ values of AS, EAS, and the isolated compounds for the nitroblue tetrazolium (NBT) superoxide scavenging activity.

Samples	IC$_{50}$ (μg/mL)	Compounds	IC$_{50}$ (μM)
AS	4.59 ± 0.68 [c]	1	19.03 ± 8.79 [b]
EAS	3.12 ± 0.75 [b]	2	16.68 ± 6.74 [b]
Allopurinol	0.10 ± 0.41 [a]	3	11.62 ± 7.86 [b]
		4	12.65 ± 11.05 [b]
		Allopurinol	3.92 ± 1.96 [a]

Values are presented as mean ± SD ($n = 3$). Values bearing different superscripts (a–c) in same columns are significantly different ($p < 0.05$).

Massive amounts of nitric oxide (NO) produced by the inducible nitric oxide synthase (iNOS) under pathological conditions, for example, inflammatory disease, are potentially harmful, especially when time-spatial regulation of the iNOS expression becomes compromised. During inflammation associated with different pathogens, NO production increases significantly and might become cytotoxic [29]. Moreover, the free radical nature of NO and its high reactivity with oxygen to produce peroxynitrite (ONOO$^-$) makes NO a potent pro-oxidant molecule, capable of inducing oxidative damage and being potentially harmful towards cellular targets [30]. Thus, the inhibition of NO production in response to inflammatory stimuli, might be a useful therapeutic strategy in inflammatory disease [31,32]. Inhibitory activities on the NO production of AS, EAS, and the four compounds were assessed. According to the results (Table 3), EAS (IC$_{50}$ = 1.14 ± 0.06 μg/mL) showed better inhibitory effects on NO production, than AS (IC$_{50}$ = 6.26 ± 0.16 μg/mL) and the positive control—NG-methyl-L-arginine acetate salt (L-NMMA) (IC$_{50}$ = 3.53 ± 0.17 μg/mL). According to the results (Table 3), most compounds showed better inhibitory effects on NO production than L-NMMA (IC$_{50}$ = 33.88 ± 27.87 μM). Compounds **2** (IC$_{50}$ = 0.78 ± 0.38 μM) and **4** (IC$_{50}$ = 2.64 ± 2.29 μM) exhibited markedly potent inhibitory effects on NO production.

Table 3. IC$_{50}$ values of AS, EAS, and the isolated compounds for the inhibitory activity on NO production.

Samples	IC$_{50}$ (μg/mL)	Compounds	IC$_{50}$ (μM)
AS	6.26 ± 0.16 [c]	1	17.81 ± 8.63 [a,b,c]
EAS	1.14 ± 0.06 [a]	2	0.78 ± 0.38 [a]
L-NMMA	3.53 ± 0.17 [b]	3	5.20 ± 2.61 [a,b]
		4	2.64 ± 2.29 [a]
		L-NMMA	33.88 ± 27.87 [b,c]

Values are presented as mean ± SD ($n = 3$). Values bearing different superscripts (a–c) in same columns are significantly different ($p < 0.05$).

EAS and AS were measured for their biological activities, and EAS was found to exhibit better activities than AS. Compounds **1–4**, isolated from EAS showed potent anti-oxidative and anti-inflammatory effects, especially **2–4**. In addition, these compounds showed cytotoxic activity against cancer cell lines [33]; however, in this study, the experiments were carried out in an amount that did not result in cytotoxicity (data not shown). In a previous study that we had carried out [34], **1–3** were greatly increased and **4** was newly formed. This seemed to have made a great contribution toward the increased efficacy of EAS.

3. Materials and Methods

3.1. General Procedure

The stationary phases for column chromatography were carried out using Sephadex LH-20 (10–25 μm, GE Healthcare Bio-Science AB, Uppsala, Sweden) and MCI-gel CHP 20P (75–150 μm, Mitsubishi Chemical, Tokyo, Japan). ODS-B gel (40–60 μm, Daiso, Osaka, Japan) was used as the stationary phase on a medium pressure liquid chromatography (MPLC) system and consisted of an injector (Waters 650E), a pump (TBP5002, Tauto Biotech, Shanghai, China), and a detector (110 UV/VIS detector, Gilson, Middleton, WI, USA). TLC analysis was carried out using precoated silica gel plates (Merck, Darmstadt, Germany) with a mixture of $CHCl_3$, CH_3OH, and H_2O (80:20:2, volume ratio) as the mobile phase. Spots on the TLC strips were detected by spraying with $FeCl_3$ and anisaldehyde-H_2SO_4 or 10% H_2SO_4, followed by heating. ^1H-(300 or 600 MHz) and ^{13}C-(150 MHz) NMR experiments, as well as 2D-NMR experiments, such as the heteronuclear single quantum coherence (HSQC) and the heteronuclear multiple bond coherence (HMBC) experiments, were performed using VNS (Varian, Palo Alto, CA, USA) and Gemini 2000 spectrometers (Varian), in the research facilities of the Chung-Ang University.

3.2. Plant Material

Barks of AS were collected from 'Kuksabong', Seoul, Republic of Korea, in January 2015 and authenticated by Professor Lee (College of Pharmacy, Chung-Ang University, Seoul, Korea). The voucher specimen (201501-AS) was placed at the Laboratory of Pharmacognosy and Natural Product-Derived Medicine at the Chung-Ang University.

3.3. Enzymatic Hydrolysis

We used Fungamyl Super AX® (Novozymes) for the hydrolysis experiments. The purchased enzyme was mixed with AS extract and distilled water, in the ratio of 3:1:1. The mixture was allowed to react at room temperature for 3 days. After the enzymatic hydrolysis, the enzyme was removed via ethyl acetate fractionation. For this, centrifugation was performed, and the supernatant obtained was mixed with an equal volume of ethyl acetate; this process was repeated thrice. The ethyl acetate layer was then evaporated to obtain EAS.

3.4. Extraction and Isolation

The barks of AS (2.8 kg) were extracted with 80% ethanol (30 L) at room temperature. After removing ethanol, the mixture was concentrated to obtain 121 g of AS extract. A part (23.27 g) of this extract was subjected to enzymatic hydrolysis using Fungamyl (to obtain EAS), followed by liquid–liquid partition using ethyl acetate. The rest of the extract was stored in the freezer and the ethyl acetate layer was then subjected to Sephadex LH-20 column chromatography and then eluted with a solvent gradient system of MeOH:H_2O (from 2:8 to 10:0), yielding eight sub-fractions (EAS-1 to 8). From fraction EAS-2, compound **1** (hirsutanonol, 283 mg) was isolated. When EAS-6 (203 mg) in the ODS gel was subjected to MPLC (flow rate: 5 mL/min) with a gradient solvent system of MeOH:H_2O (from 0:10 to 10:0), **2** (hirsutenone, 76.9 mg) was obtained. EAS-7 (1.5 g), when subjected to MCI gel open-column chromatography with a solvent gradient system of MeOH:H_2O (from 6:4 to 10:0) yielded **3** (rubranol, 504 mg) and **4** (muricarpon B, 125.8 mg).

3.5. Measurement of DPPH Radical Scavenging Activity

The antioxidant activity was evaluated on the basis of the scavenging activity of the stable DPPH free radical (Sigma, St. Louis, MO, USA). Each sample (20 µL), in anhydrous ethanol, was added to 180 µL of DPPH solution (0.2 mM, dissolved in anhydrous ethanol). After mixing gently and letting it stand for 30 min at 37 °C, in a dark environment, the absorbance was measured at 517 nm, using an enzyme-linked immunosorbent assay (ELISA) reader (TECAN, Salzburg, Austria). The free radical scavenging activity was calculated as the inhibition rate (%) = 100 − (sample O.D./control O.D.) × 100. L-ascorbic acid was used as the positive control.

3.6. Measurement of NBT Superoxide Scavenging Activity

A reaction mixture with a final volume of 632 µL/eppendorf tube was prepared with 50 mM phosphate buffer (pH 7.5) containing K-EDTA (1 mM), hypoxanthine (0.6 mM), NBT (0.2 mM) (Sigma, St. Louis, MO, USA), 20 µL of aqueous extract (distilled water for the control), and 20 µL of xanthine oxidase (1.2 U/µL) (Sigma, St. Louis, MO, USA). The xanthine oxidase was added at last. For each sample, a blank reaction was carried out by using distilled water, instead of the extract and xanthine oxidase. NBT reduction was evaluated by determining the absorbance at 612 nm, after incubation at 37 °C for 10 min. Superoxide anion scavenging activities were calculated as 100 − (sample O.D. − blank O.D.)/(control O.D. − blank O.D.) × 100, and were expressed as IC_{50} values, which were defined as the concentrations at which 50% of NBT superoxide anion was scavenged. Allopurinol was used as the positive control.

3.7. RAW264.7 Cell Culture

The murine macrophage RAW264.7 cells were purchased from the Korean Cell Line Bank. These cells were grown at 37 °C in a humidified atmosphere (5% CO_2) in Dulbecco's Modified Eagle Medium (Sigma, St. Louis, MO, USA), containing 10% fetal bovine serum, 100 IU/mL penicillin G, and 100 mg/mL streptomycin (Gibco BRL, Grand Island, NY, USA). The cells were used in the in vitro experiments, after counting with a hemocytometer.

3.8. Measurement of Inhibitory Activity on NO Production

RAW264.7 macrophage cells were cultured in a 96-well plate and incubated for 4 h at 37 °C, in a humidified atmosphere (5% CO_2). The cells were incubated in a medium containing 10 µg/mL lipopolysaccharide (Sigma) and the test samples. After incubating for an additional 20 h, the NO content was evaluated by the Griess assay. The Griess reagent (0.1% naphthylethylenediamine and 1% sulfanilamide in 5% H_3PO_4 solution; Sigma) was added to the supernatant of the cells treated with the test samples. The absorbance at 540 nm, against a standard sodium nitrite curve, was used to determine the NO content. L-NMMA was used as the positive control. NO production inhibitory activity was calculated as inhibition rate (%) = 100 − (sample O.D. − blank O.D.)/(control O.D. − blank O.D.) × 100, and was defined as IC_{50}, which was the concentration that could inhibit 50% of NO production.

3.9. Statistical Analysis

All data are expressed as the mean ± SD of three replicates. Values were analyzed by one-way analysis of variance (ANOVA) followed by Student–Newman–Keuls test using the Statistical Package for the Social Sciences (SPSS) software pack; a statistical difference was considered to be significant when the p-value was less than 0.05. Values bearing different superscripts in the same column are significantly different.

4. Conclusions

In order to evaluate the anti-oxidative and anti-inflammatory effects of the EAS and its compounds (**1–4**), DPPH radical, NBT superoxide scavenging activities, and inhibitory activity on NO production were evaluated, in vitro. According to the results, the anti-oxidative and anti-inflammatory activities of the EAS were much better than the ethanolic crude extract of AS. Isolated compounds **1–4** showed significantly better anti-oxidative and anti-inflammatory activities, compared to their respective positive controls. The contents of **1–4** were increased and this appeared to be important in increasing the efficacy of EAS. These results suggest that EAS is a new source for the development of anti-oxidative and anti-inflammatory agents.

Supplementary Materials: The following are available online at http://www.mdpi.com/1420-3049/24/10/1938/s1, Table S1: ^{1}H-NMR date of compound **1**, Table S2: ^{1}H-NMR date of compound **2**, Table S3: ^{1}H-NMR date of compound **3**, Table S4: ^{1}H- and ^{13}C-NMR date of compound **4**.

Author Contributions: Formal analysis, H.S.W.; Methodology, Y.J.H.; Supervision, M.W.L.; Writing—original draft, H.S.W.; Writing—review & editing, J.Y. and M.W.L.

Funding: This research was funded by Korea Institute of Planning and Evaluation for Technology in Food, Agriculture, Forestry and Fisheries, 117046-3.

Acknowledgments: This work was supported by the Korea Institute of Planning and Evaluation for Technology in Food, Agriculture, Forestry, and Fisheries (IPET) through the Agri-Bio industry Technology Development Program, funded by the Ministry of Agriculture, Food, and Rural Affairs (MAFRA) (117046-3).

Conflicts of Interest: The authors declare no conflict of interest.

References

1. Lee, S. *Korean Folk Medicine*; Pub. Center of Seoul National University: Seoul, Korea, 1966.
2. Asakawa, Y.; Genjida, F.; Hayashi, S.; Matsuura, T. A New Ketol from *Alunus firma* Sieb. Et Zucc.(*Betulaceae*). *Tetrahedron Lett.* **1969**, *10*, 3235–3237. [CrossRef]
3. Terazawa, M.; Okuyama, H.; Miyake, M. Isolation of hirsutanonol and hirsutenone, two new diarylheptanoids from the green bark of Keyamahannoki, *Alnus hirsuta* Turcz. *Jap. Wood Res Soc. J.* **1973**, *19*, 45–46.
4. Karchesy, J.J.; Laver, M.L.; Barofsky, D.F.; Barofsky, E. Structure of oregonin, a natural diarylheptanoid xyloside. *J. Chem. Soc. Chem. Commun.* **1974**, *16*, 649. [CrossRef]
5. Nomura, M.; Tokoroyama, T.; Kubota, T. Biarylheptanoids and other constituents from wood of Alnus japonica. *Phytochemistry* **1981**, *20*, 1097–1104. [CrossRef]
6. Asakawa, Y. Chemical Constituents of Alnus sieboldiana(BETULACEAE) II. The Isolation and Structure of Flavonoids and Stilbenes. *Chem. Soc.* **1971**, *44*, 2761–2766. [CrossRef]
7. Suga, T.; Iwata, N.; Asakawa, Y. Chemical Constituents of the Male Flower of Alnus pendula(BETULACEAE). *Chem. Soc.* **1972**, *45*, 2058–2060. [CrossRef]
8. Sakamura, F.; Ohta, S.; Aoki, T.; Suga, T. Triterpenoids from the female and male flowers of Alnus sieboldiana. *Phytochemistry* **1985**, *24*, 2744–2745. [CrossRef]
9. Suga, T.; Ohta, S.; Ohta, E.; Aoki, T. A C31-secodammarane-type triterpenic acid, 12-deoxy alnustic acid, from the female flowers of alnus pendula. *Phytochemistry* **1986**, *25*, 1243–1244. [CrossRef]
10. Ishimatsu, M.; Tanaka, T.; Nonaka, G.-I.; Nishioka, I. Alnusnins A and B from the leaves of Alnus sieboldiana. *Phytochemistry* **1989**, *28*, 3179–3184. [CrossRef]
11. Hult, K.; Berglund, P. Engineered enzymes for improved organic synthesis. *Curr. Opin. Biotechnol.* **2003**, *14*, 395–400. [CrossRef]
12. Lee, M.-W.; Kim, N.-Y.; Park, M.-S.; Ahn, K.-H.; Toh, S.-H.; Hahn, D.-R.; Kim, Y.-C.; Chung, H.-T. Diarylheptanoids with In Vitro Inducible Nitric Oxide Synthesis Inhibitory Activity from Alnus hirsuta. *Planta Medica* **2000**, *66*, 551–553. [CrossRef]
13. Choi, S.E.; Park, K.H.; Jeong, M.S.; Kim, H.H.; Lee, D.I.; Joo, S.S.; Lee, C.S.; Bang, H.; Choi, Y.W.; Lee, M.-K.; et al. Effect of Alnus japonica extract on a model of atopic dermatitis in NC/Nga mice. *J. Ethnopharmacol.* **2011**, *136*, 406–413. [CrossRef]
14. Lee, M.; Song, J.Y.; Chin, Y.-W.; Sung, S.H. Anti-adipogenic diarylheptanoids from Alnus hirsuta f. sibirica on 3T3-L1 cells. *Bioorganic Med. Chem. Lett.* **2013**, *23*, 2069–2073. [CrossRef] [PubMed]
15. Joo, S.S.; Kim, M.S.; Oh, W.S.; Lee, D.I. Enhancement of NK Cytotoxicity, Antimetastasis and Elongation Effect of Survival Time in B16-F10 Melanoma Cells by Oregonin. *Arch. Pharm. Res.* **2002**, *25*, 493–499. [CrossRef] [PubMed]
16. Ko, S.-R.; Suzuki, Y.; Choi, K.-J.; Kim, Y.-H. Enzymatic Preparation of Genuine Prosapogenin, 20(S)-Ginsenoside Rh 1, from Ginsenosides Re and Rg 1. *Biosci. Biotechnol. Biochem.* **2000**, *64*, 2739–2743. [CrossRef]
17. Ko, S.-R.; Choi, K.-J.; Suzuki, K.; Suzuki, Y. Enzymatic Preparation of Ginsenosides Rg2, Rh1, and F1. *Chem. Pharm.* **2003**, *51*, 404–408. [CrossRef]
18. Park, J.S.; Rho, H.S.; Kim, D.H.; Chang, I.S. Enzymatic Preparation of Kaempferol from Green Tea Seed and Its Antioxidant Activity. *J. Agric. Food Chem.* **2006**, *54*, 2951–2956. [CrossRef] [PubMed]

19. Guzmán-Maldonado, H.; Paredes-López, O.; Biliaderis, C.G. Amylolytic Enzymes and Products Derived from Starch: A Review. *Crit. Rev. Food Sci. Nutr.* **1995**, *35*, 373–403. [CrossRef] [PubMed]
20. D'Archivio, M.; Filesi, C.; Di Benedetto, R.; Gargiulo, R.; Giovannini, C.; Masella, R. Polyphenols, Dietary Sources and Bioavailability. *Ann. Ist. Super. Sanita* **2007**, *43*, 348.
21. Williamson, G.; Day, A.J. Biomarkers for exposure to dietary flavonoids: a review of the current evidence for identification of quercetin glycosides in plasma. *Br. J. Nutr.* **2001**, *86*, S105–S110.
22. Henrissat, B. A classification of glycosyl hydrolases based on amino acid sequence similarities. *Biochem. J.* **1991**, *280*, 309–316. [CrossRef] [PubMed]
23. Le, T.T.; Yin, J.; Lee, M. Anti-Inflammatory and Anti-Oxidative Activities of Phenolic Compounds from Alnus sibirica Stems Fermented by Lactobacillus plantarum subsp. argentoratensis. *Molecules* **2017**, *22*, 1566.
24. Yin, J.; Yoon, S.H.; Ahn, H.S.; Lee, M.W. Inhibitory Activity of Allergic Contact Dermatitis and Atopic Dermatitis-Like Skin in BALB/c Mouse through Oral Administration of Fermented Barks of Alnus sibirica. *Molecules* **2018**, *23*, 450. [CrossRef]
25. Yin, J.; Yoon, K.H.; Ahn, H.S.; Lee, M.W. Quantitative Analysis and Validation of Hirsutenone and Muricarpone B from Fermented Alnus sibirica. *Prod. Sci.* **2017**, *23*, 146. [CrossRef]
26. Kim, H.J.; Kim, K.H.; Yeom, S.H.; Kim, M.K.; Shim, J.G.; Lim, H.W.; Lee, M.W. New Diarylheptanoid from the Barks of *Alnus japonica* Steudel. *Chin. Chem. Lett.* **2005**, *16*, 1337.
27. Gonzalez-Laredo, R.F.; Chen, J.; Karchesy, Y.M.; Karchesy, J.J. Four New Diarylheptanoid Glycosides From Alnus Rubra Bark. *Prod. Lett.* **1999**, *13*, 75–80. [CrossRef]
28. Giang, P.M.; Son, P.T.; Matsunami, K.; Otsuka, H. New Diarylheptanoids from *Amomum muricarpum* E LMER. *Chem. Pharm. Bull.* **2006**, *54*, 139–140. [CrossRef]
29. Kharitonov, S.; Yates, D.; Robbin, R.; Logan-Sinclair, R.; Shinebourne, E.; Barnes, P. Increased nitric oxide in exhaled air of asthmatic patients. *Lancet* **1994**, *343*, 133–135. [CrossRef]
30. Epe, B. DNA damage by peroxynitrite characterized with DNA repair enzymes. *Nucleic Acids Res.* **1996**, *24*, 4105–4110. [CrossRef]
31. Hobbs, A.J.; Higgs, A.; Moncada, S. Inhibition of nitric oxide synthase as a potential therapeutic target. *Annu. Pharmacol. Toxicol.* **1999**, *39*, 191–220. [CrossRef] [PubMed]
32. Sautebin, L. Prostaglandins and nitric oxide as molecular targets for anti-inflammatory therapy. *Fitoterapia* **2000**, *71*, S48–S57. [CrossRef]
33. Choi, S.E.; Kim, K.H.; Kwon, J.H.; Kim, S.B.; Kim, H.W.; Lee, M.W. Cytotoxic activities of diarylheptanoids from Alnus japonica. *Arch. Pharmacal* **2008**, *31*, 1287–1289. [CrossRef]
34. Wang, H.S.; Yin, J.; Hwang, I.H.; Lee, M.W. Variation of diarylheptanoid from *Alnus sibirica* Fitch. Ex. Turcz. Processed Enzymatic Hydrolysis. *Korean J. Pharmacogn.* **2018**, *49*, 336–340.

Sample Availability: Samples of the compounds (**1–4**) are available from the authors.

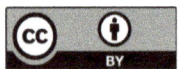

© 2019 by the authors. Licensee MDPI, Basel, Switzerland. This article is an open access article distributed under the terms and conditions of the Creative Commons Attribution (CC BY) license (http://creativecommons.org/licenses/by/4.0/).

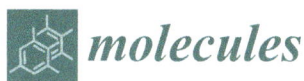

Article

Polyphenols-Rich Fruit (*Euterpe edulis* Mart.) Prevents Peripheral Inflammatory Pathway Activation by the Short-Term High-Fat Diet

Aline Boveto Santamarina [1], Giovana Jamar [1], Laís Vales Mennitti [1], Daniel Araki Ribeiro [2], Caroline Margonato Cardoso [1], Veridiana Vera de Rosso [2], Lila Missae Oyama [3] and Luciana Pellegrini Pisani [2,4,*]

[1] Programa de Pós-Graduação Interdisciplinar em Ciências da Saúde, Universidade Federal de São Paulo, Santos 11015-020, Brazil; alinesantamarina@gmail.com (A.B.S.); gi.jamar@gmail.com (G.J.); laisvmennitti@hotmail.com (L.V.M.); camargonato@gmail.com (C.M.C.)
[2] Departamento de Biociências, Universidade Federal de São Paulo, Santos 11015-020, Brazil; daribeiro@unifesp.br (D.A.R.); veriderosso@yahoo.com (V.V.d.R.)
[3] Departamento de Fisiologia, Universidade Federal de São Paulo, São Paulo 04023-062, Brazil; lmoyama@gmail.com
[4] Laboratório de Nutrição e Fisiologia Endócrina (LaNFE), Departamento de Biociências, Instituto de Saúde e Sociedade, Universidade Federal de São Paulo, Rua Silva Jardim, 136, Térreo, Vila Mathias, Santos, São Paulo 11015-020, Brazil
* Correspondence: lucianapisani@gmail.com; Tel.: +55-(13)-38783830

Academic Editor: Francesco Maione
Received: 2 April 2019; Accepted: 26 April 2019; Published: 27 April 2019

Abstract: Juçara berry is a potential inflammatory modulator, rich in dietary fiber, fatty acids, and anthocyanins. Considering this, we evaluated the high-fat diet (HFD) intake supplemented with different doses of freeze-dried juçara pulp on the TLR4 pathway. Twenty-seven male Wistar rats with ad libitum access to food and water were divided into four experimental groups: control standard chow group (C); high-fat diet control group (HFC); high-fat diet juçara 0.25% group (HFJ0.25%); and high-fat diet juçara 0.5% group (HFJ0.5%). The inflammatory parameters were analyzed by ELISA and Western blotting in liver and retroperitoneal adipose tissue (RET). The HFJ0.25% group had the energy intake, aspartate transaminase (AST) levels, and liver triacylglycerol accumulation reduced; also, the tumor necrosis factor α (TNF-α) and TNF receptor-associated factor 6 (TRAF6) expression in RET were reduced. However, there were no changes in other protein expressions in liver and adipose tissue. Adiposity and pNFκBp50 had a positive correlation in HFC and HFJ0.5%, but not in the C group and HFJ0.25%. The necrosis hepatic score did not change with treatment; however, the serum (AST) levels and the hepatic triacylglycerol were increased in HFC and HFJ0.5%. These results demonstrated that one week of HFD intake triggered pro-inflammatory mechanisms and liver injury. Additionally, 0.25% juçara prevented inflammatory pathway activation, body weight gain, and liver damage

Keywords: inflammation; short-term high-fat diet; juçara; nutraceutical food; liver; adipose tissue

1. Introduction

Western diet patterns are spread worldwide and cause the establishment of several non-communicable metabolic diseases. However, many deleterious mechanisms related to high-fat diet exposure are activated even before weight gaining reaches significant levels [1].

There is extensive literature regarding the features of long-term high-fat diet consumption, as well as its consequences for health [2]. At the same time, concerning the effects of short-term high-fat diet consumption, the literature becomes scarcer. Reports are mainly related to saturated fatty acids' (SFA) damaging action in the central nervous system and satiety control; however, the peripheral metabolic effect is slightly explored [3]. Turner et al. (2013) demonstrated a chronology of activation in inflammatory mechanisms, insulin resistance, and non-alcoholic fatty liver diseases (NAFLD), suggesting that before clinical signs, significant physiological changes may occur [4].

One of the mechanisms involved in the onset of low-grade inflammation in vitro and in vivo models of obesity is mediated by toll-like receptor 4 (TLR4) stimulated by dietary SFA. The TLR4 recognizes lipid ligands and plays an important role in non-infectious inflammatory diseases such as insulin resistance, obesity, and NAFLD. Moreover, polyunsaturated fatty acids (PUFA) ω-3 and ω-6 inhibit the inflammatory response mediated by TLR4 [5,6].

Metabolic disease control using bioactive food compounds has received attention from the scientific community and clinical practice [7]. One Brazilian native fruit with remarkable high nutritional value is juçara fruit. It contains significant amounts of dietary fiber, monounsaturated fatty acids (MUFA), and PUFA. It also has high levels of flavonoids, such as anthocyanins [8]. Therefore, it could contribute to preventing obesity, oxidative stress, and metabolic syndrome, possibly through an anti-inflammatory effect [9,10].

Although it is well known that there is an established chronic subclinical inflammatory state in obesity, only a few studies address the effect of the short-term high-fat diet and food bioactive compounds' intake. Considering the lack of studies in this field, we aim to evaluate the effectiveness of different juçara doses to prevent the deleterious effects of the short-term high-fat diet intake in the inflammatory markers and ectopic fatty liver accumulation.

2. Results

2.1. Diet Intake, Body Weight, and Tissue Weight

The average of energy intake (Kcal) along the treatment was higher in the high-fat diet control (HFC) group compared to the control (C) group ($p < 0.001$) and HFJ0.25% ($p = 0.0014$). The high-fat diet juçara 0.5% (HFJ0.5%) group had a higher energy intake compared to the C group ($p < 0.001$), and HFJ0.25% ($p = 0.029$). The HFJ0.25% group showed higher energy intake than the C group ($p = 0.0013$). The daily body weight gain was accessed day by day during the experiment. At the third day of treatment, the HFC group and HFJ0.5% had a greater body weight gain compared to the C group ($p = 0.006$ and 0.016, respectively). After six days of diet exposure, the HFJ0.5% group demonstrated an increased body weight gain comparing to the C group ($p = 0.012$). However, the other measures did not demonstrate differences among the groups regarding body weight gain (Figure 1).

Retroperitoneal and epididymal white adipose tissue (RET and EPI, respectively) absolute weights were increased in the HFC compared to the C group. Regarding the different adipose tissues evaluated, both juçara-supplemented groups (HFJ0.25% and HFJ0.5%) maintained a similarity between other groups or themselves. Liver and mesenteric white adipose tissue (MES) weight did not change among the experimental groups. The sum of white adipose tissues' weight depots (ΣWAT) was significantly increased in the HFC group compared to the control (Table 1).

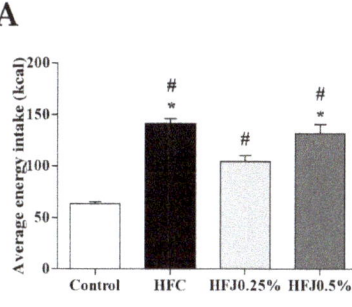
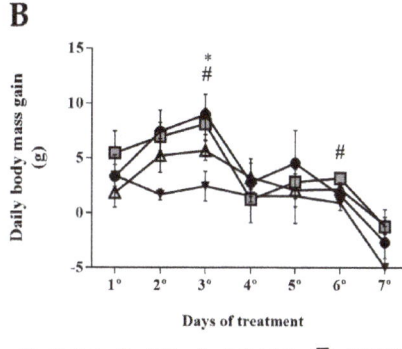

Figure 1. (**A**) Average energy intake (kcal). * $p < 0.05$ compared with the high-fat juçara 0.25% group (HFJ0.25%); # $p < 0.05$ compared with control diet by two-way ANOVA followed by the Bonferroni post-hoc test. (**B**) Daily body weight gain during the experimental period of seven days. The comparisons were performed by ANOVA for repeated measure and the Bonferroni post hoc test. # $p < 0.05$ in HFJ0.5% group compared with the control diet group; * $p < 0.05$ in high-fat diet control (HFC) group compared with the control diet group. Control standard chow (C) ($n = 6$); high-fat diet control (HFC) ($n = 7$); high-fat diet juçara 0.25% (HFJ0.25%) ($n = 7$); and high-fat diet juçara 0.5% (HFJ0.5%) ($n = 7$).

Table 1. Absolute tissue weight on different experimental groups.

	Absolute tissue weight (g)				
	Control ($n = 6$)	HFC ($n = 7$)	HFJ0.25% ($n = 7$)	HFJ0.5% ($n = 7$)	p-Vaule
Liver	10.57 ± 0.54	11.46 ± 0.66	10.23 ± 0.70	10.16 ± 0.85	-
RET	3.39 ± 0.52	6.99 ± 0.90 #	4.67 ± 0.71	4.95 ± 0.64	0.029
EPI	3.74 ± 0.38	5.67 ± 0.69 #	4.20 ± 0.61	3.94 ± 0.70	0.044
MES	3.57 ± 0.64	4.18 ± 0.44	3.44 ± 0.26	3.99 ± 0.50	-
ΣWAT	10.70 ± 1.36	16.84 ± 1.64 #	12.32 ± 1.37	12.88 ± 1.76	0.020

# $p < 0.05$ vs. control group by two-way ANOVA followed by the Bonferroni post-hoc test. The p-value is shown in the table above. Control standard chow (control); high-fat diet control (HFC); high-fat diet juçara 0.25% (HFJ0.25%); high-fat diet juçara 0.5% (HFJ0.5%). RET, retroperitoneal tissue; EPI, epididymal white adipose tissue; MES, epididymal white adipose tissue; ΣWAT, sum of white adipose tissues' weight depots.

2.2. Hepatic Ectopic Fat Accumulation

Liver histological analyses performed in hematoxylin and eosin illustrated the morphological differences among the groups (Figure 2). The necrosis histopathological score did not statistically change with the experimental treatment (Table 2). However, in the groups exposed to high-fat diet juçara 0.5%, microsteatosis in liver parenchyma was evidenced.

The hepatic triacylglycerol content in HFC and HFJ0.5% groups was increased in comparison of the C group ($p = 0.0055$ and 0.0275, respectively). Even though, HFJ0.25% did not differ from the control group, as shown in Table 3.

Accessing the serum levels of hepatic enzymes—aspartate transaminase (AST) and alanine transaminase (ALT)—there were no differences among the groups. However, the AST level was higher in the HFC and HFJ0.5% groups compared to the C group ($p = 0.044$ and 0.041, respectively). The level of AST in HFJ0.25% was similar to the C group (Table 3).

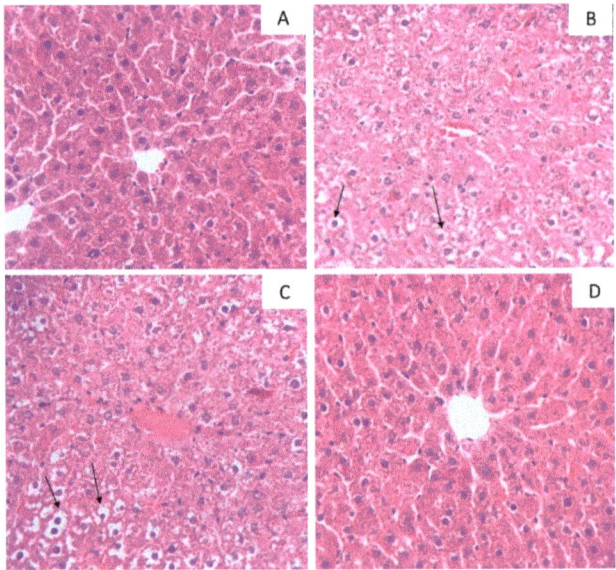

Figure 2. Photomicrographs of hepatic tissue stained by hematoxylin and eosin with a magnification of 40×. (**A**) Control standard chow (control); (**B**) high-fat diet control group (HFC); (**C**) high-fat diet juçara 0.5% group (HFJ0.5%); (**D**) high-fat diet juçara 0.25% group (HFJ0.25%). The arrows (↑) indicate the lipid droplets.

Table 2. The histopathological score in liver among the groups ($p > 0.05$).

	0	1	2	3
Control ($n = 5$)	5	0	0	0
HFC ($n = 7$)	4	3	0	0
HFJ0.5% ($n = 7$)	3	4	0	0
HFJ0.25% ($n = 7$)	5	2	0	0

The Kruskal–Wallis test was used to analyze the histopathological score among the experimental groups. Control standard chow (control); high-fat diet control (HFC); high-fat diet juçara 0.25% (HFJ0.25%); high-fat diet juçara 0.5% (HFJ0.5%).

Table 3. Hepatic enzymes analyzed in serum and liver ectopic triacylglycerol storage.

	Control ($n = 6$)	HFC ($n = 7$)	HFJ0.25% ($n = 7$)	HFJ0.5% ($n = 7$)
AST (U/L)	36.18 ± 2.77	49.43 ± 4.99 [&]	34.11 ± 7.25	49.79 ± 6.31 [&]
ALT (U/L)	16.61 ± 1.37	23.06 ± 9.89	15.41 ± 3.21	17.17 ± 4.58
TAG (mg/100mg)	129.91 ± 4.41	157.33 ± 4.92 [#]	142.59 ± 5.21	151.71 ± 2.14 [#]

AST: aspartate transaminase; ALT: alanine transaminase; TAG: triacylglycerol. [#] $p < 0.05$ vs. the control group using two-way ANOVA followed by the Bonferroni post-hoc test; [&] $p < 0.05$ vs. the control group using the t-test.

2.3. Cytokines Concentration

We observed that IL-6 increased in RET of the HFJ0.25% ($p = 0.020$) and HFJ0.5% ($p = 0.035$) groups compared to the C group. The TNF-α level in RET was increased in the HFC and HFJ0.5% groups compared to the C group ($p = 0.033$ and $p = 0.003$, respectively). In contrast, the HFJ0.25% group was similar to the C group. The IL-10 level was reduced in HFC ($p = 0.032$) and HFJ0.5% ($p = 0.009$) compared to the C group in RET (Figure 3A,C,E). Liver pro-inflammatory cytokines (IL-6 and TNF-α) did not differ among the groups, however, the anti-inflammatory cytokine (IL-10) was lower in the HFJ0.5% group than in the control ($p = 0.05$) group (Figure 3B,D,F).

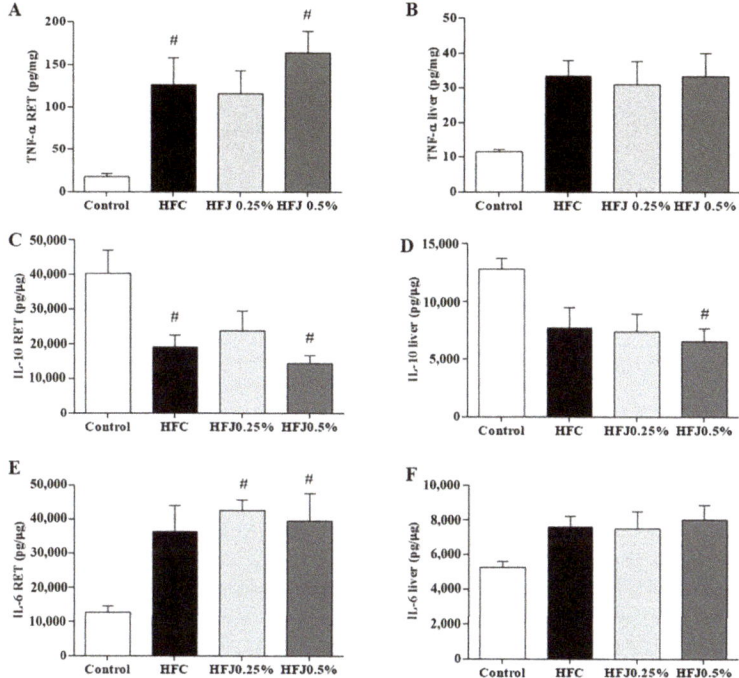

Figure 3. Cytokine levels: (**A**) TNF-α in RET; (**B**) TNF-α in liver; (**C**) IL-10 in RET; (**D**) IL-10 in liver; (**E**) IL-6 in RET; (**F**) IL-6 in liver. # $p < 0.05$ compared with the control diet by two-way ANOVA followed by the Bonferroni post-hoc test. Control standard chow (control) ($n = 6$); high-fat diet control (HFC) ($n = 7$); high-fat diet juçara 0.25% (HFJ0.25%) ($n = 7$); and high-fat diet juçara 0.5% (HFJ0.5%) ($n = 7$).

2.4. NFκB Pathway Protein Expression

The inflammatory TLR4 pathway in RET was evaluated. TNF receptor-associated factor 6 (TRAF6) protein expression was significantly reduced in the HFJ0.25% ($p = 0.048$) as in the C group ($p = 0.043$) compared to the HFC group (Figure 4A–D).

There were no differences in protein expression among TLR4 membrane receptors and their cellular signaling intermediates, such as myeloid differentiation primary response 88 (MYD88) and nuclear factor kappa-B p50 (pNFκBp50) in RET and liver. Furthermore, we did not find changes in the protein expression of the TLR4 pathway in liver (Figure 5A–D).

Analyzing the correlation between visceral adiposity (ΣWAT) and phosphorylation of hepatic NFκBp50, it is possible to note a strong positive correlation in the HFC group ($r = 0.794$; $p = 0.033$) and HFJ0.5% ($r = 0.818$; $p = 0.025$). On the other hand, the C and HFJ0.25% groups did not demonstrate this relation (Figure 6), demonstrating the higher effectiveness of the lower dose, in agreement with the results presented.

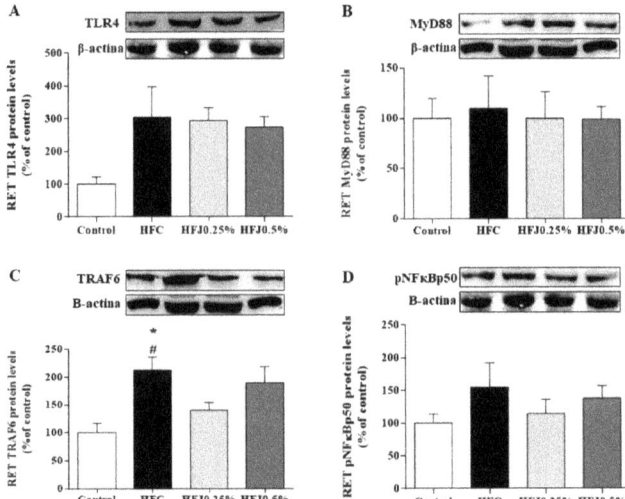

Figure 4. Protein expression of the NFκB pathway in the RET: (**A**) TLR4; (**B**) MYD88; (**C**) TRAF6; and (**D**) pNFκBp50. The housekeeping used was the β-actin expression. * $p < 0.05$ compared with the high-fat juçara 0.25% group (HFJ0.25%); # $p < 0.05$ compared with the control diet. Two-way ANOVA followed by the Bonferroni post-hoc test were performed as the statistical analyses. Control standard chow (control) ($n = 6$); high-fat diet control (HFC) ($n = 7$); high-fat diet juçara 0.25% (HFJ0.25%) ($n = 7$); and high-fat diet juçara 0.5% (HFJ0.5%) ($n = 7$).

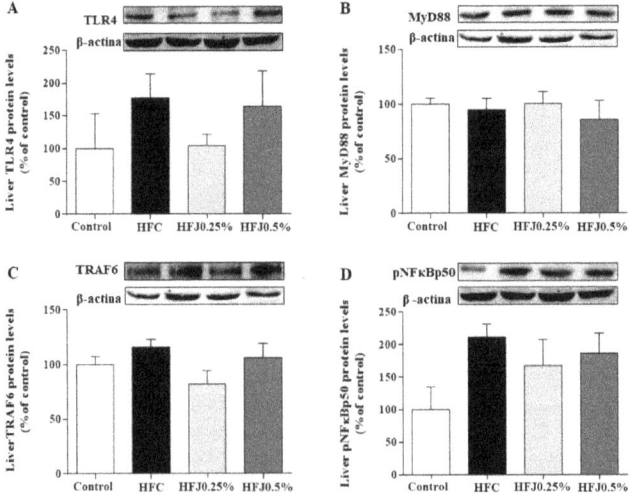

Figure 5. Protein expression of the NFκB pathway in liver: (**A**) TLR4; (**B**) MYD88; (**C**) TRAF6; and (**D**) pNFκBp50. The housekeeping was the β-actin expression. Two-way ANOVA followed by the Bonferroni post-hoc test were performed as the statistical analyses. Control standard chow (control) ($n = 6$); high-fat diet control (HFC) ($n = 7$); high-fat diet juçara 0.25% (HFJ0.25%) ($n = 7$); and high-fat diet juçara 0.5% (HFJ0.5%) ($n = 7$).

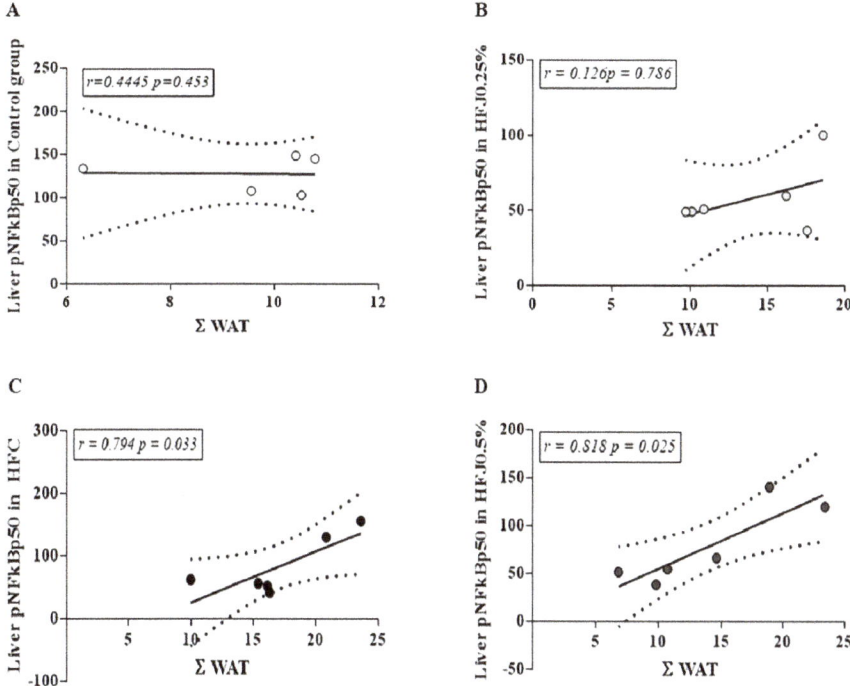

Figure 6. Correlation between ΣWAT and pNFκBp50 in liver for different experimental groups: (**A**) Control standard chow group (control); (**B**) high-fat diet juçara 0.25% (HFJ0.25%); (**C**) high-fat diet control group (HFC); (**D**) high-fat diet juçara 0.5% (HFJ0.5%). The Pearson correlation coefficient was performed considering the level of significance as $p < 0.05$ and the Pearson's r-value >0.7 for a strong correlation.

3. Discussion

The results demonstrated the influence of juçara supplementation—a fruit rich in anthocyanin and unsaturated fatty acids (MUFAs and PUFAs)—in energy intake, in adipose tissue and hepatic ectopic fat accumulation, as well as in the inflammatory profile. Regarding the TLR4 pathway, the main benefits are related to the consumption of the lower dose of the pulp.

The higher energy intake observed in the HFD chow groups compared to the control group evidence changes in eating habits due to the high energy density provided by the diet. The HFD can modulate the central regulation of appetite and satiation through intricate ways involving neuroendocrine signaling from peripheral tissues. A recent short-term HFD model study demonstrated that serum ghrelin level is high in postprandial conditions, suggesting that in HFD, the ghrelin orexigenic signal remains activated in the hypothalamus, leading to exacerbated caloric intake [11]. It is noteworthy that the HFJ0.25% group had a smaller caloric intake compared to the other HFD groups. This result can be justified by the protective hypothalamic effect promoted by the juçara supplementation due to its rich composition against the deleterious effects of HFD [12,13].

The increased adiposity (ΣWAT, RET, and EPI) in HFC indicated that our HFD model was efficient at inducing visceral fat weight gain even in a short-term diet treatment [13,14]. High-fat diet consumption is related to the pro-inflammatory mechanism stimulus, leading to chronic subclinical inflammation, promoting metabolic diseases' installation [15]. According to our findings, previous reports showed that for short-term periods, the high-fat diet is not able to promote relevant changes in body weight gain. However, the adipose pads were slightly increased, as well as the concentration of inflammatory cytokines (IL-6 and TNF-α), similar to our results [14,16,17]. These findings enforce that high-fat diet leads to deleterious pro-inflammatory pathway activation. Both groups subjected to juçara supplementation did not statistically differ from the lean group (C), in adipose depots' evaluated mass and ΣWAT. This suggests that juçara has a protective role, preventing high-fat diet's deleterious consequences in visceral adiposity gain. This can be corroborated by other short-term protocols of bioactive compounds' supplementation, which exert a metabolic protective role in experimental and clinical models [18–21]. Juçara has beneficial effects previously reported when associated with a high-fat diet, and it may be attributed to the nutritional components of juçara pulp [12,13,22].

The liver histological image illustrates, and TAG content confirms, that the lower dose of juçara (HFJ0.25%) had less injury related to high-fat diet consumption than the HFC and HFJ0.5% groups, remaining at levels similar to those observed in the control group. Furthermore, the ectopic TAG accumulation represents a trigger of NAFLD mechanisms. As a consequence, juçara consumption leads to a protective effect of the regulatory mechanisms for liver. AST and ALT levels are important liver injury markers. These enzymes can be found in hepatocytes cytoplasm and catalyze amino group transferences in the citric acid cycle. Hepatic injury is commonly related to AST and ALT release into the extracellular compartment with subsequent increase in serum. Our results demonstrate that liver integrity was preserved in the HFJ0.25% group, corroborating the reduced liver injury score observed in this group. These findings together indicate that juçara supplementation promoted a hepatic protective effect at the lower dose. Our hypothesis is supported by supplementations of anthocyanins, which protect against NAFLD in long-term high-fat feeding [23,24].

It is interesting to observe that a 0.5% juçara dose did not demonstrate greater efficiency in the modulation of cytokines involved in inflammatory profile and maintained the same level of HFC with ambiguous results in RET. IL-10 reduction in liver, only in the HFJ0.5% group, is an indicator of juçara dose excess. We postulated that high doses might exert a pro-oxidative and negative effect due to high phenolic compound and fatty acid amounts. Lecci et al. (2014) [25] corroborate this hypothesis since non-toxic polyphenol doses activated pro-apoptotic mechanisms in vitro. Despite being a physiological polyphenol and anthocyanin dose, it could exert a cytotoxic role. An in vitro adipocyte study showed that some types of polyphenols act in a pro-oxidant manner, stimulating the production of the pro-inflammatory cytokines, such as TNF-α [26]. Moreover, PUFA and MUFA have deleterious effects when consumed in substantial amounts. This highlights the importance of the fatty acid quality and polyphenol amount offered in the metabolic and inflammatory outcomes [27,28].

It has been shown that the mainly pro-inflammatory cytokines' source was the adipose tissue compared to liver in obesity and NAFLD. This enforces that peripheral tissues, such as adipose tissue, can affect disease processes in target organs [29]. This matches our results; for the effects in short-term, the adipose tissue showed greater susceptibility to the intervention for inflammatory response compared to liver.

An extensive literature review demonstrates a strong relationship between the TLR4 pathway and high-fat diet consumption in metabolic diseases [1,6]. Turner et al. (2013) have observed that changes from high-fat diet consumption occur progressively among different tissues. Although inflammatory markers in adipose tissue can be noticed after 1–3 weeks of a high-fat diet, hepatic effects are pronounced only after chronic consumption [4]. We observed no changes in TLR4, MYD88, or phosphorylated NFκB expression in RET. However, TRAF6 in RET with a dose of 0.25% was similar to the C group and reduced in comparison to the HFC group. This indicates a possible TLR4 pathway modulation mechanism, corroborating the changes observed in the cytokines' concentration in adipose tissue. Nevertheless, the diet duration was not enough to install the classic pro-inflammatory framework in liver. Analyzing the correlation between pNFκBp50 and the adiposity index (ΣWAT), the strong correlation between them in the HFC group and HFJ0.5% is noteworthy, but not in C and HFJ0.25%. This exposes two results. Firstly, it demonstrates that adiposity is strongly related to the NFκBp50 phosphorylation, and it could be attributed to high-fat diet intake and its deleterious properties [30]. Secondly, the 0.25% juçara dose was similar to the control group, showing that juçara was able to prevent the deleterious high-fat diet effects, without a correlation between this variable. NFκBp50 is an important nuclear transcription factor, which is activated by kappa B inhibitor degradation mediated by inflammatory signaling TLR4 pathways. NFκBp50's main function is to induce cytokines' production, such as TNF-α, playing a role in an inflammatory pathway [15]. The high-fat diet intake, as well as increased adiposity induce the formation of reactive oxygen species (ROS) due to the H_2O_2 production in the mitochondria and the peroxisomal oxidation in lipid metabolism; which may cause TLR4 activation [31]. Several bioactive compounds, such as anthocyanins, have been related to inhibiting ROS formation and, consequently, the TLR4 pathway activation [32]. The most relevant finding indicates that juçara effectiveness prevents the pro-inflammatory status installation. Zero-point-two-five percent of juçara associated with a high-fat diet inhibited the inflammatory response, reducing NFκBp50 phosphorylation, despite the high-fat diet's evident pro-inflammatory stimulus.

4. Materials and Methods

4.1. Short-Term High-Fat Diet

A total of 27 outbred male Wistar rats of 90-day-old were used. After one week of acclimatization, the animals were randomly divided into four experimental groups: control standard chow (C) (n = 6); high-fat diet control (HFC) (n = 7); high-fat diet juçara 0.25% (HFJ0.25%) (n = 7); and high-fat diet juçara 0.5% (HFJ0.5%) (n = 7). They received the respective diets for the acute experimental period of 7 days.

The C group was fed with standard rat commercial chow, and the composition of the experimental diets was adapted from Dornellas et al. [33] and is described in Table 4. The animals were weighed, and diet consumption was measured every day during the experimental period.

Table 4. Composition of the experimental diets used: high-fat diet control, high-fat diet juçara 0.25%, and high-fat juçara 0.5%.

Components	Diet (g/100g)			
	Control	HFC	HFJ0.25%	HFJ0.5%
Standard chow *	100	50	50	50
Sucrose	-	10	10	10
Casein	-	20	20	20
Soybean oil	-	2	2	2
Lard		18	18	18
Butyl hydroquinone	-	0.004	0.004	0.004
Juçara pulp powder	-	-	0.25	0.5
Mineral mix® §		0.5	0.5	0.5
Vitamins mix® &		1.75	1.75	1.75
Energy (Kcal/100g)	270	410	420	430

* The standard rat commercial chow used was Nuvilab CR1 (Nuvital, Brazil); § mineral mix (AIN-93M, mineral mix, Rhoster, Brazil); & vitamin mix (AIN-93M, vitamin mix, Rhoster, Brazil).

4.2. Freeze-Dried Juçara Pulp Powder

Juçara pulp was obtained from the Agro-ecological Juçara Project/Instituto de Permacultura e Ecovilas da Mata Atlântica (Ubatuba, São Paulo, Brazil) and freeze-dried into a powder. The juçara pulp powder was analyzed to confirm the pulp fruit chemo profile. For fiber content, anthocyanins' and phenolic compounds' analysis, the HPLC-PDA-MS/MS technique was performed as by Azevedo da Silva et al. (2014), and for the fatty acid analysis profile, the GC-FID-MS/MS technique was used. The results obtained in this characterization are shown in Table 5, expressed as a dry basis. The main anthocyanins and phenolic compounds detected in juçara pulp powder had already been detected in the frozen pulp [8] and are summarized in Table 5.

Table 5. The main bioactive compounds and fatty acids detected in juçara pulp powder.

Bioactive Compound	Concentration (in 100 g Dry Basis)
Cyanidin 3-rutinoside (mg)	1790.0 ± 57.5
Cyanidin 3-glucoside (mg)	740.9 ± 22.1
Total anthocyanins (mg)	2663.7 ± 76.2
Apigenin deoxyhexosyl-hexoside (mg)	224.7 ± 13.2
Luteolin deoxyhexosyl-hexoside (mg)	332.7 ± 16.8
Dihydrokaempferol-hexoside (mg)	587.6 ± 23.0
Total phenolic compounds (mg)	3976.1 ± 197.34
Total fiber (g)	28.3 ± 0.3
Fatty Acids	**(% Fatty Acids Total)**
Oleic acid (C18:1)	44.2
Linoleic acid (C18:2)	17.4
Linolenic acid (C18:3)	0.45

Test doses were chosen based on juçara pulp anthocyanin levels for physiological consumption. In this study, we proposed two different doses: 0.25% and 0.5% of juçara freeze-dried pulp diet supplementation based on previous studies with anthocyanin supplementation. It has been described that intake from 100.5–350.0 mg per day of anthocyanin is safe and improves the lipid profile and inflammatory responses [24,34].

The average daily anthocyanin intake in the upper dose (0.5%) was equivalent to 6 mg/rat/day, corresponding to a physiological and non-pharmacological dose [35]. The proportional dose for human consumption of juçara was calculated by the allometric factors proposed by the FDA in 2005 [36], considering an adult of 70 kg. The 0.5% dose corresponded to 3.3 mg of anthocyanins/kg/day, which could be obtained by consuming 100 g of fresh juçara pulp or 10 g of the same lyophilized per day. The dose of 0.25% represents 50 g of fresh juçara pulp or 5 g of the freeze-dried juçara pulp per day.

4.3. Animal Procedures

Animal procedures were approved by the Experimental Research Committee of the Universidade Federal de São Paulo (No. 5252010715), following the standards of the Brazilian Guidelines for Care and Use of Animals for Scientific Purposes and Teaching by the National Council of Animal Experimentation Control in 2013. The animals were maintained in collective cages with controlled temperature (23 ± 2 °C), humidity (60 ± 5%) and lighting (12-h light/dark) and received ad libitum water and diet.

At the end of the treatment, the animals were anesthetized with ketamine (80 mg/kg) and xylazine (10 mg/kg) and euthanized by beheading in the morning, after fasting for 12 h, between 8:00 and 10:00 Tissue samples were collected for analyses, immediately weighed, and stored at −80 °C.

4.4. Histopathological Analysis

Right lobe liver sections were collected and fixed in 10% buffered formalin for 24 h. The samples were processed and paraffin embedded. The histological sections of 4–5 μM were stained using hematoxylin and eosin for histopathological analysis.

The classification was based on score levels, considering the area of necrosis and changes such as eosinophilia, the presence of intracytoplasmic vacuoles, congestive vessels, and loss of structure established by Silva et al. [37] and described in Table 6.

Table 6. Score levels' classification considering the area of necrosis and hepatic alterations previously established by Silva et al. (2014) [37].

Score	Necrosis Area	Alterations
0	0%	Preserved structures
1	<30%	Discreet eosinophilia, the presence of intracytoplasmic vacuoles
2	≥30%	Marked eosinophilia, dilation of sinusoid space, congested vessels, and intracytoplasmic vacuoles
3	≥50%	Marked eosinophilia, congested vessels, intracytoplasmic vacuoles, karyolysis, and structural loss

4.5. Hepatic Triacylglycerol Analysis.

The liver tissue samples were homogenized and centrifuged for 5 minutes at 655.1× g at room temperature. The lipids extraction was performed as by Folch et al [38], and the total lipid extracts were evaporated under a nitrogen (N_2) atmosphere and emulsified in a 3% solution of Triton X-100 (Sigma-Aldrich, St. Louis, MO, USA). The TAG was quantified by the colorimetric method, using the Labtest® (Lagoa Santa, Minas Gerais, Brazil) commercial kit.

4.6. Hepatic Enzymes in Serum

The hepatic enzymes aspartate transaminase (AST) and alanine transaminase (ALT) in serum were measured by the colorimetric kinetic method using commercial kits (Labtest®, Lagoa Santa, Minas Gerais, Brazil).

4.7. Tissue TNF-α, IL-6, and IL-10 Concentrations

The liver and RET protein extracts were used in the commercial kits of ELISA (Duo Set ELISA, R&D Systems, Minneapolis, MN) to measure the concentrations of tumor necrosis factor-α (TNF-α), interleukin-6 (IL-6), and interleukin-10 (IL-10) following the manufacturer's recommendations.

4.8. Western Blotting Analyses

Liver and retroperitoneal adipose tissue (RET) protein samples were extracted and measured by the Bradford method. Protein samples were separated by electrophoresis on 10% SDS-polyacrylamide gels and transferred to nitrocellulose membranes. The membranes were blocked with 1% bovine serum albumin and incubated overnight with the following primary antibodies: pNFκBp50 (sc-101744) (Santa Cruz, CA, USA). The TLR4 (ab22048), MYD88 (ab2064), TRAF6 (ab33915), and β-actin (ab6276) were from ABCAM (Cambridge, U.K.).

UVITec (Cambridge, U.K.) and ECL reagent (Bio-Rad Laboratories, Hercules, CA, USA) were used to obtain the bands. Samples were quantified by ImageJ software (ImageJ, National Institute of Health, Maryland, MD, USA). The target proteins levels were normalized to β-actin expression.

4.9. Statistical Analyses

Grubb's test was performed to remove significant outliers. The interfaces between groups were accessed by one-way variance analysis followed by the Bonferroni post-hoc test for numeric variables. The Kruskal–Wallis test was used to analyze the histopathological score. The correlation levels were evaluated by the Pearson correlation coefficient (r-value < 0.7 for a strong correlation). The level of significance adopted was $p \leq 0.05$. The data were described as the mean ± SEM. Statistical analyses were performed in the software PASW Statistics software version 22.0 (IBM Corp., Armonk, NY, USA). All other tasks were performed in the Microsoft Excel (2010) program (Microsoft, Albuquerque, NM, USA).

5. Conclusions

These pieces of evidence indicate that one week of a high-fat diet is enough to trigger pro-inflammatory mechanisms in peripheral key tissues. We also concluded that the juçara dose of 0.25% is more suitable to produce positive metabolic effects, prevent body weight gain, and liver injury. It becomes clear that food should be considered in its whole and not a single nutrient. Higher doses of supplementation did not represent a more pronounced or better effect on the inflammatory, metabolic, or histological parameters. Additionally, a 0.25% dose of juçara could be considered a tool for the treatment and prevention of metabolic damage associated with a high-fat diet in liver. Nevertheless, further investigations about the effect of this powerful fruit must proceed to clarify the effects.

Author Contributions: L.P.P., V.V.d.R, D.A.R., and L.M.O. designed the study protocol. A.B.S., G.J., L.V.M., and C.M.C. conducted the experiments and analyzed the data. L.P.P. and A.B.S. critically revised the article for important intellectual content. L.P.P. and A.B.S. contributed to writing the manuscript.

Funding: This work was supported by Fundação de Amparo à Pesquisa do Estado de São Paulo, (2016/14133-0; 2015/13875-0; 2018/23623-7). L.P.P., D.A.R., V.V.d.R., and L.M.O. are recipients of the CNPq (Conselho Nacional de Desenvolvimento Científico e Tecnológico) fellowship.

Acknowledgments: The authors acknowledge Dylbert Fragoso Silvestre for technical assistance on the English language.

Conflicts of Interest: The authors declare that there is no conflict of interest regarding the publication of this paper.

References

1. Myles, I.A. Fast food fever: reviewing the impacts of the Western diet on immunity. *Nutr. J.* **2014**, *13*, 61. [CrossRef]
2. Figueiredo, P.S.; Inada, A.C.; Marcelino, G.; Cardozo, C.M.L.; de Cássia Freitas, K.; de Cássia Avellaneda Guimarães, R.; de Castro, A.P.; do Nascimento, V.A.; Hiane, P.A. Fatty acids consumption: The role metabolic aspects involved in obesity and its associated disorders. *Nutrients* **2017**, *9*, 1158. [CrossRef]
3. Shefer, G.; Marcus, Y.; Stern, N. Is obesity a brain disease? *Neurosci. Biobehav. Rev.* **2013**, *37*, 2489–2503. [CrossRef]
4. Turner, N.; Kowalski, G.M.; Leslie, S.J.; Risis, S.; Yang, C.; Lee-Young, R.S.; Babb, J.R.; Meikle, P.J.; Lancaster, G.I.; Henstridge, D.C.; et al. Distinct patterns of tissue-specific lipid accumulation during the induction of insulin resistance in mice by high-fat feeding. *Diabetologia* **2013**, *56*, 1638–1648. [CrossRef] [PubMed]
5. Rogero, M.M.; Calder, P.C. Obesity, inflammation, toll-like receptor 4 and fatty acids. *Nutrients* **2018**, *10*, 432. [CrossRef]
6. Jialal, I.; Kaur, H.; Devaraj, S. Toll-like receptor status in obesity and metabolic syndrome: A translational perspective. *J. Clin. Endocrinol. Metab.* **2014**, *99*, 39–48. [CrossRef] [PubMed]
7. Schreckinger, M.E.; Lotton, J.; Lila, M.A.; de Mejia, E.G. Berries from South America: a comprehensive review on chemistry, health potential, and commercialization. *J. Med. Food* **2010**, *13*, 233–246. [CrossRef] [PubMed]
8. Silva, N.A.D.; Rodrigues, E.; Mercadante, A.Z.; De Rosso, V.V. Phenolic compounds and carotenoids from four fruits native from the Brazilian Atlantic forest. *J. Agric. Food Chem.* **2014**, *62*, 5072–5084. [CrossRef] [PubMed]
9. Rufino, M.D.S.M.; Pérez-Jiménez, J.; Arranz, S.; Alves, R.E.; de Brito, E.S.; Oliveira, M.S.P.; Saura-Calixto, F. Açaí (Euterpe oleraceae) "BRS Pará": A tropical fruit source of antioxidant dietary fiber and high antioxidant capacity oil. *Food Res. Int.* **2011**, *44*, 2100–2106. [CrossRef]
10. Kang, J.; Thakali, K.M.; Xie, C.; Kondo, M.; Tong, Y.; Ou, B.; Jensen, G.; Medina, M.B.; Schauss, A.G.; Wu, X. Bioactivities of açaí (Euterpe precatoria Mart.) fruit pulp, superior antioxidant and anti-inflammatory properties to Euterpe oleracea Mart. *Food Chem.* **2012**, *133*, 671–677. [CrossRef]
11. Andrich, D.E.; Melbouci, L.; Ou, Y.; Leduc-Gaudet, J.P.; Chabot, F.; Lalonde, F.; Lira, F.S.; Gaylinn, B.D.; Gouspillou, G.; Danialou, G.; Comtois, A.S.; St-Pierre, D.H. Altered Feeding Behaviors and Adiposity Precede Observable Weight Gain in Young Rats Submitted to a Short-Term High-Fat Diet. *J. Nutr. Metab.* **2018**, *2018*. [CrossRef] [PubMed]

12. Jamar, G.; Santamarina, A.B.; Mennitti, L.V.; de Cássia Cesar, H.; Oyama, L.M.; de Rosso, V.V.; Pisani, L.P. Bifidobacterium spp. reshaping in the gut microbiota by low dose of juçara supplementation and hypothalamic insulin resistance in Wistar rats. *J. Funct. Foods* **2018**, *46*, 212–219. [CrossRef]
13. Santamarina, A.B.; Jamar, G.; Mennitti, L.V.; de Rosso, V.V.; Cesar, H.C.; Oyama, L.M.; Pisani, L.P. The Use of Juçara (Euterpe edulis Mart.) Supplementation for Suppression of NF-κB Pathway in the Hypothalamus after High-Fat Diet in Wistar Rats. *Mol. (Baselswitz.)* **2018**, *23*, 1814. [CrossRef]
14. Wiedemann, M.S.F.; Wueest, S.; Item, F.; Schoenle, E.J.; Konrad, D. Adipose tissue inflammation contributes to short-term high-fat diet-induced hepatic insulin resistance. *Am. J. Physiol. -Endocrinol. Metab.* **2013**, *305*, E388–E395. [CrossRef]
15. Estadella, D.; da Penha Oller do Nascimento, C.M.; Oyama, L.M.; Ribeiro, E.B.; Dâmaso, A.R.; de Piano, A. Lipotoxicity: Effects of Dietary Saturated and Transfatty Acids. *Mediat. Inflamm.* **2013**, *2013*, 1–13. [CrossRef] [PubMed]
16. Das, N.; Sikder, K.; Bhattacharjee, S.; Majumdar, S.B.; Ghosh, S.; Majumdar, S.; Dey, S. Quercetin alleviates inflammation after short-term treatment in high-fat-fed mice. *Food Funct.* **2013**, *4*, 889. [CrossRef] [PubMed]
17. Magri-Tomaz, L.; Melbouci, L.; Mercier, J.; Ou, Y.; Auclair, N.; Lira, F.S.; Lavoie, J.M.; St-Pierre, D.H. Two weeks of high-fat feeding disturb lipid and cholesterol molecular markers. *Cell Biochem. Funct.* **2018**, *36*, 387–393. [CrossRef] [PubMed]
18. Most, J.; Goossens, G.H.; Jocken, J.W.E.; Blaak, E.E. Short-term supplementation with a specific combination of dietary polyphenols increases energy expenditure and alters substrate metabolism in overweight subjects. *Int. J. Obes.* **2014**, *38*, 698–706. [CrossRef] [PubMed]
19. Nogueira, L.D.P.; Nogueira Neto, J.F.; Klein, M.R.S.T.; Sanjuliani, A.F. Short-term Effects of Green Tea on Blood Pressure, Endothelial Function, and Metabolic Profile in Obese Prehypertensive Women: A Crossover Randomized Clinical Trial. *J. Am. Coll. Nutr.* **2017**, *36*, 108–115. [CrossRef] [PubMed]
20. Lyall, K.A.; Hurst, S.M.; Cooney, J.; Jensen, D.; Lo, K.; Hurst, R.D.; Stevenson, L.M. Short-term blackcurrant extract consumption modulates exercise-induced oxidative stress and lipopolysaccharide-stimulated inflammatory responses. *Am. J. Physiol. -Regul. Integr. Comp. Physiol.* **2009**, *297*, R70–R81. [CrossRef] [PubMed]
21. Mullan, A.; Delles, C.; Ferrell, W.; Mullen, W.; Edwards, C.A.; McColl, J.H.; Roberts, S.A.; Lean, M.E.; Sattar, N. Effects of a beverage rich in (poly)phenols on established and novel risk markers for vascular disease in medically uncomplicated overweight or obese subjects: A four week randomized trial. *Atherosclerosis* **2016**, *246*, 169–176. [CrossRef]
22. Oyama, L.M.; Silva, F.P.; Carnier, J.; De Miranda, D.A.; Santamarina, A.B.; Ribeiro, E.B.; Oller Do Nascimento, C.M.; De Rosso, V.V. Juçara pulp supplementation improves glucose tolerance in mice. *Diabetol. Metab. Syndr.* **2016**, *8*, 1–8. [CrossRef]
23. Liu, Y.; Wang, D.; Zhang, D.; Lv, Y.; Wei, Y.; Wu, W.; Zhou, F.; Tang, M.; Mao, T.; Li, M.; Ji, B. Inhibitory Effect of Blueberry Polyphenolic Compounds on Oleic Acid-Induced Hepatic Steatosis in Vitro. *J. Agric. Food Chem.* **2011**, *59*, 12254–12263. [CrossRef] [PubMed]
24. Valenti, L.; Riso, P.; Mazzocchi, A.; Porrini, M.; Fargion, S.; Agostoni, C. Dietary anthocyanins as nutritional therapy for nonalcoholic fatty liver disease. *Oxidative Med. Cell. Longev.* **2013**, *2013*. [CrossRef]
25. Lecci, R.; Logrieco, A.; Leone, A. Pro-Oxidative Action of Polyphenols as Action Mechanism for their Pro-Apoptotic Activity. *Anti-Cancer Agents Med. Chem.* **2014**, *14*, 1363–1375. [CrossRef]
26. Hatia, S.; Septembre-Malaterre, A.; Le Sage, F.; Badiou-Bénéteau, A.; Baret, P.; Payet, B.; Lefebvre D'hellencourt, C.; Gonthier, M.P. Evaluation of antioxidant properties of major dietary polyphenols and their protective effect on 3T3-L1 preadipocytes and red blood cells exposed to oxidative stress. *Free Radic. Res.* **2014**, *48*, 387–401. [CrossRef] [PubMed]
27. Blachnio-Zabielska, A.; Baranowski, M.; Zabielski, P.; Gorski, J. Effect of high fat diet enriched with unsaturated and diet rich in saturated fatty acids on sphingolipid metabolism in rat skeletal muscle. *J. Cell. Physiol.* **2010**, *225*, 786–791. [CrossRef] [PubMed]
28. Buettner, R.; Parhofer, K.G.; Woenckhaus, M.; Wrede, C.E.; Kunz-Schughart, L.A.; Schölmerich, J.; Bollheimer, L.C. Defining high-fat-diet rat models: Metabolic and molecular effects of different fat types. *J. Mol. Endocrinol.* **2006**, *36*, 485–501. [CrossRef] [PubMed]
29. Gerner, R.R.; Wieser, V.; Moschen, A.R.; Tilg, H. Metabolic inflammation: role of cytokines in the crosstalk between adipose tissue and liver. *Can. J. Physiol. Pharm.* **2013**, *91*, 867–872. [CrossRef]

30. Lira, F.S.; Rosa, J.C.; Dos Santos, R.V.; Venancio, D.P.; Carnier, J.; Sanches, P.D.L.; Do Nascimento, C.M.O.; De Piano, A.; Tock, L.; Tufik, S.; et al. Visceral fat decreased by long-term interdisciplinary lifestyle therapy correlated positively with interleukin-6 and tumor necrosis factor-α and negatively with adiponectin levels in obese adolescents. *Metab. Clin. Exp.* **2011**, *60*, 359–365. [CrossRef] [PubMed]
31. Fernández-Sánchez, A.; Madrigal-Santillán, E.; Bautista, M.; Esquivel-Soto, J.; Morales-González, Á.; Esquivel-Chirino, C.; Durante-Montiel, I.; Sánchez-Rivera, G.; Valadez-Vega, C.; Morales-González, J.A. Inflammation, oxidative stress, and obesity. *Int. J. Mol. Sci.* **2011**, *12*, 3117–3132. [CrossRef] [PubMed]
32. Jayarathne, S.; Koboziev, I.; Park, O.H.; Oldewage-Theron, W.; Shen, C.L.; Moustaid-Moussa, N. Anti-Inflammatory and Anti-Obesity Properties of Food Bioactive Components: Effects on Adipose Tissue. *Prev. Nutr. Food Sci.* **2017**, *22*, 251–262. [CrossRef]
33. Dornellas, A.P.S.; Watanabe, R.L.H.; Pimentel, G.D.; Boldarine, V.T.; Nascimento, C.M.O.; Oyama, L.M.; Ghebremeskel, K.; Wang, Y.; Bueno, A.A.; Ribeiro, E.B. Deleterious effects of lard-enriched diet on tissues fatty acids composition and hypothalamic insulin actions. *Prostaglandins Leukot. Essent. Fat. Acids* **2015**, *102–103*, 21–29. [CrossRef]
34. Karlsen, A.; Retterstøl, L.; Laake, P.; Paur, I.; Kjølsrud-Bøhn, S.; Sandvik, L.; Blomhoff, R. Anthocyanins Inhibit Nuclear Factor-κB Activation in Monocytes and Reduce Plasma Concentrations of Pro-Inflammatory Mediators in Healthy Adults. *J. Nutr.* **2007**, *137*, 1951–1954. [CrossRef]
35. Graf, D.; Seifert, S.; Jaudszus, A.; Bub, A.; Watzl, B. Anthocyanin-Rich Juice Lowers Serum Cholesterol, Leptin, and Resistin and Improves Plasma Fatty Acid Composition in Fischer Rats. *PLOS ONE* **2013**, *8*, 1–5. [CrossRef] [PubMed]
36. Center for Drug Evaluation and Research Guidance for Industry: Estimating the Maximum Safe Starting Dose in Initial Clinical Trials for Therapeutics in Adult Healthy Volunteers. *Us Dep. Health Hum. Serv.* **2005**, 1–27. [CrossRef]
37. Da Silva, V.H.P.; de Moura, C.F.G.; Ribeiro, F.A.P.; Cesar, A.; Pereira, C.D.S.; Silva, M.J.D.; Vilegas, W.; Ribeiro, D.A. Genotoxicity and cytotoxicity induced by municipal effluent in multiple organs of Wistar rats. *Environ. Sci. Pollut. Res.* **2014**, *21*, 13069–13080. [CrossRef] [PubMed]
38. Folch, J.; Lees, M.; Sloane, G.H. A simple method for the isolation and purification of total lipides from animal tissues. *J. Biol. Chem.* **1953**, *226*, 497–509. [CrossRef]

Sample Availability: Not available.

© 2019 by the authors. Licensee MDPI, Basel, Switzerland. This article is an open access article distributed under the terms and conditions of the Creative Commons Attribution (CC BY) license (http://creativecommons.org/licenses/by/4.0/).

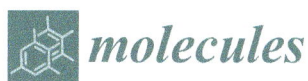

Article

Antineuroinflammatory Activities and Neurotoxicological Assessment of Curcumin Loaded Solid Lipid Nanoparticles on LPS-Stimulated BV-2 Microglia Cell Models

Palanivel Ganesan [1,2,†], Byungwook Kim [2,3,†], Prakash Ramalaingam [4,5,†], Govindarajan Karthivashan [2], Vishnu Revuri [6], Shinyoung Park [2], Joon Soo Kim [2], Young Tag Ko [5,*] and Dong-Kug Choi [1,2,*]

1. Department of Integrated Bioscience-Biomedical Chemistry, College of Biomedical and Health Science, Konkuk University, Chungju 27478, Korea; palanivel67@gmail.com
2. Nanotechnology Research Center and Department of Integrated Bioscience-Biotechnology, Konkuk University, Chungju 27478, Korea; kbwxfile@gmail.com (B.K.); karthivashan@gmail.com (G.K.); ifresha@nate.com (S.P.); kgfdkr@gmail.com (J.S.K.)
3. Department of Medical & Molecular Genetics, Stark Neurosciences Research Institute, Indiana University School of Medicine, Indianapolis, IN 46202, USA
4. Department of Pharmaceutical Sciences, Philadelphia College of Pharmacy, University of the Sciences, Philadelphia, PA 19104, USA; ramprabaprakash@gmail.com
5. College of Pharmacy, Gachon University, Incheon 406-799, Korea
6. Department of Green Bio engineering Korea National University of Transportation, Daehakro 750, Chungju 27469, Korea; vishnurevuri91@gmail.com
* Correspondence: youngtakko@gachon.ac.kr (Y.T.K.); choidk@kku.ac.kr (D.-K.C.); Tel.: +82-43-840-3610 (D.-K.C.); Fax: +82-43-840-3872 (D.-K.C.)
† Equally contributed authors.

Academic Editors: Francesco Maione and Thomas J. Schmidt
Received: 12 December 2018; Accepted: 19 March 2019; Published: 25 March 2019

Abstract: Curcumin, which is a potential antineuroinflammatory and neuroprotective compound, exhibits poor bioavailability in brain cells due to its difficulty in crossing the blood–brain barrier and its rapid metabolism during circulation, which decreases its efficacy in treating chronic neuroinflammatory diseases in the central nervous system. The bioavailability and potential of curcumin can be improved by using a nanodelivery system, which includes solid lipid nanoparticles. Curcumin-loaded solid lipid nanoparticles (SLCN) were efficiently developed to have a particle size of about 86 nm and do not exhibit any toxicity in the endothelial brain cells. Furthermore, the curcumin-loaded solid lipid nanoparticles (SLCN) were studied to assess their efficacy in BV-2 microglial cells against LPS-induced neuroinflammation. The SLCN showed a higher inhibition of nitric oxide (NO) production compared to conventional curcumin in a dose-dependent manner. Similarly, the mRNA and proinflammatory cytokine levels were also reduced in a dose-dependent manner when compared to those with free curcumin. Thus, SLCN could be a potential delivery system for curcumin to treat microglia-mediated neuroinflammation.

Keywords: lipopolysaccharide; solid lipid nanoparticle; curcumin; antineuroinflammation; toxicity; SEM

---

1. Introduction

Neurodegenerative diseases, such as Parkinson's disease (PD) or Alzheimer's disease, are age-related chronic illnesses that are characterized by the loss of neurons and activation of microglia in brain cells [1,2]. Numerous studies have confirmed that neuroinflammation is a major factor of the degeneration in nigral neurons that are important characteristics of neurodegenerative diseases [3]. Neuroinflammation leads to the activation of microglia and results in a higher production of inflammatory markers, including nitric oxide, TNF-α, IL-1β, and IL-6 [4–7]. The suppression of inflammatory markers using natural phytoextracts is in great demand for delaying neuroinflammation and its related diseases.

Phytoextracts have been used for generations as traditional treatments for neurodegenerative diseases [8–11]. Curcumin is a major bioactive compound that is found in turmeric powder and it is used in traditional Indian and Chinese medicine due to its various health enhancing effects to treat the inflammation associated with chronic diseases [12–16]. Furthermore, several in vitro and in vivo mechanisms have determined for the antineuroinflammatory pathway of curcumin. Its efficacy is still limited due to its low solubility, higher degradation by enzymes, lower absorption, and faster elimination [17–21]. To improve the properties and biological activity, novel lipid-based delivery vehicles are in greater demand [22], such as solid lipid nanoparticles (SLN).

SLN delivery systems are highly efficient delivery systems for phytocompounds with less absorption and poorly bioavailability, such as curcumin, resveratrol etc. [23,24], due to their size and higher stability. Recently, some researchers studied the curcumin-loaded SLN and observed an enhancement in antitumor activity in vitro [25]. Furthermore, there was enhanced delivery of curcumin-loaded SLN to cells without altering the integrity of the cellular junction [26]. SLN is in greater demand compared to other nanodelivery systems due to its lower toxicity, ability to hold larger lipophilic compounds, and higher bioavailability and solubility [27–29]. SLNs were also reported to adhere to the endothelial cells of the blood–brain barrier (BBB) due to the surface adsorption of blood proteins, such as apolipoproteins and can effectively shuttle drugs across BBB. This was proved in a previous study, in which SLN was found to effectively shuttle the hydrophilic trypanocidal drug diminazene across the BBB. Our previous research confirmed that the curcumin-loaded SLN increased the bioavailability of curcumin in various organs, including the brain [30]. We further controlled the release of orally administered curcumin by developing a modified chitosan coated SLN that enhanced the bioavailability of curcumin [31–34]. To our knowledge, only a few studies have reported on the antineuroinflammatory role of curcumin-loaded SLN against lipopolysaccharide (LPS)-induced neuroinflammation in vitro and the molecular mechanism of its targeted pathways. Curcumin-loaded SLN is an important means to deliver curcumin to microglial cells in a highly bioactive way. Thus, the present study focused on the antineuroinflammatory mechanism of curcumin-loaded SLN (SLCN) and its possible pathway in LPS-induced microglial cells.

2. Results

2.1. Physical Properties of SLN and SLCN

The particle size of SLN and SLCN, PDI and zeta potential are shown in Table 1. The particle size of the SLCN was slightly higher compared to that of SLN, which means that the addition of curcumin slightly increased the particle size of the SLCN. However, the particle size was found to be lower than 100 nm and this could facilitate a higher bioavailability of curcumin to the cells. The EE and LC of SLCN were 98.8% and 3%, respectively. A very high lipophilic behaviour of curcumin (log P (Octanol/water partition coefficient) = 3.29) resulted in the higher intake of curcumin in the SLN solid lipid core, which is made up of only lipids. There were no traces of curcumin after centrifugation for EE and LC determination, with 98.8% of curcumin recovered from the SLN. The higher encapsulation might be due to the ability of SLN to strongly accommodate the lipophilic curcumin. We were able to confirm that curcumin has higher encapsulation efficiency in the SLN.

Table 1. Physical properties of solid lipid nanoparticles (SLN) and curcumin-loaded solid lipid nanoparticles (SLCN).

Formulations	Particle size (nm)	PDI	Zeta Potential (mV)	EE (%)	LC (%)
SLN	83.16 ± 1.24	0.27 ± 0.02	−24.29 ± 1.66	-	-
SLCN	86.60 ± 9.85	0.29 ± 0.02	−22.15 ± 1.32	98.8 ± 1.00	3.01

SLN: solid lipid nanoparticle; SLN: Curcumin loaded solid lipid nanoparticle; PDI: poly dispersity index; EE: Encapsulation efficiency; and LC: Loading capacity.

2.2. Scanning Electron Microscopy (SEM) of SLCN

Furthermore, we confirmed the particle size of the dispersed SLCN in SEM and found that the SLCN has a uniform particle size of less than 100 nm with a spherical shape (Figure 1).

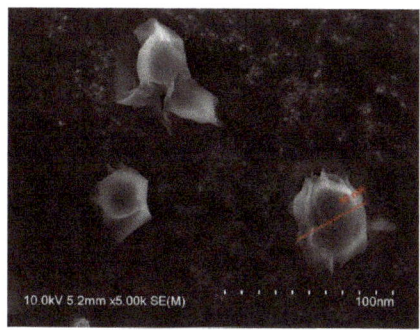

Figure 1. SEM micrograph of SLCN.

2.3. Cellular Toxicity Studies

The cell viability of the SLN and SCLN was compared between that in bEnd3 cells or NiH/3T3 cells, which is shown in Figure 2. The increase of about 100 μg/mL in the concentration of SLCN in brain endothelial cells showed no cellular toxicity while the increase of about 500 μg/mL in the NIH/3T3 cells showed no cellular toxicity for both SLN and SLCN.

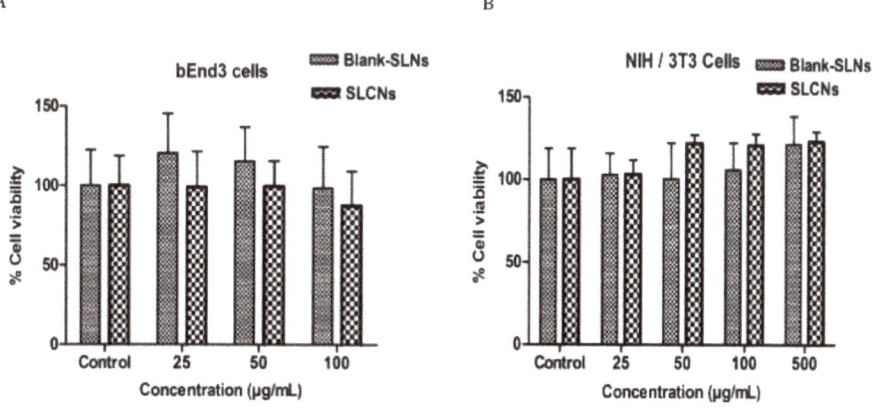

Figure 2. Cell viability of SLN and SLCN in bEnd3 cells (**a**) or NIH/3T3 cells (**b**).

2.4. Effect of SLCN on NO Production in LPS-Stimulated BV2 Cells

Most of the naturally-derived candidates were reported to be safe with negligible/null toxicity. Considering the potential of toxicity involved during formulation process in this study, we evaluated the cytotoxic effects of SLCN, base curcumin and/or LPS in BV2 cells. The cells were pretreated with SLCN (18 and 36 μg/mL) and base curcumin (36 μg/mL) for 1 h before the addition of LPS (100 ng/mL). The incubation with LPS alone markedly increased the NO production in the BV2 cells compared to the control (17.86 ± 0.98 μM; Figure 3A; ###$p < 0.001$ vs. untreated group). However, the pretreatment with SLCN and base curcumin prevented this increase in the levels of NO production in LPS-stimulated BV2 cells (Figure 3A; **$p < 0.01$ and ***$p < 0.001$ vs. LPS-treated group). Moreover, SLCN resulted in a significantly greater inhibition of NO compared to base curcumin for the same concentration (Figure 3A; \$\$$p < 0.01$ vs. SLCN-treated group). The cell viability was determined using an MTT assay. According to the results of our study, both drugs and LPS treated cells exhibited minimal/null toxic effects at the selected concentrations (Figure 3B).

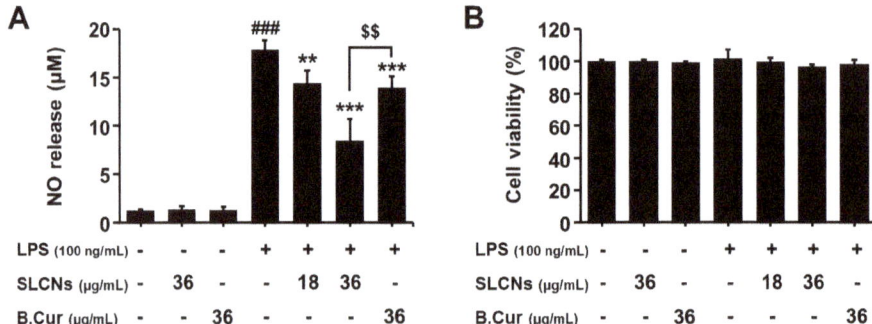

Figure 3. Effect of SLCN and base curcumin on NO production and cell viability in lipopolysaccharide LPS-stimulated BV2 cells. BV2 cells were pretreated with the indicated concentrations (18 and 36 μg/mL) of SLCN and base curcumin (B.Cur) for 1 h before incubation with LPS (100 ng/mL) for 24 h. Nitrite was measured using the Griess reaction (**A**). The cell viability was evaluated using the MTT assay (**B**). Results are displayed as a percentage of untreated groups. ###$p < 0.001$, vs. untreated group; **$p < 0.01$ and ***$p < 0.001$ vs. LPS-treated group; \$\$$p < 0.01$ vs. SLCN-treated group (one-way ANOVA; n = 4).

2.5. SLCN Attenuated iNOS and COX-2 mRNA Expressions in LPS-Stimulated BV2 Cells

BV2 cells were induced with LPS (100 ng/mL) in the presence or absence of SLCN and base curcumin at various concentrations (18 and 36 μg/mL, 36 μg/mL, respectively). LPS treatment significantly increased the iNOS and COX-2 mRNA levels (###$p < 0.001$ vs. untreated group) but pretreatment with SLCN and base curcumin at the indicated concentrations inhibited this LPS-induced mRNA expression of iNOS and COX-2 (Figure 4; **$p < 0.01$ and ***$p < 0.001$ vs. LPS-treated group). Furthermore, SLCN improved the COX-2 mRNA level compared to the base curcumin at the same concentration (Figure 4; \$$p < 0.05$ vs. SLCN-treated group). As discussed earlier, this can be attributed to the enhanced drug delivery potential of SLN. Thereby, as reported in earlier studies, the relatively enhanced bioavailability of curcumin released from SLCN is likely responsible for its higher suppression of iNOS and COX-2 mRNA expressions compared to its free form.

2.6. SLCN Inhibited the Production of Proinflammatory Cytokines in LPS-Induced BV2 Cells

RT-PCR results demonstrated elevated mRNA levels of these cytokines at 6 h after LPS treatment (###$p < 0.001$ vs. untreated group). Pretreatment with SLCN significantly inhibited the LPS-induced production of IL-1β, IL-6 and TNF-α (Figure 5; **$p<0.01$ and ***$p<0.001$ vs. LPS group). Furthermore,

SLCN resulted in a greater reduction in the IL-6 and TNF-α mRNA levels compared to the base curcumin at the same concentration (Figure 5; $^\$p < 0.05$ and $^{\$\$}p < 0.01$ vs. SLCN-treated group). Thus, our results indicate that SLCN inhibited the expression of proinflammatory mediators and associated cytokines involved in the inflammatory process.

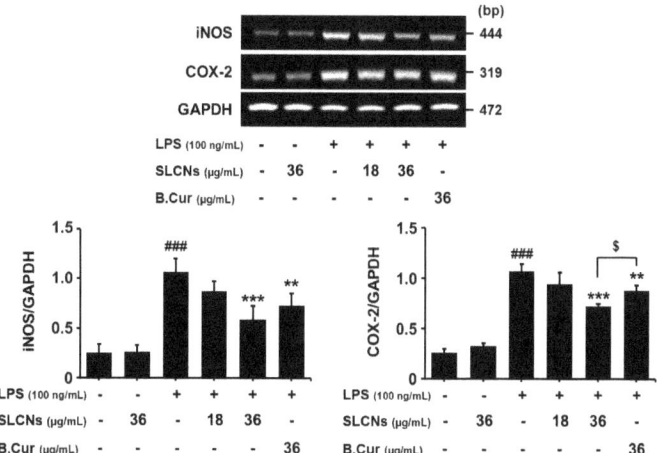

Figure 4. SLCN attenuates iNOS and COX-2 mRNA levels in LPS-stimulated BV2 cells. BV2 cells were pretreated with the indicated concentrations of SLCN and base curcumin for 1 h before being incubated with LPS (100 ng/mL) for 6 h (RT-PCR). Total RNA was prepared and analysed for iNOS and COX-2 gene expression by RT-PCR. Quantification data are shown in the lower panel. ###$p < 0.001$ vs. untreated group; **$p < 0.01$ and ***i < 0.001 vs. LPS-treated group; $$p < 0.05$ vs. SLCN-treated group (one-way ANOVA; n = 3).

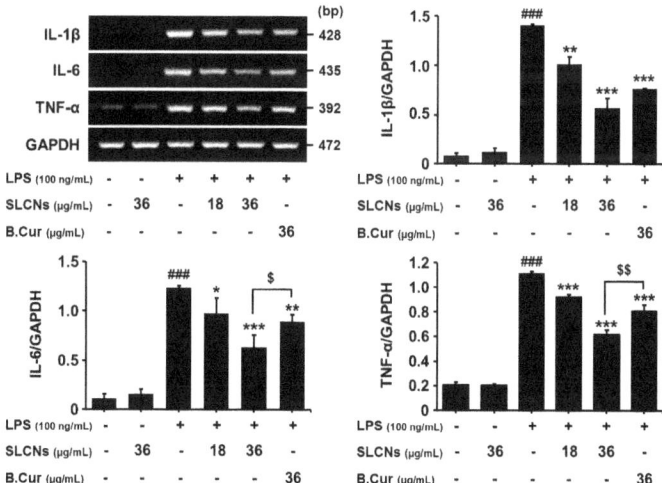

Figure 5. SLCN decreases the production of proinflammatory cytokines. Cells were pretreated with the indicated doses of SLCN and base curcumin for 1 h before LPS (100 ng/mL) treatment. The mRNA levels of TNF-α, IL-1β, IL-6 and GAPDH were determined via RT-PCR. There was a representative densitometry analysis of TNF-α, IL-1β and IL-6 compared with GAPDH mRNA, respectively. ###$E < 0.001$ vs. untreated group; *$p < 0.05$, **$p < 0.01$ and ***$p < 0.001$ vs. LPS-treated group; $p < 0.05$ and $$$p < 0.01$ vs. SLCN-treated group (one-way ANOVA; n = 3).

3. Discussion

The research aim of this study was to enhance the delivery of curcumin to the brain cells and to study the possible antineuroinflammatory molecular mechanisms and neurotoxicological effects of the curcumin loaded in SLN. SLCN created with different lipids had higher particle sizes [30], which confirmed that the lipids in SLN play a significant role in determining the particle size of the SLCN. The incorporation of curcumin also causes a slight increase in the PDI and the zeta potential of the SLCN, with similar results observed in other studies [19,30]. The higher encapsulation might be due to the ability of SLN to strongly accommodate the lipophilic curcumin. The results were consistent with our previous studies [32]. Furthermore, the toxicity evaluation showed that a higher concentration of curcumin loaded in SLN resulted in lower toxicity towards the brain endothelial cells. Similar results were also shown in other studies with a higher concentration of SLCN, which showed no cellular toxicity [34].

Furthermore, we studied the antineuroinflammatory mechanism of curcumin-loaded SLN in LPS-induced BV2 microglial cells. The macrophage-like microglia are the resident innate immune cells of central nervous system, which form the first-line defense to the CNS from the invading candidates via several inflammatory signaling pathways [35]. The activation of microglial cells, either acute or chronic, release several proinflammatory signals and cytotoxic factors, such as nitric oxide, cytokines and ROS, to efficiently eradicate the invaded neuronal cells and safeguard the spread of disease conditions. Despite this, the glial cells were also reported to facilitate neuroprotective properties to regulate and resolve the inflammatory conditions by promoting several anti-inflammatory mediators and cytoactive growth factors to repair the cells. Thus, it plays a dual role in both the destruction and protection of neuronal cells. The homeostasis of the neuroinflammation is balanced by a feedback loop, which limits the collateral damage inflicted by the inflammatory response. However, the imbalance of this inflammatory homeostasis leads to an overproduction of NO, which subsequently cascades several neuroinflammatory disorders. This is consistent with previous studies where the nanolipid drug formulations exhibit better NO inhibitory activity in LPS-stimulated macrophages compared to its free form. This is likely due to the enhanced drug delivery potential. Although most of the naturally-derived candidates were reported to be safe with negligible/null toxicity, considering the potential toxicity involved during the formulation process in this study, we evaluated the cytotoxic effects of SLCN, base curcumin and/or LPS in BV2 cells. The cell viability was determined using an MTT assay. According to the results of our study, both drugs and LPS treated cells exhibited minimal/null toxic effects at the selected concentrations.

At the inflammation site, the activated microglial cells were reported to elevate the proinflammatory mediators that are commonly generated by the inducible isoforms of NO synthase (iNOS) and cyclooxygenase-2 (COX-2) enzymes. Several scientific evidences reported that the inducible forms of iNOS and COX-2 facilitates the inflammatory conditions by the production of surplus NO and prostaglandins (PG), respectively, which are highly cytotoxic. Interestingly, the induction of both iNOS and COX 2 were bound to the transcriptional regulation. In our study, the relatively enhanced bioavailability of curcumin released from SLCN is likely responsible for its higher suppression of iNOS and COX-2 mRNA expression compared to its free from. The activated microglial cell releases proinflammatory mediators (iNOS and COX 2) and further facilitates the transcriptional cascades to elevate the supply of downstream proinflammatory cytokines, such as IL-1β, IL-6 and TNF-α [36]. These released proinflammatory cytokines were reported to synergistically exacerbate the inflammatory milieu together with NO and PGs by activating the neighboring glial cells and astrocytes. Thus, they play pivotal roles in microglia-mediated inflammation. It was previously reported that LPS induction substantially elevates the upsurge of proinflammatory cytokines (IL-1β, IL-6 and TNF-α) via the MAPK signaling pathway in BV-2 glial cells. Relatively, the candidates that suppress the expression of these proinflammatory cytokines were reported to show substantial neuroprotective effects against several inflammatory induced neurodegenerative disorders [37]. This is consistent with previous study findings where the active drug candidates loaded into nanoparticles resulted in substantial suppression of proinflammatory cytokines and exhibited relatively higher antineuroinflammatory effects than their free forms. Another recent study showed that curcumin exerts an antiinflammatory effect by downregulating the PI3k/Akt signaling pathway and NF-κB (nuclear factor kappa-light-chain-enhancer of activated B cells) protein levels [38]. This could possibly be attributed to the downregulation of mRNA expression of proinflammatory cytokines by SLCN in our current study. It is also noteworthy that a previous study report states that SLN itself does not impact the viability and inflammatory effects of macrophages [39]. Thus, our results indicate that curcumin-loaded SLCN inhibited the expression of proinflammatory mediators and associated cytokines involved in the inflammatory process. The possible antiinflammatory mechanism of the SLCN in LPS that stimulated BV-2 microglial cells is depicted in Figure 6.

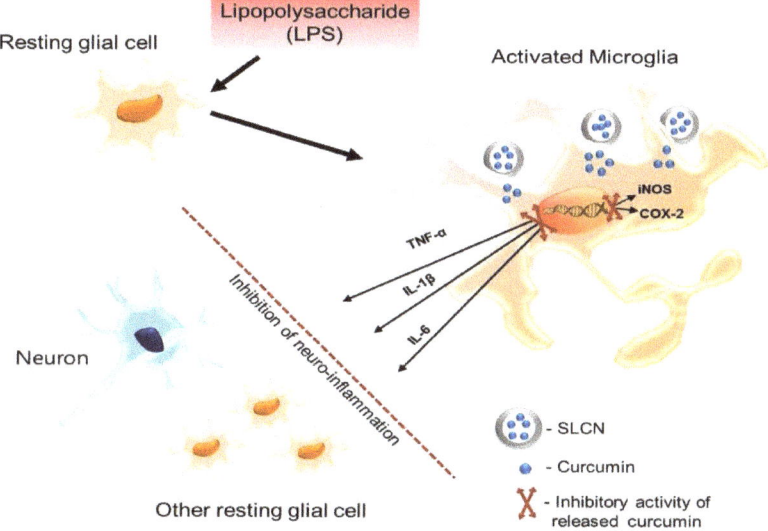

Figure 6. Postulated SLCN antineuroinflammatory mechanism of action in LPS-stimulated BV2 cells.

4. Materials and Methods

4.1. Materials

Curcumin (*C. longa. Linn*) was obtained from TCI Co., Ltd. (Tokyo, Japan), Lipopolysaccharide (LPS, E. coli 0111:B4), dimethyl sulfoxide (DMSO), sulfanilamide, N-(1-naphthyl)-ethylenediamine dihydrochloride 3-(4,5-dimethylthiazol-2-yl)-2,5-diphenyltetrazolium bromide (MTT) and Tween-20 were purchased from Sigma–Aldrich (St. Louis, MO, USA). Foetal bovine serum (FBS), Dulbecco's Modified Eagle Medium (DMEM), penicillin-streptomycin (P-S), trypsin/EDTA (TE), TRIzol and other cell culture plates were obtained from Gibco-BRL (Rockville, MD, USA).

4.2. Solid Lipid Curcumin Nanoparticle Formulation and Optimization

The formulation of curcumin-loaded SLCN was prepared using high shear homogenization and ultrasonication techniques, with the different lipid formulations of SLCN used as shown in Table 1. This was conducted according to the modified method of Ramalingam and Ko Briefly, different ratios of precirol, palmitic acid and gelucire were heated to 85 °C to complete solubilize the lipid. After the lipid was completely melted, curcumin was added to the lipid phase. The aqueous phase containing Tween 80 was added to the lipid phase and homogenized using Ultra- Turrax homogenizer (IKA-Werke, Staufen, Germany) at around 11,000 rpm for 5 min. The curcumin or free preemulsion was further ultrasonicated for 5 min using a probe sonicator (Vibracell VCX130; Sonics, Newtown, CT, USA). The obtained SLCN was cooled for 30 min and lyophilized before being stored at 4 °C for further experiments.

4.3. Particle Size, Zeta Potential and Polydispersity Index

The particle size, zeta potential and polydispersity index (PDI) of SLN and SLCN was measured using an ELSZ-1000 zeta potential and particle size analyser (Photal OTSUKA Electronics, Tokyo, Japan). The SLCN efficiency of EE and LC was measured according to the modified method as described by Ramalingam and Ko [30]. For SEM, 10 µL of the 0.1 mg/mL SLN sample was added to the silica grid, dried, sputter coated with platinum and further used for HR-SEM analysis (High Resolution Field Emission Scanning Electron Microscope JSM-7610F, JEOL Ltd., Akishima, Tokyo, Japan).

4.4. Cell Toxicity Studies

Cellular toxicity studies of SLCN and SLN were carried out and compared using two different cells, such as NIH/3T3 and brain endothelial cells, using an MTT assay.

4.5. Cell Culture, NO Release Assay and Cell Viability

BV2 cells were cultured in DMEM supplemented with 5% FBS and 100 U/mL P-S before being maintained in a humidified incubator in an 5% CO_2 atmosphere. In all experiments, cells were seeded at a density of 5×10^5 cells/mL and were pretreated for 1 h with the indicated concentrations of curcumin-loaded solid lipid nanoparticles (SLCN) and base curcumin before being incubated in a medium containing LPS (100 ng/mL). The LPS-induced release of NO in the culture medium was determined and the cell viability of the cultured cells was measured. Briefly, the seeded cells were treated with different concentrations of SLCN (18 and 36 µg/mL) and 36 µg/mL of base curcumin, which was followed by incubation with LPS for 24 h. After incubation with LPS for 24 h, 50 µL of each culture medium was mixed with 50 µL of Griess reagent. Nitrite levels were determined using a microplate reader at 540 nm (Tecan Trading AG, Switzerland) and nitrite concentrations were calculated by reference to a standard curve generated by the known concentrations of sodium nitrite. The cell viability was measured by adding 0.5 mg/mL of MTT to each well. After incubation for another 4 h at 37 °C and 5% CO2, the medium was removed from each well and the formazan crystals that formed were dissolved in DMSO. The absorbance was determined at 540 nm using a microplate reader (Tecan Trading AG).

4.6. Reverse Transcription-Polymerase Chain Reaction (RT-PCR) Viability

BV2 microglia cells were plated overnight in 6-well culture plates and were pretreated for 1 h with the indicated concentrations of SLCN (18 and 36 µg/mL) and base curcumin (36 µg/mL) before incubation in a medium containing LPS (100 ng/mL). The total RNA was extracted using TRIZOL (Invitrogen). RNA (1 µg) was reverse-transcribed using ReverTra Ace-α kit (Toyobo, Osaka, Japan) according to the manufacturer's instructions. The inducible nitric oxide synthase, cyclooxygenase type 2 (COX-2), tumour necrosis factor-alpha (TNF-α), interleukin 1β (IL-1β), IL-6 and glyceraldehyde 3-phosphate dehydrogenase (GAPDH) genes were amplified from the cDNA via polymerase chain reaction (PCR). cDNA was amplified by PCR using the specific primers mentioned in Table 2. PCR was performed using an initial step of denaturation (5 min at 94 °C), 20–27 cycles of amplification (94 °C for 30 s, 54–58 °C for 1 min and 72 °C for 1 min) and an extension (72 °C for 5 min). PCR products were analysed on 1.5% agarose gels with EtBr stained. The mRNA of GAPDH served as an internal control for sample loading and mRNA integrity. The band intensity was quantified via a densitometry analysis using multi-gauge software V3.1 (Fujifilm, Tokyo, Japan).

Table 2. Primer sets used for RT-PCR.

Gene		Primer Sequence	Size (bp)	Accession
iNOS	Forward	5′-CTTGCAAGTCCAAGTCTTGC-3′	369	NM_010927
	Reverse	5′-GTATGTGTCTGCAGATGTGCTG-3′		
COX-2	Forward	5′-ACATCCCTGAGAACCTGCAGT-3′	414	NM_011198
	Reverse	5′-CCAGGAGGATGGAGTTGTTGT-3′		
IL-1β	Forward	5′-CATATGAGCTGAAAGCTCTCCA-3′	385	NM_008361
	Reverse	5′-GACACAGATTCCATGGTGAAGTC-3′		
IL-6	Forward	5′-GGAGGCTTAATTACACATGTT-3′	435	NM_031168
	Reverse	5′-TGATTTCAAAGATGAATTGGAT-3′		
TNF-α	Forward	5′-TTCGAGTGACAAGCCTGTAGC-3′	390	NM_013693
	Reverse	5′-AGATTGACCTCAGCGCTGAGT-3′		
GAPDH	Forward	5′-CCAGTATGACTCCACTCACG-3′	378	GU214026
	Reverse	5′-CCTTCCACAATGCCAAAGTT-3′		

4.7. Statistical Analysis

The values given are means ± S.E.M. of at least three separate experiments conducted in triplicate. The comparisons between groups were analyzed using a one-way analysis of variance (ANOVA) followed by Tukey's multiple comparison test using software GraphPad Prism V6.01 (GraphPad Software Inc., San Diego, CA, USA)

5. Conclusions

The antineuroinflammatory potential of curcumin-loaded solid lipid nanoparticles was studied in this work. SLCN effectively and dose-dependently reduced the NO release in LPS-induced BV-2 microglial cells, which potentially occurred via the regulation of proinflammatory cytokines and associated mediators. Interestingly, the curcumin released from SLN exhibited a relatively higher inflammation-suppressive activity compared to its free form, which can be likely attributed towards the sustained release and enhanced bioavailability of SLN. Thus, further studies on fabrication and functionalization of SLCN can effectively pave the way to develop novel drug candidates to treat inflammation-mediated neurodegenerative disorders.

Author Contributions: P.G., B.K. and P.R. designed the experiments. J.S.K., B.K., V.R. and G.K. performed and analysed the experiments. Y.T.K. read and approved the final manuscripts. D.K.C. supervised the overall work and directed experimental sections.

Funding: This study was supported by the Basic Science Research Program through the National Research Foundation of Korea (NRF), funded by the Ministry of Education, Science and Technology (NRF-2017R1C1B2010276 and 2017R1A2A2A07001035).

Conflicts of Interest: The authors declare no conflict of interest.

References

1. Chernoff, N.; Hill, D.J.; Diggs, D.L.; Faison, B.D.; Francis, B.M.; Lang, J.R.; Larue, M.M.; Le, T.T.; Loftin, K.A.; Lugo, J.N.; et al. A critical review of the postulated role of the non-essential amino acid, β-N-methylamino-L-alanine, in neurodegenerative disease in humans. *J. Toxicol. Environ. Health Part B Crit. Rev.* **2017**. [CrossRef]
2. Wood, H. Neurodegenerative disease: Halting neurodegeneration—Are repurposed drugs the answer? *Nat. Rev. Neurol.* **2017**, *13*, 317. [CrossRef]
3. Visalli, G.; Currò, M.; Iannazzo, D.; Pistone, A.; Pruiti Ciarello, M.; Acri, G.; Testagrossa, B.; Bertuccio, M.P.; Squeri, R.; Di Pietro, A. In vitro assessment of neurotoxicity and neuroinflammation of homemade MWCNTs. *Environ. Toxicol. Pharmacol.* **2017**. [CrossRef]
4. Cai, Q.; Li, Y.; Pei, G. Polysaccharides from Ganoderma lucidum attenuate microglia-mediated neuroinflammation and modulate microglial phagocytosis and behavioural response. *J. Neuroinflamm.* **2017**. [CrossRef]

5. Chen, R.; Zhao, L.D.; Liu, H.; Li, H.H.; Ren, C.; Zhang, P.; Guo, K.T.; Zhang, H.X.; Geng, D.Q.; Zhang, C.Y. Fluoride Induces Neuroinflammation and Alters Wnt Signaling Pathway in BV2 Microglial Cells. *Inflammation* **2017**. [CrossRef]
6. Regen, F.; Hellmann-Regen, J.; Costantini, E.; Reale, M. Neuroinflammation and Alzheimer's Disease: Implications for Microglial Activation. *Curr. Alzheimer Res.* **2017**. [CrossRef]
7. Gao, X.; Wu, B.; Fu, Z.; Zhang, Z.; Xu, G. Carvedilol abrogates hypoxia-induced oxidative stress and neuroinflammation in microglial BV2 cells. *Eur. J. Pharmacol.* **2017**. [CrossRef]
8. Bassani, T.B.; Turnes, J.M.; Moura, E.L.R.; Bonato, J.M.; Cóppola-Segovia, V.; Zanata, S.M.; Oliveira, R.M.M.W.; Vital, M.A.B.F. Effects of curcumin on short-term spatial and recognition memory, adult neurogenesis and neuroinflammation in a streptozotocin-induced rat model of dementia of Alzheimer's type. *Behav. Brain Res.* **2017**. [CrossRef]
9. Zaky, A.; Bassiouny, A.; Farghaly, M.; El-Sabaa, B.M. A Combination of Resveratrol and Curcumin is Effective Against Aluminum Chloride-Induced Neuroinflammation in Rats. *J. Alzheimer's Dis.* **2017**. [CrossRef]
10. Ullah, F.; Liang, A.; Rangel, A.; Gyengesi, E.; Niedermayer, G.; Münch, G. High bioavailability curcumin: An anti-inflammatory and neurosupportive bioactive nutrient for neurodegenerative diseases characterized by chronic neuroinflammation. *Arch. Toxicol.* **2017**, *91*, 1623–1634. [CrossRef]
11. Xiao, L.; Ding, M.; Fernandez, A.; Zhao, P.; Jin, L.; Li, X. Curcumin alleviates lumbar radiculopathy by reducing neuroinflammation, oxidative stress and nociceptive factors. *Eur. Cells Mater.* **2017**. [CrossRef]
12. Begum, A.N.; Jones, M.R.; Lim, G.P.; Morihara, T.; Kim, P.; Heath, D.D.; Rock, C.L.; Pruitt, M.A.; Yang, F.; Hudspeth, B.; et al. Curcumin Structure-Function, Bioavailability, and Efficacy in Models of Neuroinflammation and Alzheimer's Disease. *J. Pharmacol. Exp. Ther.* **2008**. [CrossRef]
13. Ray, B.; Lahiri, D.K. Neuroinflammation in Alzheimer's disease: Different molecular targets and potential therapeutic agents including curcumin. *Curr. Opin. Pharmacol.* **2009**, *9*, 434–444. [CrossRef]
14. Tiwari, V.; Chopra, K. Protective effect of curcumin against chronic alcohol-induced cognitive deficits and neuroinflammation in the adult rat brain. *Neuroscience* **2013**. [CrossRef]
15. Tegenge, M.A.; Rajbhandari, L.; Shrestha, S.; Mithal, A.; Hosmane, S.; Venkatesan, A. Curcumin protects axons from degeneration in the setting of local neuroinflammation. *Exp. Neurol.* **2014**. [CrossRef]
16. Liu, Z.-J.; Li, Z.-H.; Liu, L.; Tang, W.-X.; Wang, Y.; Dong, M.-R.; Xiao, C. Curcumin Attenuates Beta-Amyloid-Induced Neuroinflammation via Activation of Peroxisome Proliferator-Activated Receptor-Gamma Function in a Rat Model of Alzheimer's Disease. *Front. Pharmacol.* **2016**. [CrossRef]
17. Takahashi, M.; Uechi, S.; Takara, K.; Asikin, Y.; Wada, K. Evaluation of an oral carrier system in rats: Bioavailability and antioxidant properties of liposome-encapsulated curcumin. *J. Agric. Food Chem.* **2009**. [CrossRef]
18. Munjal, B.; Pawar, Y.B.; Patel, S.B.; Bansal, A.K. Comparative oral bioavailability advantage from curcumin formulations. *Drug Deliv. Transl. Res.* **2011**. [CrossRef]
19. Pawar, Y.B.; Munjal, B.; Arora, S.; Karwa, M.; Kohli, G.; Paliwal, J.K.; Bansal, A.K. Bioavailability of a lipidic formulation of curcumin in healthy human volunteers. *Pharmaceutics* **2012**. [CrossRef]
20. Vitaglione, P.; Barone Lumaga, R.; Ferracane, R.; Radetsky, I.; Mennella, I.; Schettino, R.; Koder, S.; Shimoni, E.; Fogliano, V. Curcumin bioavailability from enriched bread: The effect of microencapsulated ingredients. *J. Agric. Food Chem.* **2012**. [CrossRef]
21. Wan, S.; Sun, Y.; Qi, X.; Tan, F. Improved Bioavailability of Poorly Water-Soluble Drug Curcumin in Cellulose Acetate Solid Dispersion. *AAPS PharmSciTech* **2012**. [CrossRef]
22. Hua, S.; Wu, S.Y. The use of lipid-based nanocarriers for targeted pain therapies. *Front. Pharmacol.* **2013**, *4*, 143. [CrossRef]
23. Ganesan, P.; Ramalingam, P.; Karthivashan, G.; Ko, Y.T.; Choi, D.-K. Recent developments in solid lipid nanoparticle and surface-modified solid lipid nanoparticle delivery systems for oral delivery of phyto-bioactive compounds in various chronic diseases. *Int. J. Nanomed.* **2018**, *13*. [CrossRef] [PubMed]
24. Gothai, S.; Ganesan, P.; Park, S.-Y.; Fakurazi, S.; Choi, D.-K.; Arulselvan, P. Natural phyto-bioactive compounds for the treatment of type 2 diabetes: Inflammation as a target. *Nutrients* **2016**, *8*. [CrossRef]
25. Sun, J.; Bi, C.; Chan, H.M.; Sun, S.; Zhang, Q.; Zheng, Y. Curcumin-loaded solid lipid nanoparticles have prolonged in vitro antitumour activity, cellular uptake and improved in vivo bioavailability. *Colloids Surf. B Biointerfaces* **2013**. [CrossRef] [PubMed]

26. Guri, A.; Gülseren, I.; Corredig, M. Utilization of solid lipid nanoparticles for enhanced delivery of curcumin in cocultures of HT29-MTX and Caco-2 cells. *Food Funct.* **2013**. [CrossRef] [PubMed]
27. Clemente, N.; Ferrara, B.; Gigliotti, C.; Boggio, E.; Capucchio, M.; Biasibetti, E.; Schiffer, D.; Mellai, M.; Annovazzi, L.; Cangemi, L.; et al. Solid Lipid Nanoparticles Carrying Temozolomide for Melanoma Treatment. Preliminary In Vitro and In Vivo Studies. *Int. J. Mol. Sci.* **2018**. [CrossRef]
28. Paranjpe, M.; Müller-Goymann, C.C. Nanoparticle-mediated pulmonary drug delivery: A review. *Int. J. Mol. Sci.* **2014**, *15*, 5852–5873. [CrossRef]
29. Serini, S.; Cassano, R.; Corsetto, P.A.; Rizzo, A.M.; Calviello, G.; Trombino, S. Omega-3 PUFA loaded in resveratrol-based solid lipid nanoparticles: Physicochemical properties and antineoplastic activities in human colorectal cancer cells in vitro. *Int. J. Mol. Sci.* **2018**. [CrossRef]
30. Ramalingam, P.; Ko, Y.T. Enhanced oral delivery of curcumin from N-trimethyl chitosan surface-modified solid lipid nanoparticles: Pharmacokinetic and brain distribution evaluations. *Pharm. Res.* **2015**. [CrossRef] [PubMed]
31. Ramalingam, P.; Ko, Y.T. Improved oral delivery of resveratrol from N-trimethyl chitosan-g-palmitic acid surface-modified solid lipid nanoparticles. *Colloids Surf. B Biointerfaces* **2016**. [CrossRef]
32. Ramalingam, P.; Yoo, S.W.; Ko, Y.T. Nanodelivery systems based on mucoadhesive polymer coated solid lipid nanoparticles to improve the oral intake of food curcumin. *Food Res. Int.* **2016**. [CrossRef]
33. Ramalingam, P.; Ko, Y.T. A validated LC-MS/MS method for quantitative analysis of curcumin in mouse plasma and brain tissue and its application in pharmacokinetic and brain distribution studies. *J. Chromatogr. B Anal. Technol. Biomed. Life Sci.* **2014**. [CrossRef] [PubMed]
34. Ramalingam, P.; Ko, Y.T. Validated LC-MS/MS method for simultaneous quantification of resveratrol levels in mouse plasma and brain and its application to pharmacokinetic and brain distribution studies. *J. Pharm. Biomed. Anal.* **2016**. [CrossRef] [PubMed]
35. Bessis, A.; Béchade, C.; Bernard, D.; Roumier, A. Microglial control of neuronal death and synaptic properties. *Glia* **2007**, *55*, 233–238. [CrossRef]
36. Sorrenti, V.; Contarini, G.; Sut, S.; Dall'Acqua, S.; Confortin, F.; Pagetta, A.; Giusti, P.; Zusso, M. Curcumin prevents acute neuroinflammation and long-term memory impairment induced by systemic lipopolysaccharide in mice. *Front. Pharmacol.* **2018**. [CrossRef] [PubMed]
37. Solaro, R.; Chiellini, F.; Battisti, A. Targeted delivery of protein drugs by nanocarriers. *Materials* **2010**, *3*, 1928–1980. [CrossRef]
38. Cianciulli, A.; Calvello, R.; Porro, C.; Trotta, T.; Salvatore, R.; Panaro, M.A. PI3k/Akt signalling pathway plays a crucial role in the anti-inflammatory effects of curcumin in LPS-activated microglia. *Int. Immunopharmacol.* **2016**. [CrossRef] [PubMed]
39. Schöler, N.; Hahn, H.; Müller, R.H.; Liesenfeld, O. Effect of lipid matrix and size of solid lipid nanoparticles (SLN) on the viability and cytokine production of macrophages. *Int. J. Pharm.* **2002**. [CrossRef]

Sample Availability: Samples of the compounds (SLCN) are available from the authors.

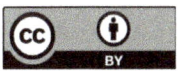

© 2019 by the authors. Licensee MDPI, Basel, Switzerland. This article is an open access article distributed under the terms and conditions of the Creative Commons Attribution (CC BY) license (http://creativecommons.org/licenses/by/4.0/).

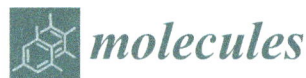

Article

Theaflavins Improve Memory Impairment and Depression-Like Behavior by Regulating Microglial Activation

Yasuhisa Ano *, Rena Ohya, Masahiro Kita, Yoshimasa Taniguchi and Keiji Kondo

Research Laboratories for Health Science & Food Technologies, Kirin Company Ltd., Kanazawa-ku, Yokohama-shi, Kanagawa 236-0004, Japan; Rena_Ohya@kirin.co.jp (R.O.); Masahiro_Kita@kirin.co.jp (M.K.); Yoshimasa_Taniguchi@kirin.co.jp (Y.T.); kondok@kirin.co.jp (K.K.)
* Correspondence: Yasuhisa_Ano@kirin.co.jp; Tel.: +81-45-330-9007

Received: 8 January 2019; Accepted: 27 January 2019; Published: 28 January 2019

Abstract: Inflammation in the brain is associated with various disorders including Alzheimer's disease and depression. Thus, inflammation has received increasing attention regarding preventive approaches to such disorders. Epidemiological investigations have reported that drinking tea reduces the risk of dementia and depression. Theaflavins, a polyphenol found in black tea, are known to have anti-oxidative and anti-inflammation effects, but the effects of theaflavins on cognitive decline and depression induced by inflammation have not been investigated. To address this research gap, the present study assessed whether theaflavins could protect synapses and dendrites damaged by inflammation and prevent concomitant memory impairment and depression-like behavior in mice. Intracerebroventricular injection with lipopolysaccharide (LPS) induces neural inflammation associated with reduced spontaneous alternations in the Y-maze test and increased immobility in the tail suspension test, indicating impaired spatial memory and depression-like behavior, respectively. Oral administration with theaflavins prevented these behavioral changes induced by LPS. Theaflavins also suppressed productions of inflammatory cytokines and prevented dendritic atrophy and spine loss in the brain. Notably, theaflavins have a stronger anti-inflammatory effect than other polyphenols such as catechin, chlorogenic acid, and caffeic acid. These results suggest that theaflavins can suppress neural inflammation and prevent the symptoms of inflammation-related brain disorders.

Keywords: black tea polyphenol; depression; inflammation; memory; microglia; neuroprotection; theaflavins

---

1. Introduction

Inflammation in the brain is associated with various brain disorders and may accelerate their pathologies [1–4]. Recent studies have revealed the involvement of microglia, which regulate immune response and inflammation in the brain [5], in brain disorders. Microglia play a key role in maintaining the neuroenvironment by removing pathogens, waste products, and old synapses via phagocytosis and by promoting synapse extension [6]. These functions of microglia decline due to various factors including aging and stress [7,8]. In the brains of patients with Alzheimer's disease and depression, microglia are excessively activated and produce reactive oxygen species and inflammatory cytokines that can damage neurons, leading to cognitive decline [9] and psychiatric syndromes [10]. Regulation of neuroinflammation and microglia are, thus, of increasing interest for prevention and as therapeutic targets [11,12].

Epidemiological studies have reported that the consumption of tea has preventive effects on psychiatric disorders, including depression [13] and cognitive decline leading to dementia [14,15]. An epidemiological survey in Finland reported that people who consume black tea score lower on the Beck Depression Inventory and have lower rates of depression [16], whereas another epidemiological study reported that tea reduces the risk of anxiety and depressive mood [17]. Higher tea consumption is also associated with a significant reduction in the risk of cognitive disorders [14,15]. Moreover, a French cohort showed that the intake of a combination of polyphenols from specific plant products—including tea and red wine—was associated with lower dementia risk [14].

In the case of green tea, polyphenols such as epicatechin, epigallocatechin, and epigallocatechin-3-gallate (EGCG) may be beneficial compounds. Recent reports have shown that green tea polyphenol improves cognitive decline and depression in preclinical studies [18,19]. In an experiment using obese mice model, EGCG improved high-fat- and high-fructose-induced cognitive impairment via regulation of the ERK/CREB/BDNF pathway [20]. An experiment using lipopolysaccharide (LPS)-induced memory-impaired mice showed that EGCG prevented the production of pro-inflammatory cytokines and memory impairment [21]. Black tea is the most widely consumed tea worldwide and is rich in polyphenol compounds, especially theaflavins. Theaflavins are antioxidant polyphenols with a reddish color formed by the condensation of flavan-3-ols in tea leaves during the fermentation of black tea [22,23]. Theaflavins are composed of theaflavin (TF1), theaflavin-3-monogallate (TF2a), theaflavin-3'-monogallate (TF2b), and theaflavin-3,3'-digallate (TF3). Theaflavins are reported to have anti-hyperglycemia [24], anti-inflammation [25], anti-viral [26,27], and anti-inflammatory activities [25]. On the other hand, the effects of theaflavins administered orally on cognitive decline and depression-like behavior induced by inflammation have not been investigated. To address this research gap, the present study assessed whether theaflavins administered orally could protect synapses and dendrites damaged induced by inflammation and prevent concomitant memory impairment and depression-like behavior in mice. In addition, the effects of theaflavins on primary microglia and neuronal cells were evaluated.

2. Results

2.1. Effects of Theaflavins on Memory Impairment and Depression Induced by Inflammation

To evaluate the effects of theaflavins on memory impairment induced by inflammation, mice received an injection with LPS to the lateral ventricle of the brain and were subjected to the Y-maze test. LPS treatment significantly reduced spontaneous alternations in the Y-maze, indicating impairment in spatial working memory compared with phosphate buffered saline (PBS) treatment indicated as LPS(-) (Figure 1a). LPS did not change arm entries (data not shown). Administration theaflavins once daily for 3 days significantly attenuated the LPS-induced reduction in spontaneous alternations compared with the control treatment (Figure 1a). Next, to evaluate the effects of theaflavins on depression-like behavior, mice with LPS injection to the lateral ventricle of the brain were subjected to the tail suspension test (TST). LPS significantly increased the immobility time during suspension, indicating that LPS induced a depression-like behavior (Figure 1b). Theaflavins administration significantly reduced the immobility time compared with the control treatment (Figure 1b). These results indicate that theaflavins improved memory impairment and depression-like behavior induced by LPS. On the other hand, theaflavins did not change the spontaneous alternation of Y-maze test and immobility time of TST in mice without the injection with LPS (Figure 1c,d, respectively).

To evaluate the effects of theaflavins on inflammation induced by the LPS injection to the brain, the amounts of cytokines and chemokines in the hippocampus were measured by a multiplex system. The amounts of tumor necrosis factor (TNF)-α and IL-1β in the hippocampus of LPS-treated mice were significantly increased compared with those in the PBS-treated mice (Figure 1e,f, respectively). Furthermore, administration of theaflavins reduced the amounts of TNF-α and IL-1β in the LPS-treated mice (Figure 1e,f, respectively).

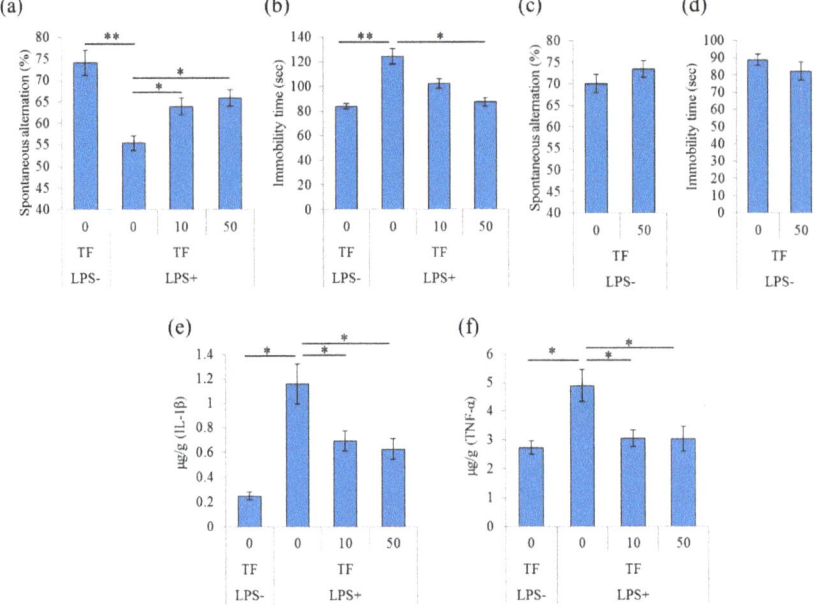

Figure 1. Effects of theaflavins on cognitive decline and depression-like behavior induced by lipopolysaccharide (LPS). (**a–d**), Crl:CD1 mice were orally administered 0, 10, or 50 mg/kg of theaflavins (TF) for 3 days and intracerebroventricularly injected with PBS or 10 µg LPS 1 h after the last administration. The mice were subjected to the spontaneous alternation test and tail suspension test at 1 day and after LPS injection. Spontaneous alternations and arm entries in the Y-maze to evaluate spatial memory (**a**); immobility time in the tail suspension test 1 day after LPS (**b**). Crl:CD1 mice were orally administered 0 or 50 mg/kg of theaflavins (TF) for 3 days and subjected to the spontaneous alternation test (**c**) and tail suspension test (**d**). (**e,f**), Crl:CD1 mice were orally administered 0, 10, or 50 mg/kg of TF for 3 days and intracerebroventricularly injected with phosphate buffered saline (PBS) or 10 µg LPS 1 h after the last administration. Amounts of IL-1β (**e**) and tumor necrosis factor (TNF)-α (**f**) in the hippocampus 24 h after LPS injection, respectively. Data are mean ± SE of 10 mice per group. The p values shown were calculated using the Student's t-test (LPS [−] vs. [+] at 0 mg/kg TF) and one-way ANOVA followed by Dunnett's test (LPS [+] at 0 mg/kg TF vs. LPS [+] at 10 and 30 mg/kg TF). * $p < 0.05$ and ** $p < 0.01$.

To evaluate the effects of theaflavins on neural dendrites in LPS-treated mice, dendrites were analyzed by Golgi staining. LPS injection to the brain significantly reduced the number of apical dendrites of pyramidal neurons and spines along those dendrites in the CA1 region of the hippocampus compared with the control treatment, but this effect of LPS was significantly prevented by treatment with theaflavins (Figure 2a,b). This theaflavins-induced prevention from the LPS-induced dendritic atrophy and spine loss was also observed in the prefrontal cortex (Figure 2c,d). These results suggest that administration of theaflavins reduced LPS-induced inflammation in the brain and the concomitant dendritic atrophy of pyramidal neurons in the hippocampus and prefrontal cortex.

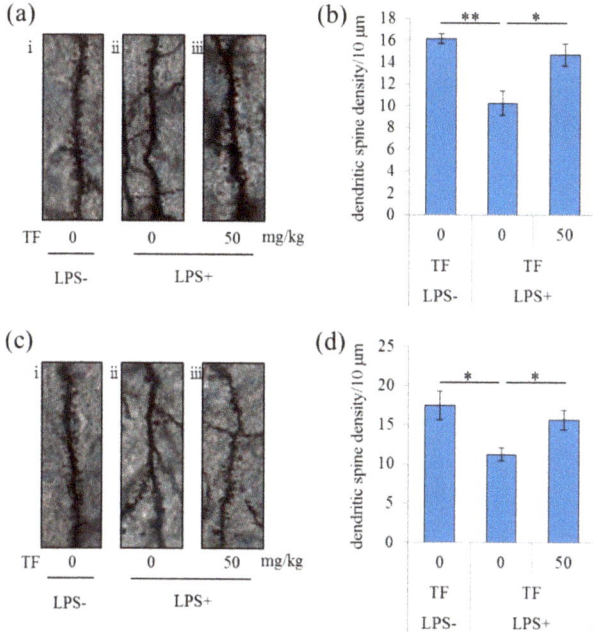

Figure 2. Effects of theaflavins on LPS-induced changes in dendritic spine density. Crl:CD1 mice were orally administered 0 or 50 mg/kg of theaflavins (TF) for 3 days and intracerebroventricularly injected with PBS or 0.3 mg/kg LPS 1 h after the last administration. The brain was subjected to Golgi staining 1 day after LPS injection. (**a,c**) Representative photomicrographs of Golgi-stained neurons in the CA1 of the hippocampus (a-i, ii, iii) and prefrontal cortex (c-i, ii, iii) of mice without LPS, with LPS and 0 mg/kg TF, with LPS and 50 mg/kg TF, respectively. Number of dendritic spines per 10 μm in the CA1 (**b**) and prefrontal cortex (**d**). Data are mean ± SE of 10 mice per group. The p values shown were calculated using the Student's t-test. * $p < 0.05$ and ** $p < 0.01$.

2.2. Effects of Theaflavins on the Inflammatory Response of Cultured Microglia

To evaluate the effects of theaflavins on primary microglia, the levels of cytokines and chemokines in the supernatant of microglial culture treated with LPS were quantified by enzyme-linked immune sorbent assay (ELISA) or a multiplex system. Theaflavins at a concentration of 10 to 30 μM significantly reduced TNF-α production in the supernatant of a microglial culture treated with LPS (Figure 3a) without apparent cytotoxicity or cell proliferation (data not shown). Next, to measure cytokine production, the percentages of TNF-α- and macrophage inflammatory proteins (MIP)-1α-producing cells in CD11b-positive microglia were analyzed using flow cytometry. Treatment with theaflavins at 10 and 30 μM significantly reduced the percentages of TNF-α- and MIP-1α-producing microglia compared with the control treatment (Figure 3b,c, respectively). This result suggests that theaflavins suppressed inflammatory responses of microglia.

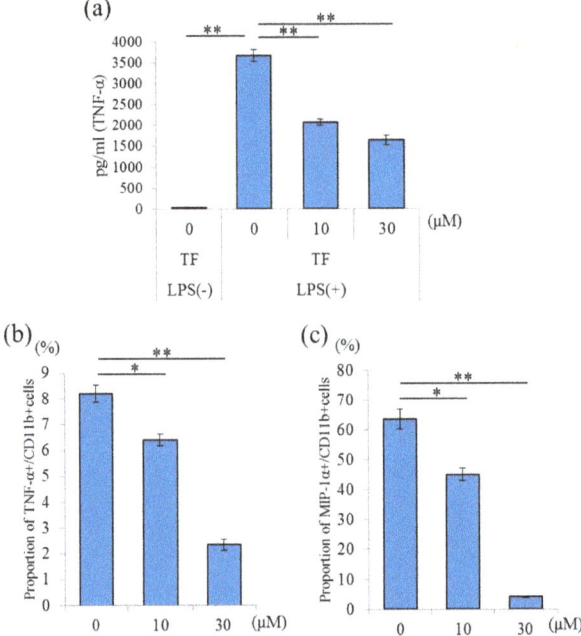

Figure 3. Effects of in vitro theaflavins (TF) treatment on microglial anti-inflammatory activity. (**a**), Amount of TNF-α in the supernatant of microglia pretreated with 0, 10, or 30 μM TF and treated with 5 ng/mL LPS and 0.5 ng/mL IFN-γ. (**b**,**c**) Intracellular cytokine production in microglia pretreated with 0, 10, or 30 μM TF and treated with a leukocyte activation-cocktail with BD GolgiPlug. Scatter plots and percentages of macrophage inflammatory proteins (MIP)-1α- and TNF-α-producing cells in CD11b-positive cells, respectively. Columns and bars represent the means and SEs of triplicate wells per sample, respectively. The p values shown were calculated using the Student's t-test (LPS [−] vs. [+] at 0 μM TF) and one-way ANOVA followed by Dunnett's test (LPS [+] at 0 μM TF vs. LPS [+] at 10 and 30 μM TF). * $p < 0.05$ and ** $p < 0.01$.

2.3. Theaflavins-Induced Suppression of Neurotoxic Effects of Activated Microglia

To examine whether theaflavins attenuate the neurotoxic effects of substances released from LPS-stimulated microglia differentiated neuronal, Neuro2A cells were cultured with a conditioned medium of microglia cultured with LPS. The lengths of neurites are shown in Figure 4a–c. A conditioned medium of LPS-stimulated microglia significantly decreased the length of neurites, whereas this effect was not observed with a conditioned medium of non-stimulated microglia (Figure 4d). Treatment of microglia with theaflavins before LPS stimulation attenuated the reduction in neurite length induced by a conditioned medium of LPS-stimulated microglia (Figure 4d). Direct treatment of Neuro2A cells with theaflavins at 30 μM had no effects on the growth of neurites (data not shown). These results show that theaflavins attenuated the neurotoxic effect of LPS-stimulated microglia.

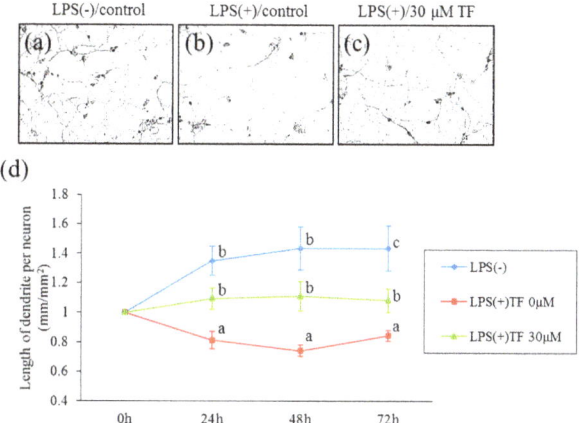

Figure 4. Effects of the conditioned medium of microglial culture treated with theaflavins on neuroprotection. (**a**–**c**), Morphological changes of the neuronal dendrites in Neuro-2A cells. Differentiated Neuro-2A were cultured with the supernatant of microglia with PBS as a vehicle (**a**) and with LPS and interferon (IFN)-γ after pretreatment with 0 or 30 μM theaflavins (**b**,**c**, respectively). (**d**), Length of the dendrites per neuron (mm/mm^2) after 0–72 h of culture. Bars represent the SE of three wells per sample. The p values shown were calculated using the Student's t-test (LPS [−] vs. [+] at 0 μM TF) and one-way ANOVA followed by Dunnett's test (LPS [+] at 0 μM TF vs. LPS [+] at 30 μM TF). Different letters indicate significant differences between groups ($p < 0.05$).

To compare the anti-inflammatory activity of theaflavins with those of other polyphenols, microglia were treated with theaflavins, catechin, EGCG, chlorogenic acid, or caffeic acid at concentrations of 0, 1, 3, 10, and 30 μM before LPS treatment. Pretreatment with theaflavins, catechin, and EGCG decreased LPS-induced production of TNF-α of microglia in a concentration dependent manner, whereas pretreatment with chlorogenic acid and caffeic acid had marginal effects (Figure 5). Theaflavins and EGCG reduced LPS-induced production of TNF-α to similar levels, whereas the effect was smaller with catechin. These results indicate that the anti-inflammatory effects of theaflavins on microglia are stronger than those of common polyphenols, but comparable to those of EGCG.

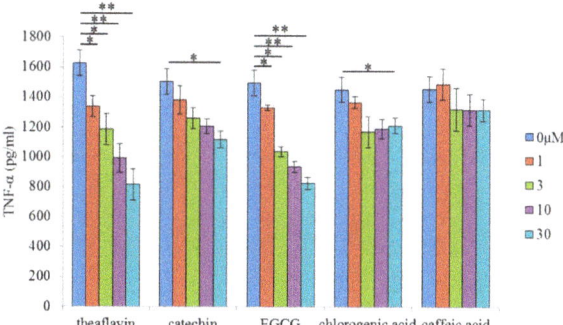

Figure 5. Effects of in vitro treatment with polyphenols on microglial anti-inflammatory activity. Amount of TNF-α in the supernatant of microglia pretreated with 0, 1, 3, 10, or 30 μM theaflavins, catechin, epigallocatechin-3-gallate (EGCG), chlorogenic acid, or caffeic acid and treated with 5 ng/mL LPS and 0.5 ng/mL IFN-γ. Columns and bars represent the means and SEs of three wells per sample, respectively. p-values shown in the graph were calculated by one-way ANOVA followed by the Dunnett's test. * $p < 0.05$ and ** $p < 0.01$.

3. Discussion

The present study showed that the black tea polyphenol theaflavins suppress inflammatory responses in the brain and attenuate concomitant cognitive impairment and depression-like behavior. Theaflavins suppressed production of pro-inflammatory cytokines in murine and human microglia, and hence neurotoxic effects of activated microglia. This finding is consistent with epidemiological studies reporting that tea consumption suppresses cognitive decline and depressive symptoms [13–15]. The anti-inflammatory effect of theaflavins was stronger than those of other polyphenols like catechin in green tea and chlorogenic acid and caffeic acid in coffee, but it was equivalent to that of EGCG in green tea. Since EGCG has been reported to suppress pro-inflammatory cytokines in the brain and depression-like behavior in mice [21], the effects of theaflavins and EGCG may be comparable.

Inflammation in the brain is associated with cognitive dysfunction and psychiatric conditions as well as motor disorders and chronic fatigue [28]. In the present study, LPS injection to the brain induced dendritic atrophy of pyramidal neurons in prefrontal cortex and hippocampus, and pretreatment with theaflavins reduced the dendritic atrophy. Dendritic atrophy is associated with cognitive decline [29] and depression [30]. It has been reported that intracerebroventricular administration of LPS induces dendritic changes in the hippocampus and prefrontal cortex and depressive-like behavior, whereas suppression of inflammation can improve these impairments [31,32]. Because the hippocampus and prefrontal cortex are involved in spatial working memory [33] and depression [34], the neuroprotective effects of theaflavins in these areas may attenuate cognitive impairment and depression. Consistently, pretreatment of microglia with theaflavins attenuated neurotoxic effects of a conditioned medium of LPS-stimulated microglia, as measured by neurite shortening. It has also been reported that microglia activated by LPS produce large amounts of reactive oxygen species (ROS) and pro-inflammatory cytokines, leading to neuronal damage [35]. It is reported that theaflavins inhibit IκB kinase (IKK) and nuclear factor-κB (NF-κB) activation, which is supposed to suppress the inflammatory response of microglia against LPS stimulation [36]. Taken together, these findings support the neuroprotective effects of theaflavins through attenuating inflammation in the brain.

Theaflavin is supposed not to enter into the brain via blood–brain barrier, because in case of EGCG, almost EGCG was detected in the intestine and blood, and EGCG was detectable in the brain, but the level in the brain was much lower than other organs [37]. This report suggests that theaflavins display the anti-inflammatory effects in the intestine and blood, but not directly in the brain. On the other hand, in the present study, we used the model mice injected with LPS. Acute brain inflammation damages the blood–brain barrier and more peripheral monocytes and microglia infiltrate into the brain [38,39]. Especially, it is reported that infiltrated neutrophils and monocytes rather than resident microglia are major inflammatory cells in LPS-injected brain [40]. In the LPS-injected model mice, theaflavin itself or monocyte affected by theaflavin in the peripheral tissue might be delivered to the brain. Further study needs to evaluate the blood–brain permeability in the normal mice and mice with brain inflammation.

This study is subject to several limitations. The amount evaluated in the present study (10 mg/kg) is equivalent to 486 mL of tea for a human weighing 60 kg according to the following calculation. This amount is a little more than the typical daily intake. Based on the formula human equivalent dose (HED) (mg/kg) = Animal does (mg/kg) × (Animal Km/Human Km), where Human Km = 37, Mouse Km = 3 [41,42], mouse dose 10 mg/kg equals to human 0.81 mg/kg, that is, 48.6 mg theaflavins for a human weighing 60 kg. As tea contains approximately 100 mg/L theaflavins [43,44], 48.6 mg theaflavins is equivalent to 486 mL of tea for a human weighing 60 kg. However, as LPS treatment in the brain induces acute inflammation that is more severe than that in chronic inflammatory diseases such as dementia, the effective amount of theaflavins for memory impairment and depression-like behavior may be less than that used in the present study. Further research is needed to evaluate the effective amount of theaflavins for chronic inflammatory diseases. In addition, we need to analyze in the further study whether theaflavins enter the brain through the blood–brain barrier or act on the vagal nerve, leading to prevention from cognitive decline and depression.

Overall, our findings of the neuroprotective effects of theaflavins are consistent with previous epidemiological studies suggesting that consuming tea is beneficial for preventing cognitive decline and depression. Further study will elucidate the effects of theaflavins on animal models or patients of chronic diseases.

4. Materials and Methods

4.1. Preparation of Pure Theaflavins

TF40, a crude theaflavins extract containing about 40% w/w theaflavins, was purchased from Yaizu Suisankagaku Industry (Shizuoka, Japan). After being dissolved in 50% EtOH, TF40 (20 g) was repeatedly subjected to reversed-phase preparative high-performance liquid chromatography (HPLC; column: 150 × 22 mm id, 5 µm, Alltima C18 column; Systech, Tokyo, Japan); solvent: H_2O/H_3PO_4 (85%), 100/1 (v/v) (solvent A) and acetonitrile (solvent B), linear gradient from 20% to 70% B; flow rate: 22.8 mL/min. Each fraction containing TF1, TF2a, TF2b, and TF3 described in Figure 6 was pooled and combined before acetonitrile was evaporated using a rotary evaporator. Next, theaflavins were extracted with ethyl acetate from the residual aqueous solution. and the organic solvent was evaporated. The residue was dissolved in a small amount of EtOH and added to water. The resulting suspension was lyophilized, yielding an orange, uniform powder (5.7 g). The purity of the theaflavins estimated by HPLC was more than 97%. Purified TFs were composed of 1.0% of TF1, 36.9% of TF2a, 14.7% of TF2b, and 44.6% of TF3.

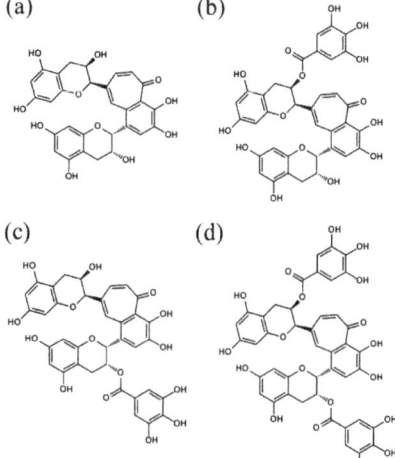

Figure 6. Chemical structures of theaflavins. Structures of theaflavin (TF1) (**a**), theaflavin 3-O-gallate (TF2a) (**b**), theaflavin 3'-O-gallate (TF2b) (**c**) and theaflavin 3,3'-O-digallate (TF3) (**d**). This is a figure, Schemes follow the same formatting. If there are multiple panels, they should be listed as: (**a**) Description of what is contained in the first panel; (**b**) Description of what is contained in the second panel.

4.2. Animals

Pregnant C57BL/6J mice and six-week-old Crl:CD1(ICR) male mice were purchased from Charles River Japan (Tokyo, Japan) and maintained at the Kirin Co. Ltd. All experiments were approved by the Animal Experiment Committee of Kirin Co. Ltd. and conducted in strict accordance with their guidelines in 2016–2017. The Approved ID was AN10339-Z00 and AN10623-Z00. All efforts were made to minimize the suffering. The mice were fed a standard rodent diet (CE-2; CLEA Japan,

Tokyo, Japan) and maintained at room temperature (23 ± 1 °C) under a constant 12-h light/dark cycle (light period from 8:00 a.m. to 8:00 p.m.).

4.3. Neural Inflammation Induced by LPS

Crl:CD1 mice were orally administered 0, 10, or 50 mg/kg of theaflavins dissolved in distilled water (10 mL/kg) once a day for 3 days. One hour after the last administration, the mice were deeply anesthetized with sodium pentobarbital (Kyoritsu Seiyaku, Tokyo, Japan) and intracerebroventricularly injected with 10 μg of LPS (L7895; Sigma-Aldrich, St. Louis, MO, USA), in accordance with previous work [45]. Briefly, LPS dissolved in PBS or PBS (for sham-operated controls) was injected into the cerebral ventricle as previously described [45]. Briefly, a micro-syringe with a 27-gauge stainless steel needle, 2 mm in length, was used for the microinjection. The needle was inserted unilaterally 1 mm to the right and left of the midline point equidistant from each eye in both left and right hemispheres, at an equal distance between the eyes and ears, and perpendicular to the plane of the skull (anteroposterior, −0.22 mm from the bregma; lateral). LPS was delivered gradually within 30 s. The needle was withdrawn after waiting 30 s. Twenty-four hours later, the hippocampus and frontal cortex of the corresponding hemisphere were homogenized in Tris-buffered saline buffer (Wako, Tokyo, Japan) containing a protease inhibitor cocktail (BioVision, Milpitas, CA, USA) with a multi-beads shocker (Yasui Kikai, Osaka, Japan). After centrifugation at 50,000× g for 20 min, the supernatants were collected. The total protein concentration of each supernatant was measured using a bicinchoninic acid (BCA) protein assay kit (ThermoScientific, Yokohama, Japan). To evaluate inflammation in the brain, the amounts of cytokines and chemokines in the supernatants were quantified using a multiplex system (Biopoex; Bio-Rad, Hercules, CA, USA). The other hemisphere was used for morphological analysis of the dendrites. Brain sections at the bregma −2.06 mm were prepared and stained using the FD Rapid GolgiStain Kit (FD Neuro Technologies, Columbia, MD, USA) following the manufacturer's instructions. Spines were counted within the CA1, and the prefrontal cortex dendrites were counted starting from their point of origin from the primary dendrite, as previously described [32]. For spine density measurements, all areas containing 50 to 100 μm of secondary dendrites from the neuron were used.

In the experiment evaluating cognitive function and depression, mice were orally administered 0, 10, or 50 mg/kg theaflavins daily for 3 days, and 1 h after the last administration, mice were intracerebroventricularly injected with 10 μg of LPS. Twenty-four hours after LPS treatment, the mice were subjected to the tail suspension test (TST) and the spontaneous alternation test, as described below.

4.4. Tail Suspension Test

The TST was used to assess behavioral despair, which is a feature of depression. Each mouse was individually suspended by its tail using adhesive tape in a box for 6 min while being video recorded. The video was carefully scored for total time of immobility during suspension. Mice were considered immobile only when they hung passively and were completely motionless.

4.5. Spontaneous Alternation Test

The spontaneous alternation test was performed as previously described [46,47]. A three-arm Y-maze (25 cm long × 5 cm wide × 20 cm high) with equal angles between all arms constructed from dark black polyvinyl plastic was used. Each mouse was initially placed in one arm, and the sequence and number of arm entries were counted for 8 min. The alternation score (%) for each mouse was defined as the ratio of the actual number of alternations to the possible number (defined as the total number of arm entries minus two) multiplied by 100, i.e., % Alternation = [(Number of alternations)/(Total arm entries − 2)] × 100.

4.6. Primary Murine Microglia Cell Culture

Primary microglial cells were isolated from the brains of newborn C57BL/6J mice (<7 days old) via magnetic cell sorting after conjugation with anti-CD11b antibodies (Miltenyi Biotec, Bergisch Gladbach, Germany), as previously described [48]. The isolated CD11b-positive cells (>90% pure as evaluated by flow cytometry) were plated in poly-D-lysine (PDL)-coated 96-well plates (BD Biosciences, Billerica, MA, USA) and cultured in DMEM/F-12 (Gibco, Carlsbad, CA, USA) medium supplemented with 10% fetal bovine serum (FBS; Gibco) and 100 U/mL penicillium/streptomycin (Sigma-Aldrich). Microglia isolated from newborn C57BL/6J mice were plated at a density of 30,000 per well in a PDL-coated plate.

To measure inflammatory cytokine production in the supernatant, microglia were treated with theaflavins, catechin (Sigma-Aldrich), EGCG (Sigma-Aldrich), chlorogenic acids (Sigma-Aldrich), or caffeic acid (Sigma-Aldrich) for 12 h, and then treated with LPS (5 ng/mL; Sigma-Aldrich) and interferon-γ (IFN-γ, 0.5 ng/mL; R&D systems, Minneapolis, MN, USA) for 12 h. After stimulation, the supernatants were assayed using a Bio-Plex assay system (Bio-Rad).

To measure intracellular cytokines, microglia were treated with the test samples for 12 h, then treated with a leukocyte activation-cocktail with BD GolgiPlug^{TM} (BD Biosciences, San Jose, CA, USA) for 12 h, and then assessed using the BD Cytofix/Cytoperm Fixation/Permeabilization kit (BD Biosciences) as described in the previous study [49]. The cells were then stained with the anti-MIP-1α-PE (eBioscience, San Diego, CA, USA), anti-TNF-α-FITC (eBioscience), and anti-CD11b-APC-Cy7 (BD Biosciences) antibodies. The cells were finally analyzed with a flow cytometer (FACSCantoII; BD Biosciences). Each sample was assayed in three wells.

4.7. Neurotoxicity Assay

To evaluate the effects of the microglial culture supernatant treated with theaflavins and LPS, a neurotoxicity assay was conducted as described in our previous work [50]. The mouse neuroblastoma Neuro2A cell line (ATCC CCL-131) was maintained in minimum essential medium (MEM, Gibco) medium supplemented with 10% FBS (Gibco), non-essential amino acids (Gibco), and 100 U/mL penicillin/streptomycin (Sigma-Aldrich). Neuro2A cells were plated at a density of 4000 cells per well in a 96-well cell culture plate (Essen Bioscience, Welwyn Garden City, UK). After 24 h, FBS was added at a final concentration of 1% along with all-trans retinoic acid (Wako) to a final concentration of 10 μM to induce the Neuro2A to differentiate into neuronal cells. After removing the medium, the cells were incubated with microglial culture supernatant. Microglial culture supernatants were prepared as follows: first, microglia from newborn C57BL/6J mice were plated and pretreated with 0 or 30 μM theaflavins for 12 h, followed by 5 ng/mL LPS and 0.5 ng/mL interferon (IFN)-γ for 12 h. Quantitative live cell imaging was performed to assess the length of the dendrites in the Neuro2A cells using an IncuCyte Zoom real-time imaging system (Essen Biosciences, Ann Arbor, MI, USA). Images were obtained every 24 h at 20× magnification in the phase-contrast mode. The length of the neuronal dendrites per neuron was determined using IncuCyte Neurotrack Software (Essen Biosciences). Each sample was assayed in three wells.

4.8. Statistical Analysis

Data are presented as the mean with error bars indicating the standard error (SE). Data were analyzed by Student's *t*-test and one-way analysis of variance (ANOVA) followed by Dunnett's test, as indicated in the figure legends. All statistical analyses were performed using the Ekuseru–Toukei 2012 software program (Social Survey Research Information, Tokyo, Japan). A *p*-value < 0.05 was considered statistically significant.

Author Contributions: Y.A. designed and conducted most of the experiments, analyzed the results, and wrote most of the paper. R.O. performed the behavioral evaluation. M.K. performed the neurotoxicity assay. Y.T. conducted the preparation of the theaflavins used in the present study. K.K. supervised this research.

Acknowledgments: We appreciate Prof. Tomoyuki Furuyashiki (Kobe University, Japan) for giving us valuable comments on our manuscript.

Conflicts of Interest: Y.A., R.O., M.K., Y.T., and K.K. are employed by Kirin Company Ltd. The authors declare that they have no other conflicts of interest with the content of this article.

References

1. Heppner, F.L.; Ransohoff, R.M.; Becher, B. Immune attack: The role of inflammation in Alzheimer disease. *Nat. Rev. Neurosci.* **2015**, *16*, 358–372. [CrossRef]
2. Miller, A.H.; Raison, C.L. The role of inflammation in depression: From evolutionary imperative to modern treatment target. *Nat. Rev. Immunol.* **2016**, *16*, 22–34. [CrossRef]
3. Abbott, A. Depression: The radical theory linking it to inflammation. *Nature* **2018**, *557*, 633–634. [CrossRef]
4. Montoya, J.G.; Holmes, T.H.; Anderson, J.N.; Maecker, H.T.; Rosenberg-Hasson, Y.; Valencia, I.J.; Chu, L.; Younger, J.W.; Tato, C.M.; Davis, M.M. Cytokine signature associated with disease severity in chronic fatigue syndrome patients. *Proc. Natl. Acad. Sci. USA* **2017**, *114*, e7150–e7158. [CrossRef] [PubMed]
5. Li, Q.; Barres, B.A. Microglia and macrophages in brain homeostasis and disease. *Nat. Rev. Immunol.* **2018**, *18*, 225–242. [CrossRef] [PubMed]
6. Weinhard, L.; di Bartolomei, G.; Bolasco, G.; Machado, P.; Schieber, N.L.; Neniskyte, U.; Exiga, M.; Vadisiute, A.; Raggioli, A.; Schertel, A.; et al. Microglia remodel synapses by presynaptic trogocytosis and spine head filopodia induction. *Nat. Commun.* **2018**, *9*, 1228. [CrossRef] [PubMed]
7. Nie, X.; Kitaoka, S.; Tanaka, K.; Segi-Nishida, E.; Imoto, Y.; Ogawa, A.; Nakano, F.; Tomohiro, A.; Nakayama, K.; Taniguchi, M.; et al. The Innate Immune Receptors TLR2/4 Mediate Repeated Social Defeat Stress-Induced Social Avoidance through Prefrontal Microglial Activation. *Neuron* **2018**, *99*, 464–479.e467. [CrossRef]
8. Spittau, B. Aging Microglia-Phenotypes, Functions and Implications for Age-Related Neurodegenerative Diseases. *Front. Aging Neurosci.* **2017**, *9*, 194. [CrossRef] [PubMed]
9. Salter, M.W.; Stevens, B. Microglia emerge as central players in brain disease. *Nat. Med.* **2017**, *23*, 1018–1027. [CrossRef]
10. Reus, G.Z.; Fries, G.R.; Stertz, L.; Badawy, M.; Passos, I.C.; Barichello, T.; Kapczinski, F.; Quevedo, J. The role of inflammation and microglial activation in the pathophysiology of psychiatric disorders. *Neuroscience* **2015**, *300*, 141–154. [CrossRef] [PubMed]
11. Akiyama, H.; Barger, S.; Barnum, S.; Bradt, B.; Bauer, J.; Cole, G.M.; Cooper, N.R.; Eikelenboom, P.; Emmerling, M.; Fiebich, B.L.; et al. Inflammation and Alzheimer's disease. *Neurobiol. Aging* **2000**, *21*, 383–421. [CrossRef]
12. Kohler, O.; Krogh, J.; Mors, O.; Benros, M.E. Inflammation in Depression and the Potential for Anti-Inflammatory Treatment. *Curr. Neuropharmacol.* **2016**, *14*, 732–742. [CrossRef]
13. Chan, S.P.; Yong, P.Z.; Sun, Y.; Mahendran, R.; Wong, J.C.M.; Qiu, C.; Ng, T.P.; Kua, E.H.; Feng, L. Associations of Long-Term Tea Consumption with Depressive and Anxiety Symptoms in Community-Living Elderly: Findings from the Diet and Healthy Aging Study. *J. Prev. Alzheimer's Dis.* **2018**, *5*, 21–25.
14. Lefevre-Arbogast, S.; Gaudout, D.; Bensalem, J.; Letenneur, L.; Dartigues, J.F.; Hejblum, B.P.; Feart, C.; Delcourt, C.; Samieri, C. Pattern of polyphenol intake and the long-term risk of dementia in older persons. *Neurology* **2018**, *90*, e1979–e1988. [CrossRef] [PubMed]
15. Liu, X.; Du, X.; Han, G.; Gao, W. Association between tea consumption and risk of cognitive disorders: A dose-response meta-analysis of observational studies. *Oncotarget* **2017**, *8*, 43306–43321. [CrossRef] [PubMed]
16. Hintikka, J.; Tolmunen, T.; Honkalampi, K.; Haatainen, K.; Koivumaa-Honkanen, H.; Tanskanen, A.; Viinamaki, H. Daily tea drinking is associated with a low level of depressive symptoms in the Finnish general population. *Eur. J. Epidemiol.* **2005**, *20*, 359–363. [CrossRef] [PubMed]
17. Pan, C.W.; Ma, Q.; Sun, H.P.; Xu, Y.; Luo, N.; Wang, P. Tea Consumption and Health-Related Quality of Life in Older Adults. *J. Nutr. Health Aging* **2017**, *21*, 480–486. [CrossRef]
18. Guo, Y.; Zhao, Y.; Nan, Y.; Wang, X.; Chen, Y.; Wang, S. (−)-Epigallocatechin-3-gallate ameliorates memory impairment and rescues the abnormal synaptic protein levels in the frontal cortex and hippocampus in a mouse model of Alzheimer's disease. *Neuroreport* **2017**, *28*, 590–597. [CrossRef]

19. Zhu, W.L.; Shi, H.S.; Wei, Y.M.; Wang, S.J.; Sun, C.Y.; Ding, Z.B.; Lu, L. Green tea polyphenols produce antidepressant-like effects in adult mice. *Pharmacol. Res.* **2012**, *65*, 74–80. [CrossRef] [PubMed]
20. Mi, Y.; Qi, G.; Fan, R.; Qiao, Q.; Sun, Y.; Gao, Y.; Liu, X. EGCG ameliorates high-fat- and high-fructose-induced cognitive defects by regulating the IRS/AKT and ERK/CREB/BDNF signaling pathways in the CNS. *FASEB J. Off. Publ. Fed. Am. Soc. Exp. Biol.* **2017**, *31*, 4998–5011. [CrossRef] [PubMed]
21. Lee, Y.J.; Choi, D.Y.; Yun, Y.P.; Han, S.B.; Oh, K.W.; Hong, J.T. Epigallocatechin-3-gallate prevents systemic inflammation-induced memory deficiency and amyloidogenesis via its anti-neuroinflammatory properties. *J. Nutr. Biochem.* **2013**, *24*, 298–310. [CrossRef] [PubMed]
22. Yang, Z.; Jie, G.; Dong, F.; Xu, Y.; Watanabe, N.; Tu, Y. Radical-scavenging abilities and antioxidant properties of theaflavins and their gallate esters in H2O2-mediated oxidative damage system in the HPF-1 cells. *Toxicol. In Vitro Int. J. Publ. Assoc. BIBRA* **2008**, *22*, 1250–1256. [CrossRef]
23. Wu, Y.Y.; Li, W.; Xu, Y.; Jin, E.H.; Tu, Y.Y. Evaluation of the antioxidant effects of four main theaflavin derivatives through chemiluminescence and DNA damage analyses. *J. Zhejiang Univ. Sci. B* **2011**, *12*, 744–751. [CrossRef]
24. Maron, D.J.; Lu, G.P.; Cai, N.S.; Wu, Z.G.; Li, Y.H.; Chen, H.; Zhu, J.Q.; Jin, X.J.; Wouters, B.C.; Zhao, J. Cholesterol-lowering effect of a theaflavin-enriched green tea extract: A randomized controlled trial. *Arch. Intern. Med.* **2003**, *163*, 1448–1453. [CrossRef]
25. Wu, Y.; Jin, F.; Wang, Y.; Li, F.; Wang, L.; Wang, Q.; Ren, Z.; Wang, Y. In vitro and in vivo anti-inflammatory effects of theaflavin-3,3'-digallate on lipopolysaccharide-induced inflammation. *Eur. J. Pharmacol.* **2017**, *794*, 52–60. [CrossRef] [PubMed]
26. De Oliveira, A.; Prince, D.; Lo, C.Y.; Lee, L.H.; Chu, T.C. Antiviral activity of theaflavin digallate against herpes simplex virus type 1. *Antivir. Res.* **2015**, *118*, 56–67. [CrossRef] [PubMed]
27. Liu, S.; Lu, H.; Zhao, Q.; He, Y.; Niu, J.; Debnath, A.K.; Wu, S.; Jiang, S. Theaflavin derivatives in black tea and catechin derivatives in green tea inhibit HIV-1 entry by targeting gp41. *Biochim. Biophys. Acta* **2005**, *1723*, 270–281. [CrossRef]
28. Nakatomi, Y.; Mizuno, K.; Ishii, A.; Wada, Y.; Tanaka, M.; Tazawa, S.; Onoe, K.; Fukuda, S.; Kawabe, J.; Takahashi, K.; et al. Neuroinflammation in Patients with Chronic Fatigue Syndrome/Myalgic Encephalomyelitis: An (1)(1)C-(R)-PK11195 PET Study. *J. Nucl. Med. Off. Publ. Soc. Nucl. Med.* **2014**, *55*, 945–950. [CrossRef]
29. Koleske, A.J. Molecular mechanisms of dendrite stability. *Nat. Rev. Neurosci.* **2013**, *14*, 536–550. [CrossRef]
30. Qiao, H.; Li, M.X.; Xu, C.; Chen, H.B.; An, S.C.; Ma, X.M. Dendritic Spines in Depression: What We Learned from Animal Models. *Neural Plast.* **2016**, *2016*, 8056370. [CrossRef]
31. Lawson, M.A.; Parrott, J.M.; McCusker, R.H.; Dantzer, R.; Kelley, K.W.; O'Connor, J.C. Intracerebroventricular administration of lipopolysaccharide induces indoleamine-2,3-dioxygenase-dependent depression-like behaviors. *J. Neuroinflamm.* **2013**, *10*, 87. [CrossRef]
32. Zhang, J.C.; Wu, J.; Fujita, Y.; Yao, W.; Ren, Q.; Yang, C.; Li, S.X.; Shirayama, Y.; Hashimoto, K. Antidepressant effects of TrkB ligands on depression-like behavior and dendritic changes in mice after inflammation. *Int. J. Neuropsychopharmacol.* **2014**, *18*. [CrossRef] [PubMed]
33. Broadbent, N.J.; Squire, L.R.; Clark, R.E. Spatial memory, recognition memory, and the hippocampus. *Proc. Natl. Acad. Sci. USA* **2004**, *101*, 14515–14520. [CrossRef]
34. Koenigs, M.; Grafman, J. The functional neuroanatomy of depression: Distinct roles for ventromedial and dorsolateral prefrontal cortex. *Behav. Brain Res.* **2009**, *201*, 239–243. [CrossRef] [PubMed]
35. Block, M.L.; Zecca, L.; Hong, J.S. Microglia-mediated neurotoxicity: Uncovering the molecular mechanisms. *Nat. Rev. Neurosci.* **2007**, *8*, 57–69. [CrossRef]
36. Ukil, A.; Maity, S.; Das, P.K. Protection from experimental colitis by theaflavin-3,3'-digallate correlates with inhibition of IKK and NF-kappaB activation. *Br. J. Pharmacol.* **2006**, *149*, 121–131. [CrossRef] [PubMed]
37. Ostrowska, J.Ł.W.; Augustyniak, A.; Skrzydlewska, E. Green and Black Tea in Brain Protection. *Oxidative Stress Neurodegener. Disord.* **2007**, 581–605. [CrossRef]
38. London, A.; Cohen, M.; Schwartz, M. Microglia and monocyte-derived macrophages: Functionally distinct populations that act in concert in CNS plasticity and repair. *Front. Cell. Neurosci.* **2013**, *7*, 34. [CrossRef] [PubMed]

39. Varvel, N.H.; Neher, J.J.; Bosch, A.; Wang, W.; Ransohoff, R.M.; Miller, R.J.; Dingledine, R. Infiltrating monocytes promote brain inflammation and exacerbate neuronal damage after status epilepticus. *Proc. Natl. Acad. Sci. USA* **2016**, *113*, E5665–E5674. [CrossRef]
40. Ji, K.A.; Yang, M.S.; Jeong, H.K.; Min, K.J.; Kang, S.H.; Jou, I.; Joe, E.H. Resident microglia die and infiltrated neutrophils and monocytes become major inflammatory cells in lipopolysaccharide-injected brain. *Glia* **2007**, *55*, 1577–1588. [CrossRef]
41. Reagan-Shaw, S.; Nihal, M.; Ahmad, N. Dose translation from animal to human studies revisited. *FASEB J. Off. Publ. Fed. Am. Soc. Exp. Biol.* **2008**, *22*, 659–661. [CrossRef] [PubMed]
42. Nair, A.B.; Jacob, S. A simple practice guide for dose conversion between animals and human. *J. Basic Clin. Pharm.* **2016**, *7*, 27–31. [CrossRef] [PubMed]
43. Liang, Y.; Lu, J.; Zhang, L.; Wu, S.; Wu, Y. Estimation of black tea quality by analysis of chemical composition and colour difference of tea infusions. *Food Chem.* **2003**, *80*, 283–290. [CrossRef]
44. Nakamura-Sugimoto, Y.; Takahashi, Y.; Kageyama, S. Development of Functional Tea Drink. 2012. Available online: https://www.tiit.or.jp/userfiles/file/report2012-16.pdf (accessed on 25 Januray 2019).
45. Ano, Y.; Ozawa, M.; Kutsukake, T.; Sugiyama, S.; Uchida, K.; Yoshida, A.; Nakayama, H. Preventive effects of a fermented dairy product against Alzheimer's disease and identification of a novel oleamide with enhanced microglial phagocytosis and anti-inflammatory activity. *PLoS ONE* **2015**, *10*, e0118512. [CrossRef] [PubMed]
46. Ano, Y.; Ayabe, T.; Kutsukake, T.; Ohya, R.; Takaichi, Y.; Uchida, S.; Yamada, K.; Uchida, K.; Takashima, A.; Nakayama, H. Novel lactopeptides in fermented dairy products improve memory function and cognitive decline. *Neurobiol. Aging* **2018**, *72*, 23–31. [CrossRef]
47. Ano, Y.; Hoshi, A.; Ayabe, T.; Ohya, R.; Uchida, S.; Yamada, K.; Kondo, K.; Kitaoka, S.; Furuyashiki, T. Iso-alpha-acids, the bitter components of beer, improve hippocampus-dependent memory through vagus nerve activation. *FASEB J. Off. Publ. Fed. Am. Soc. Exp. Biol.* **2019**. [CrossRef]
48. Ano, Y.; Dohata, A.; Taniguchi, Y.; Hoshi, A.; Uchida, K.; Takashima, A.; Nakayama, H. Iso-alpha-acids, Bitter Components of Beer, Prevent Inflammation and Cognitive Decline Induced in a Mouse Model of Alzheimer's Disease. *J. Biol. Chem.* **2017**, *292*, 3720–3728. [CrossRef]
49. Ano, Y.; Takaichi, Y.; Uchida, K.; Kondo, K.; Nakayama, H.; Takashima, A. Iso-alpha-Acids, the Bitter Components of Beer, Suppress Microglial Inflammation in rTg4510 Tauopathy. *Molecules* **2018**, *23*, 3133. [CrossRef]
50. Ano, Y.; Kutsukake, T.; Hoshi, A.; Yoshida, A.; Nakayama, H. Identification of a novel dehydroergosterol enhancing microglial anti-inflammatory activity in a dairy product fermented with Penicillium candidum. *PLoS ONE* **2015**, *10*, e0116598. [CrossRef]

Sample Availability: Samples of the compounds theaflavins are available from the authors.

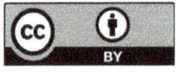

© 2019 by the authors. Licensee MDPI, Basel, Switzerland. This article is an open access article distributed under the terms and conditions of the Creative Commons Attribution (CC BY) license (http://creativecommons.org/licenses/by/4.0/).

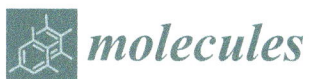

Article

20-Hydroxy-3-Oxolupan-28-Oic Acid Attenuates Inflammatory Responses by Regulating PI3K–Akt and MAPKs Signaling Pathways in LPS-Stimulated RAW264.7 Macrophages

Yufeng Cao [1,2,†], Fu Li [3,†], Yanyan Luo [2,†], Liang Zhang [2], Shuya Lu [2], Rui Xing [2], Bingjun Yan [2], Hongyin Zhang [4,*] and Weicheng Hu [2,*]

1. Institute of Life Sciences, Jiangsu University, Zhenjiang 212013, China; 17851567661@163.com
2. Jiangsu Collaborative Innovation Center of Regional Modern Agriculture & Environmental protection/Jiangsu Key Laboratory for Eco-Agricultural Biotechnology around Hongze Lake, Huaiyin Normal University, Huaian 223300, China; lyy122525@163.com (Y.L.); liangzhang_xj@163.com (L.Z.); lushuyawork@163.com (S.L.); xingrui0707@163.com (R.X.); 15380617203@163.com (B.Y.)
3. Key Laboratory of Mountain Ecological Restoration and Bioresource Utilization and Ecological Restoration Biodiversity Conservation Key Laboratory of Sichuan Province, Chengdu Institute of Biology, Chinese Academy of Sciences, Chengdu 610041, China; lifu@cib.ac.cn
4. School of Food and Biological Engineering, Jiangsu University, Zhenjiang 212013, China
* Correspondence: hu_weicheng@163.com (W.H.); zhanghongyin126@126.com (H.Z.); Tel: +86-517-8352-5992 (W.H.); +865-118-879-0211 (H.Z)
† These authors equally contributed to this work.

Received: 19 December 2018; Accepted: 21 January 2019; Published: 22 January 2019

Abstract: 20-Hydroxy-3-oxolupan-28-oic acid (HOA), a lupane-type triterpene, was obtained from the leaves of *Mahonia bealei*, which is described in the Chinese Pharmacopeia as a remedy for inflammation and related diseases. The anti-inflammatory mechanisms of HOA, however, have not yet been fully elucidated. Therefore, the objective of this study was to characterize the molecular mechanisms of HOA in lipopolysaccharide (LPS)-stimulated RAW264.7 cells. HOA suppressed the release of nitric oxide (NO), pro-inflammatory cytokine tumor necrosis factor α (TNF-α), and interleukin 6 (IL-6) in LPS-stimulated RAW264.7 macrophages without affecting cell viability. Quantitative real-time reverse-transcription polymerase chain reaction (RT-qPCR) analysis indicated that HOA also suppressed the gene expression of inducible NO synthase (iNOS), TNF-α, and IL-6. Further analyses demonstrated that HOA inhibited the phosphorylation of upstream signaling molecules, including p85, PDK1, Akt, IκBα, ERK, and JNK, as well as the nuclear translocation of nuclear factor κB (NF-κB) p65. Interestingly, HOA had no effect on the LPS-induced nuclear translocation of activator protein 1 (AP-1). Taken together, these results suggest that HOA inhibits the production of cytokine by downregulating iNOS, TNF-α, and IL-6 gene expression via the downregulation of phosphatidylinositol 3-kinase (PI3K)/Akt and mitogen-activated protein kinases (MAPKs), and the inhibition of NF-κB activation. Our findings indicate that HOA could potentially be used as an anti-inflammatory agent for medical use.

Keywords: inflammation; nitric oxide; macrophage; NF-κB; lupane-type triterpene

1. Introduction

The inflammatory response is initiated in living tissues in defense of harmful stimuli, including invading microorganisms, irritants, or noxious chemicals [1]. Physiologically, the inflammatory response provides the benefit of removing invading pathogenic microorganisms, including exogenous stimuli, and promoting the repair of damaged tissues [2,3]. However, prolonged inflammation can lead to long-term, severe inflammatory reactions that can enhance the pathological processes of various inflammatory diseases, such as arthritis, Alzheimer's disease, septic shock, type 2 diabetes, and cardiovascular diseases [4,5]. Macrophages are major inflammatory and immune effector cells that play crucial roles in producing cytokines, chemokines, and inflammatory mediators, including nitric oxide (NO), prostaglandin E_2, hydrolytic enzymes, and pro-inflammatory cytokines, such as tumor necrosis factor α (TNF-α), interleukin 1β (IL-1β) and interleukin 6 (IL-6) [6,7]. These pathophysiological changes initiate signal transducers, such as phosphoinositide 3-kinase (PI3K)-Akt, mitogen-activated protein kinases (MAPKs), or Janus kinase/signal transducer and activator of transcription (JAK-STATs) to boost the activation and nuclear translocation of transcription factors, such as nuclear factor κB (NF-κB), activator protein 1 (AP-1), and STATs [8,9].

Any substances that suppress the regulation of these mediators are therefore important for the treatment and prevention of inflammation and related diseases. The pro-inflammatory NF-κB pathway is central to the regulation of inflammation. NF-κB is found to be chronically active in many inflammatory diseases [10,11]. Thus, the development of a potential anti-inflammatory drug derived from natural products based on NF-κB target isolation is a promising avenue for research.

Mahonia bealei (Fort.) Carr is a member of the Berberidanceae family and is widely distributed in mountainous areas of southern China. *M. bealei* is included in the Chinese Pharmacopeia as a folk medicine for the treatment of dysentery, jaundice, periodontitis, and bloody urine [12]. Its leaves, which are consumed traditionally in China as a bitter tea, engage in antioxidant, anti-proliferation, anti-inflammatory, anti-bacterial, and anti-influenza activities [13–15]. Pharmacological testing of the leaves has been conducted mainly on extracts of the plant and its chemical constituents and their pharmacological activities have yet to be investigated. Previous studies of the active components of this plant have focused primarily on alkaloids, such as epiberberine, berberine, and jatrorrhizine, because they were thought to be responsible for its anti-inflammatory effects [16,17]. However, activity of *M. bealei* non-alkaloids and their underlying mechanisms have yet to be fully defined.

In our previous work, we found that the dichloromethane fraction from *M. bealei* leaves exerted an anti-inflammatory effect both in vitro and in vivo [13]. However, the active compounds in this extract remain unclear. Hence, biological activity guided separation was carried out to search for the active individuals. As a result, a lupane-type triterpene, 20-hydroxy-3-oxolupan-28-oic acid (HOA) (Figure 1) was found to exhibit significant anti-inflammatory effects and NF-κB inhibitory effects (unpublished data). To the best of our knowledge, the biological activities of HOA are unknown. Therefore, as part of our ongoing investigation, this study was conducted to investigate the anti-inflammatory properties and molecular mechanisms underlying the anti-inflammatory properties of HOA.

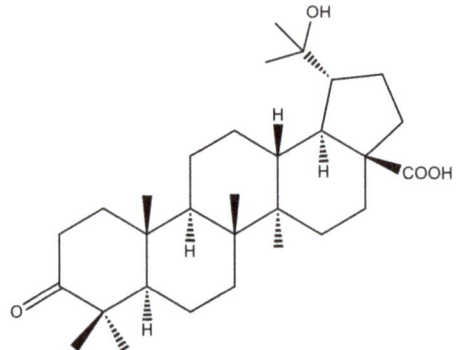

Figure 1. The structure of 20-hydroxy-3-oxolupan-28-oic acid (HOA).

2. Results

2.1. Effects of HOA on the Viability of RAW264.7 Cells

To evaluate the cytotoxic effects of HOA on RAW264.7 cells, cells were incubated with various concentrations of HOA (5, 10, 20, 30, 40, 50, and 100 µM) for 24 h. The result of an MTT assay showed that HOA had no significant cytotoxic effects at concentrations up to 40 µM (Figure 2A). However, cell viability began to decrease to below 90% when the HOA concentration was increased to 50 µM. Accordingly, we limited the concentration of HOA in subsequent experiments to below 50 µM.

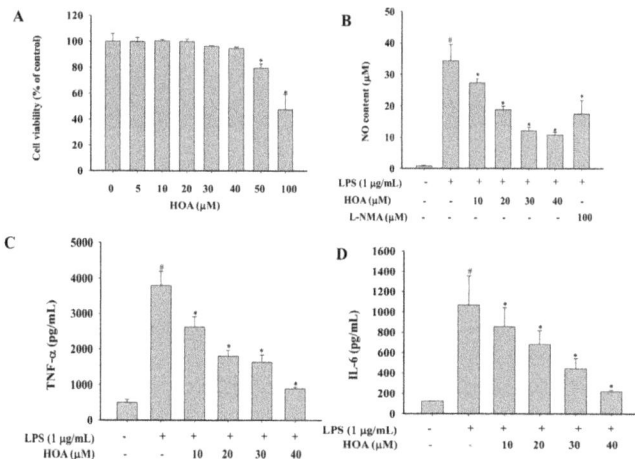

Figure 2. Anti-inflammatory effect of HOA on LPS-induced RAW264.7 cells. (**A**) RAW264.7 cells were treated with various concentrations of HOA for 24 h. The cell viability was determined by MTT assay, as described in section of Materials and Methods. (**B–D**) Cells were pretreated with various concentrations of HOA for 30 min and treated with lipopolysaccharide (LPS) for an additional 24 h. The NO content was determined by Griess reagent and the production of cytokines were measured by cytometric bead array (CBA) kit using the flow cytometry. The data are presented as means ± SD (n = 3). * indicates a significant difference between LPS group and HOA+LPS groups ($p < 0.05$). # indicates a difference between LPS group and the control group ($p < 0.05$).

2.2. Effect of HOA on NO Production and Pro-Inflammatory Cytokine Production in LPS-Stimulated RAW264.7 Cells

In the present study, we first investigated the inhibitory effect of HOA on NO in lipopolysaccharide (LPS)-treated cells. The cells were pre-treated with different concentrations of HOA (10, 20, 30, and 40 µM) for 30 min before adding LPS (1 µg/mL), when a NO detection assay was performed. NO production was 41.76-fold higher in RAW264.7 cells after 24 h of LPS stimulation than in the control group. L-NMMA, an inhibitor of NO that we used as a positive control and also suppressed NO production to 17.46 µM at 100 µM. HOA was found more potent to inhibit NO generation to 27.32, 18.76, 12.06, and 10.79 µM at concentrations of 10, 20, 30, and 40 µM, respectively. In the current study, concentrations of TNF-α and IL-6 in culture supernatants of RAW264.7 cells were detected using a cytometric bead array (CBA) kit. LPS stimulation significantly upregulated the concentrations of pro-inflammatory cytokines (Figure 2C,D). In contrast, treatment with HOA significantly inhibited the levels of TNF-α and IL-6 that were induced by LPS. These results indicate that HOA exerts anti-inflammatory activity via the suppression of NO production and pro-inflammatory cytokines in LPS-stimulated RAW264.7 cells.

2.3. Effect of HOA on Morphology of LPS-Stimulated RAW264.7 Cells

Morphological changes in RAW264.7 cells were assessed with scanning electron microscopy (SEM). The untreated control group RAW264.7 cells were round, with smooth cell edges without pseudopodia (Figure 3), whereas those stimulated with LPS (1 µg/mL) for 10 min had characteristics of activation of macrophage, such as increase in cell size and elongated pseudopodia. Following HOA treatment, the changes in morphological structure of cells were ameliorated.

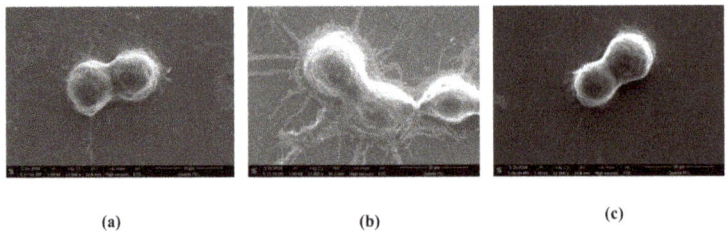

(a) (b) (c)

Figure 3. Photograph of RAW264.7 cells after incubation with LPS and HOA under scanning electron microscopy (SEM). (a) Control; (b) LPS treatment; (c) LPS and HOA treatment.

2.4. Effect of HOA on Expression of Pro-Inflammatory Cytokines in LPS-Stimulated RAW264.7 Cells

To further determine whether HOA-mediated inhibition of inflammation was involved in the modulation of the inducible NO synthase (iNOS), IL-6, and TNF-α gene expression at the transcriptional level, RAW264.7 cells were pretreated with different concentrations of HOA for 30 min and stimulated with LPS (1 µg/mL) for 6 h and analyzed by reverse-transcription polymerase chain reaction (RT-qPCR). As shown in Figure 4, RT-qPCR revealed that iNOS, IL-6, and TNF-α mRNAs expression levels were low in unstimulated RAW264.7 cells. However, mRNA expression levels were sharply increased by LPS treatment and significantly inhibited by HOA treatment except iNOS expression at 20 µM. Furthermore, western blot was carried out to confirm that iNOS expression was significantly inhibited both at 20 and 40 µM. These results suggest that the inhibitory effect of HOA on iNOS, TNF-α, and IL-6 secretion following LPS stimulation is attributable to downregulation of expression of iNOS, TNF-α, and IL-6.

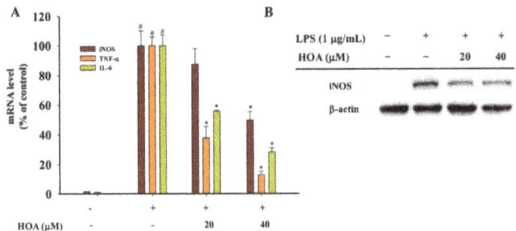

Figure 4. The effect of HOA on LPS-induced pro-inflammatory cytokines expression in RAW264.7 cells. (**A**) Cells were plated at a density of 5×10^6 cells/dish in 60-mm culture dishes and treated with LPS and HOA for 6 h. After preparation of the nuclear fraction, the mRNA expression levels of inducible NO synthase (iNOS), tumor necrosis factor α (TNF-α), and interleukin 6 (IL-6) were measured using reverse-transcription polymerase chain reaction (RT-qPCR). The data are presented as means ± SD (n = 3). * indicates a significant difference between LPS group and HOA+LPS groups ($p < 0.05$). # indicates a significant difference between LPS group and the control group ($p < 0.05$). (**B**) Cells were plated at a density of 5×10^6 cells/dish in 60-mm culture dishes and treated with LPS and HOA for indicated time points. After preparation of the total protein, the expression of iNOS was measured by western blot.

2.5. Effects of HOA on the Regulation of Transcription Factors and Its Upstream Signalling Pathway

We examined the effects of HOA on NF-κB/AP-1 translocation into the nuclei of LPS-treated RAW264.7 cells. Macrophages were treated with HOA for 30 min, followed by stimulation with LPS (1 µg/mL) for 10 min and 30 min. HOA suppressed LPS-induced nuclear localization of p65, a major NF-κB subunit, at 10 min and 30 min (Figure 5A). However, HOA did not affect the translation of c-Jun and c-Fos. To further validate the inhibition NF-κB translocation in the LPS-induced inflammatory response, we observed the immunofluorescence intensity of p65 by immunofluorescence staining through a confocal microscope. LPS induced a clear immunofluorescence signal of p65 translocation from the cytoplasm to the nucleus (Figure 5B). Pretreatment with 40 µM HOA dramatically decreased p65 translocation from the cytoplasm to the nucleus. Taken together, these results suggest that HOA attenuates the LPS-stimulated expression of iNOS, TNF-α, and IL-6 by inhibiting NF-κB activation. To assess the modulation of the signaling cascade related to NF-κB expression inhibition, we determined the conserved family of signal transduction enzymes involved in the PI3K/Akt and MAPK pathway. Intriguingly, HOA inhibited the phosphorylation of p85, PDK1, Akt, IκBα, ERK, and JNK in LPS-treated RAW264.7 cells compared with cells treated with LPS alone (Figure 6A,B). We also investigated the functional effect of the PI3K-Akt inhibitor. Pre-incubation of RAW264.7 cells with PI3K-Akt inhibitor significantly inhibited the upregulation of luciferase activity in NF-κB stimulated by LPS in a dose-dependent manner (Figure 6B).

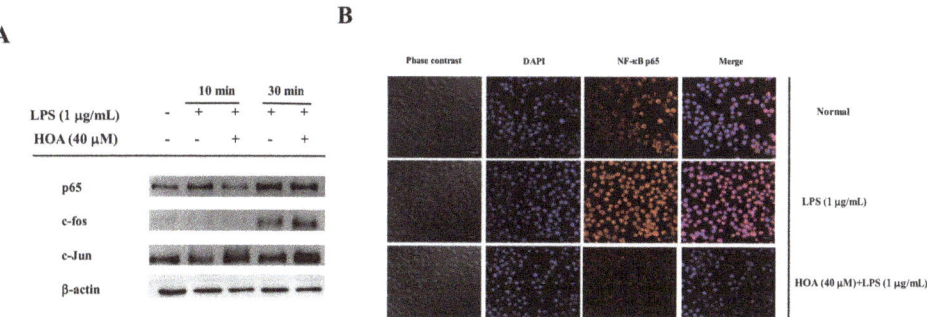

Figure 5. Effect of HOA on translocation of transcription factors in LPS-induced RAW264.7 cells. (**A**) Cells were plated at a density of 5×10^6 cells/dish in 60-mm culture dishes and treated with LPS and HOA for indicated time points. After preparation of the nuclear fraction, the protein expression levels of p65, c-Jun, and c-Fos were measured. (**B**) The localization of NF-κB p65 in the cytoplasm and nuclear were visualized by a confocal microscopy.

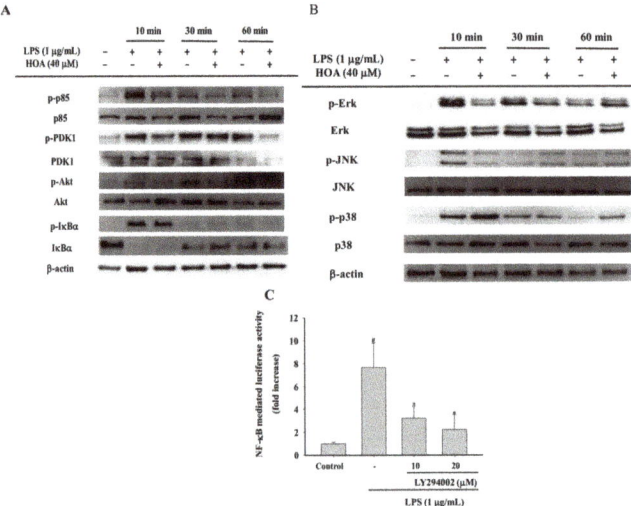

Figure 6. Effects of HOA on LPS-induced activation of PI3K/Akt and MAPKs signaling pathways. (**A**) Cells were plated at a density of 5×10^6 cells/dish in 60-mm culture dishes and treated with LPS and HOA for indicated time points. After preparation of the total protein, the phosphorylated and total forms of PDK1, p85, and Akt were measured by western blot. (**B**) Cells were plated at a density of 5×10^6 cells/dish in 60-mm culture dishes and treated with LPS and HOA for indicated time points. After preparation of the total protein, the phosphorylated and total forms of ERK, JNK, and p38 were measured by western blot. (**C**) Inhibitory effects of LY294002 on LPS-induced NF-κB-luc activity in RAW264.7 cells. Results are representative of three experiments. * indicates a significant difference between LPS group and LY294002 + LPS groups ($p < 0.05$). # indicates a significant difference between LPS group and the control group ($p < 0.05$).

3. Discussion

The pathology of inflammation is initiated by complex processes triggered by microbial pathogens, such as LPS, a prototypical endotoxin that is a component of the outer membranes of gram-negative bacteria [18]. LPS-stimulated macrophages produce reactive nitrogen species (RNS), reactive oxygen species (ROS), and pro-inflammation molecules and cytokines, such as IL-1β, MCP-1, IL-6, and TNF-α, through the TLR4-mediated signaling pathway [19,20]. Therefore, LPS-stimulated TLR4-mediated inflammatory mediators and cytokines have been widely used as excellent models for screening anti-inflammatory drugs and elucidating their underlying mechanisms [21]. The pro-inflammatory NF-κB pathway is central to the regulation of inflammation, and NF-κB is chronically active in many inflammatory diseases [22]. Therefore, it is regarded as a key contributor to the alleviation of inflammatory disorders. To date, numerous natural products have been considered as potential anti-inflammatory agents that can strongly scavenge inflammatory mediators [23–25].

Lupane-type triterpenoids are distributed among many plant families. Previous studies have shown that several lupane triterpenes exhibit a wide range of pharmacological effects and engage in important biological activities, especially those involving anti-inflammation, liver protection, anti-tumor processes, and immune system regulation [26–28]. Based on our previous activity-guide isolation work, this work was undertaken to clarify the anti-inflammatory potential of HOA on LPS-stimulated RAW264.7 macrophages and its potential mechanisms.

RNS play an important role in regulating multiple molecular targets related to acute and chronic inflammation [29,30]. NO is endogenous RNS and signaling molecules with a short half-life that is largely released at inflammatory sites and modulates various pathophysiological conditions [31]. Acute and chronic inflammation is induced by NO overproduction, which contributes to the damage of many biological molecules, in turn amplifying inflammation to cause cell death by inducing apoptosis [32]. For these reasons, increased attention is being paid to the development of natural agents for target therapies [33–35]. Several pro-inflammatory cytokines, including TNF-α, GM-CSF, IL-6, and IL-1β, are secreted at an early stage and play a critical role in inflammatory-related diseases [36]. TNF-α can regulate the cytokine cascade to stimulate the release of other pro-inflammatory cytokines, such as IL-1β and IL-6, which, in turn, enhance the recruitment of leukocytes to the site of inflammation [37]. IL-6 is a multifunctional cytokine that aggravates the pathogenic processes of autoimmune and inflammatory diseases, such as rheumatoid arthritis, multiple sclerosis, Castleman disease, and fever [38]. Therefore, agents derived from natural compounds that can block the production of these pro-inflammatory mediators could be developed as anti-inflammatory drug candidates. The result of an MTT assay showed that HOA had no significant cytotoxic effects at concentrations up to 40 µM (Figure 2A). Accordingly, the concentrations of HOA used in subsequent experiments were below 50 µM. The present data revealed that HOA significantly inhibited the production of NO, TNF-α, and IL-6 without affecting the cell viability in LPS-stimulated RAW264.7 cells (Figure 2A–D). The secretion of immune-related chemokines and cytokines requires a complicated signaling cascade for the transcriptional activation of inflammatory genes [39]. NO is regulated by three isoforms of NOS, including iNOS, neuronal NOS (nNOS), and endothelial NOS (eNOS). Of these, nNOS and eNOS are related to Ca^{2+}/calmodulin activity, whereas iNOS is key enzyme producing an overabundance of NO when induced by bacterial products, such as LPS [40]. Therefore, blocking NO and cytokine production by inhibiting mRNA expression may be a useful approach to the development of novel anti-inflammatory agents [41,42]. In our investigation, we found HOA could significantly inhibit the mRNA expression of iNOS, TNF-α, and IL-6, which was associated with inhibition of the production of NO and proinflammatory cytokines (Figure 4). It was similar to other natural compounds, such as xanthotoxin, cnidilide, and cirsimarin [43–45].

NF-κB and AP-1 are ubiquitous transcription factors that are activated during the inflammatory response to LPS to trigger the transcription of pro-inflammatory mediators and associated target genes, such as iNOS, COX-2, and TNF-α [46,47]. Previous literature showed that numerous compounds like poligalen, flavokawain A, and melittin inhibit cytokine production through inhibition nuclear translocation of AP-1 and NF-κB [25,48,49]. Interestingly, we found that HOA could attenuate the nuclear translocation of LPS-induced NF-κB p65 in RAW264.7 cells, whereas it did not affect the nuclear translocation of AP-1 (Figure 5A). The IKK kinase complex is the core element of the NF-κB cascade [50]. As the final confluence point of the inflammation signal, NF-κB participates in the regulation of TNF-α, IL-6, IL-1β, and other inflammatory mediators and plays a very important role in the inflammatory response [30]. In the absence of external stimuli, NF-κB is present in the cytoplasm in an inactive state through the formation of the NF-κB-IκBα complex with IκBs α/β). When cells are stimulated by external conditions, such as LPS, pro-inflammatory factors, and oxidative stress, the conformation of IκBs changes and it is degraded by ATP-dependent proteasomes, releasing Rel protein; a nuclear localization signal then activates NF-κB [51]. Activated NF-κB rapidly translocates into the nucleus after it is detached from IκBα and binds to the target gene κB locus to induce transcription of the target gene [52]. The upstream signaling molecules, including p85/PI3K, PDK1, Akt, ERK, JNK, and p38, are activated by LPS and have been demonstrated to play a vital role in NF-κB activation [53,54]. Additional experiments were carried out to investigate the upstream signaling molecules that could control the activation NF-κB. Similarly, the result showed that inhibiting PI3K can eliminate the phosphorylation of Akt, accompanied by inhibiting the phosphorylation of the proteins from IκBα (Figure 6A) and ultimately inhibiting the activation of NF-κB. Interestingly, the HOA remarkably suppressed the phosphorylation of ERK and JNK at early time point (Figure 6B). These results suggested that HOA inhibits LPS-induced phosphorylation of PI3K/Akt and MAPKs, and activation of NF-κB that similar to other anti-inflammatory agents, such as phlorofucofuroeckol A, cordycepin, and miyabenol A [55–57].

In summary, our findings showed for the first time that HOA, a lupane-type triterpene, inhibited the LPS-induced release of pro-inflammatory mediators by downregulating the PI3K/Akt and MAPKs signaling pathways. Large quantities of HOA are currently being prepared using a preparative HPLC method, and in vivo efficacy testing is being conducted to further understand the molecular mechanisms of HOA.

4. Materials and Methods

4.1. Chemicals and Reagents

HOA was isolated from the leaves of *M. bealei* in our lab and the purity of HOA was about 97% determined by high purity liquid chromatography (HPLC) with content of 0.0163% of the dry matter. The spectroscopic data (^{1}H-NMR, ^{13}C-NMR, and MS data) of HOA were well in accordance with the data reported in the literature [58]. Moreover, (3-4,5-dimethylthiazol-2-yl)-2,5-diphenyltetrazolium bromide (MTT), DAPI, sodium nitrite, dimethyl sulfoxide (DMSO), lipopolysaccharide (LPS), N-1-napthylethylenediamine dihydrochloride, and sulfanilamide were obtained from Sigma-Aldrich (St. Louis, MO, USA). NG-monomethyl-L-arginine (L-NMMA) was available from Beyotime (Haimen, Jiangsu, China). RPMI medium 1640 was purchased from Sigma-Aldrich (Irvine, UK). TRIzol Reagent for isolation of mRNA was obtained from Ambion (Austin, TX, USA). The fetal bovine serum (FBS) was from Corning (Medford, MA, USA). Penicillin–streptomycin solution (10,000 unit/10,000 µg/mL) was purchased from Invitrogen-Gibco (Carlsbad, CA, USA). Prolong Gold anti-fade reagent was obtained from Biomeda (Foster City, CA, USA). Protease and phosphatase inhibitors cocktail tablets were bought from Roche (Mannheim, Germany). SYBR real-time PCR kit was purchased from Bio-Rad (Hercules, CA, USA). The cytometric bead array (CBA) kit was purchased from BD (San Diego, CA, USA). The primary antibodies against p-Erk, Erk, p-JNK, JNK, p-p38, p38, p-PDK1, PDK1, PI3 kinase p85, p-Akt, Akt, p-IκBα, IκBα, c-Jun, c-Fos, NF-κB p65, and COX-2 were purchased from Cell Signalling Technology (Beverly, MA, USA). The other primary antibody including p-PI3 kinase p85/p55 was provided by Abcam (Cambridge, MA, USA). Secondary antibody goat anti-rabbit IgG H&L and goat anti-mouse antibodies were acquired from Abcam (Cambridge, MA, USA). All of the other chemicals and solvents were of analytical reagent grade.

4.2. Cell Culture and Cell Cytotoxicity Assay

RAW264.7 cell line was obtained from the American Type Culture Collection (Rockville, MD, USA). RAW264.7 cells were grown in RPMI 1640 medium supplemented with 10% (v/v) FBS and 1% antibiotics (v/v) (100 U/mL penicillin 100 µg/mL and streptomycin) and preserved in CO$_2$ incubator (SANYO, Tokyo, Japan). Cytotoxicity of HOA against RAW264.7 cells was evaluated by a conventional MTT assay, as previously described. Briefly, cells (1×10^6 cells/well) were cultured for 18 h in a 96-well plate and treated with different concentrations of HOA for an additional 24 h. The optical density (OD) was measured at 550 nm using a microplate reader (Tecan Infinite M200 Pro, Männedorf, Switzerland).

4.3. Determination of NO, TNF-α, and IL-6 Content

RAW264.7 macrophage cells were seeded in 96-well plate at a concentration of 1×10^6 cells/mL (100 µL/well) and 18 h. RAW264.7 cells pretreated with HOA or L-NMMA for 30 min were incubated with LPS (1 µg/mL) for 24 h. The NO content was determined by Griess reagent as described previously [59]. The secretion of TNF-α and IL-6 was measured using the flow cytometry (C6 Plus, BD Sceinces, Sparks, MD, USA), according to the manufacturer's guidelines.

4.4. Scanning Electron Microscopy (SEM)

RAW264.7 cells were seeded onto glass coverslips in 6-well plates at a density of 2×10^6 cells/mL (2 mL/well) for 18 h. RAW264.7 cells pretreated with HOA for 30 min were incubated with LPS (1 µg/mL) for 10 min. Hereafter, the cells were fixed in 2.5% glutaraldehyde for 1 h at 4 °C.

Next, the cells were washed with PBS three times (5 min each time) and dewatered using 30%, 50%, 70%, 90%, and 100% ethanol gradients two times (5 min each time). The fixed cells were observed with SEM (FEI Quanta 450 FEG, Hillsboro, OR, USA).

4.5. Quantitative Real-Time Reverse-Transcription Polymerase Chain Reaction (RT-qPCR) Analysis

RAW264.7 macrophage cells were seeded in 60-mm culture dishes at a density of 5×10^6 cells/well for 18 h. RAW264.7 cells pretreated with HOA for 30 min were incubated with LPS (1 µg/mL) for 6 h. Total RNA was isolated from cells using TRIzol reagent according to the standard protocol. Four micrograms of RNA were reverse transcribed to cDNA using RevertAid First Strand cDNA Synthesis Kit and respective gene expression was determined by CFX-96™ Real-Time instrument (Bio-Rad, Hercules, CA, USA) using the $2^{-\Delta\Delta Ct}$ method. The primers used were from Sangon Biotech (Shanghai, China) and were described in Table 1.

Table 1. The primer sequences for RT-qPCR.

Gene Name	Primer Squence (5'-3')
iNOS	F: CATTGATCTCCGTGACAGCC R: CATGCTACTGGAGGTGGGTG
IL-6	F: TGGGACTGATGCTGGTGACAAC R: AGCCTCCGACTTGTGAAGTGGT
TNF-α	F: TGCCTATGTCTCAGCCTCTTC
	R: GAGGCCATTTGGGAACTTCT
GAPDH	F: CACTCACGGCAAATTCAACGGCACA R: GACTCCACGACATACTCAGCAC

4.6. Western Blot Analysis

RAW264.7 macrophage cells were seeded in 60-mm culture dishes at a density of 5×10^6 cells/well for 18 h. RAW264.7 cells pretreated with HOA for 30 min were incubated with LPS (1 µg/mL) for the indicated time points. Commercial kits according to the manufacturer's instructions prepared the whole cell and nuclear lysates. Western blot analysis was performed as previously reported using the indicated antibodies [60].

4.7. Immunofluorescence and Confocal Microscopy

RAW264.7 macrophage cells were seeded sterile cover slips at a concentration of 1×10^6 cells/mL (2 mL/well) and placed in 35 mm petri dishes for 18 h. RAW264.7 cells pretreated with HOA for 30 min were incubated with LPS (1 µg/mL) for 10 min. The cells were washed three times with cold PBS, fixed in 4.0% paraformaldehyde for 15 min, and permeabilized with 0.5% Triton X-100 for 10 min. After that, the cells were blocked with 3% BSA/PBS for 1 h. Cells were then incubated with an NF-κB p65 antibody diluted in 3% BSA/PBS for 2 h. After incubation, cell were washed three times for 5 min with PBS, and incubated with Donkey Anti-Rabbit IgG H&L (Alexa Fluor® 4647) (Abcam, Cambridge, MA, USA) secondary antibody diluted in 3% BSA/PBS for 1 h. Cells were stained with 1 µg/mL DAPI solution and images were captured using a LSM700 confocal laser scanning microscope (Zeiss, Jena, Germany).

4.8. Transfections and Luciferase Assay

RAW264.7 macrophage cells were seeded in 12-well plate at a density of 5×10^4 cells/well for 18 h. RAW264.7 cells were then transfected with plasmids containing NF-κB using Lipofectamine 2000 (Invitrogen, Carlsbad, CA, USA). After 24 h, cells were pretreated with LY294002 for 30 min and then incubated with LPS (1 µg/mL) for additional of 24 h. The luciferase activity was carried out using the commercial kit from (Promega, Madison, WI, USA) according to the manufacturer's instruction.

4.9. Data Analysis

All analyses were performed using SPSS 19.0 package (SPSS Inc., Chicago, IL, USA) for Windows 7. Values shown represent the mean ± standard derivation (SD). Differences among samples were compared using a Duncan's multiple range test and *p*-values less than 5% were considered statistically different.

Author Contributions: All the authors listed below were involved in the study and they have approved the manuscript submission. Y.C., F.L., and Y.L. participated in the main experiment and edited the manuscript. F.L. participated in experimental design, data collection, and statistical analysis. Y.L., L.Z., S.L., R.X., and B.Y. participated in the experiment and provided literature. H.Z. and W.H. proposed the research concept, supervised the research, and were responsible for the revision and review of manuscripts.

Funding: This study was supported financially by National Natural Science Foundation of China (31600281), Natural Science Foundation of Jiangsu Province (BK20171269), and Qing Lan Project of Jiangsu Province.

Conflicts of Interest: The authors claim no conflict of interests.

Abbreviations

AP-1, activator protein 1; CBA, cytometric bead array; DMSO, dimethyl sulfoxide; eNOS, endothelial NOS; FBS, fetal bovine serum; HOA, 20-Hydroxy-3-oxolupan-28-oic acid; HPLC, High Purity Liquid Chromatography; IL-6, interleukin 6; iNOS, inducible NO synthase; IL-1β, interleukin-1β; JAK-STATs, Janus kinase/signal transducer and activator of transcription; L-NMMA, NG-monomethyl-L-arginine; LPS, lipopolysaccharide; MTT, (3-4,5-dimethylthiazol-2-yl)-2,5-diphenyltetrazolium bromide; MAPKs, mitogen-activated protein kinase; NF-κB, nuclear factor-κB; NO, nitric oxide; PGE_2, prostaglandin E2; PI3K, phosphatidylinositide 3-kinase; RNS, radical nitrogen species; ROS, reactive oxygen species; SEM, scanning electron microscopy; TNF-α, tumor necrosis factor-α.

References

1. Branzk, N.; Gronke, K.; Diefenbach, A. Innate lymphoid cells, mediators of tissue homeostasis, adaptation and disease tolerance. *Immunol. Rev.* **2018**, *286*, 86–101. [CrossRef] [PubMed]
2. Perez-Lopez, A.; Behnsen, J.; Nuccio, S.P.; Raffatellu, M. Mucosal immunity to pathogenic intestinal bacteria. *Nat. Rev. Immunol.* **2016**, *16*, 135–148. [CrossRef] [PubMed]
3. Belkai, Y.; Hand, T.W. Role of the microbiota in immunity and inflammation. *Cell* **2014**, *157*, 121–141. [CrossRef]
4. Ahmed, S.M.U.; Luo, L.; Namani, A.; Namani, A.; Wang, X.J.; Tang, X. Nrf2 signalling pathway: Pivotal roles in inflammation. *Bba-Mol. Basis Dis.* **2016**, *1863*, 585–597. [CrossRef] [PubMed]
5. Lavieri, R.; Rubartelli, A.; Carta, S. Redox stress unbalances the inflammatory cytokine network: Role in autoinflammatory patients and healthy subjects. *J. Leukoc. Biol.* **2016**, *99*, 79–86. [CrossRef] [PubMed]
6. Zhang, L.; Wang, C. Inflammatory response of macrophages in infection. *HBPD Int.* **2014**, *13*, 138–152. [CrossRef]
7. Wang, T.; He, C. Pro-inflammatory cytokines: The link between obesity and osteoarthritis. *Cytokine Growth Factor Rev.* **2018**, *44*, 38–54. [CrossRef] [PubMed]
8. Arora, S.; Dev, K.; Agarwal, B.; Das, P. Macrophages: Their role, activation and polarization in pulmonary diseases. *Immunobiology* **2017**, *223*, 383–396. [CrossRef] [PubMed]
9. Zhou, D.; Huang, C.; Lin, Z.; Zhan, S.; Kong, L.; Fang, C.; Li, J. Macrophage polarization and function with emphasis on the evolving roles of coordinated regulation of cellular signalling pathways. *Cell. Signal.* **2013**, *26*, 192–197. [CrossRef] [PubMed]
10. Park, M.H.; Hong, J. Roles of NF-κB in cancer and inflammatory diseases and their therapeutic approaches. *Cells* **2016**, *5*, 15. [CrossRef] [PubMed]
11. Zhang, Q.; Lenardo, M.J.; Baltimore, D. 30 Years of NF-κB: A blossoming of relevance to human pathobiology. *Cell* **2017**, *168*, 37–57. [CrossRef] [PubMed]
12. He, J.; Mu, Q. The medicinal uses of the genus *Mahonia* in traditional Chinese medicine: An ethnopharmacological, phytochemical and pharmacological review. *J. Ethnopharmacol.* **2015**, *175*, 668–683. [CrossRef] [PubMed]

13. Hu, W.; Wu, L.; Qiang, Q.; Ji, L.; Wang, X.; Luo, H.; Wu, H.; Jiang, H.; Wang, G.; Shen, T. The dichloromethane fraction from *Mahonia bealei* (Fort.) Carr. leaves exerts an anti-inflammatory effect both in vitro and in vivo. *J. Ethnopharmacol.* **2016**, *188*, 134–143. [CrossRef] [PubMed]
14. Zhang, L.; Zhu, W.; Zhang, Y.; Yang, B.; Fu, Z.; Li, X.; Tian, J. Proteomics analysis of *Mahonia bealei* leaves with induction of alkaloids via combinatorial peptide ligand libraries. *J. Proteom.* **2014**, *110*, 59–71. [CrossRef]
15. Hu, W.; Yu, L.; Wang, M.H. Antioxidant and antiproliferative properties of water extract from *Mahonia bealei* (Fort.) Carr. Leaves. *Food Chem. Toxicol.* **2011**, *49*, 799–806. [CrossRef] [PubMed]
16. Zeng, X.; Dong, Y.; Sheng, G.; Dong, X.; Sun, X.; Fu, J. Isolation and structure determination of anti-influenza component from *Mahonia bealei*. *J. Ethnopharmacol.* **2006**, *108*, 317–319. [CrossRef] [PubMed]
17. Zhang, S.L.; Li, H.; He, X.; Zhang, R.Q.; Sun, Y.H.; Zhang, C.F.; Wang, C.Z.; Yuan, C.S. Alkaloids from *Mahonia bealei* posses anti-H+/K+-ATPase and anti-gastrin effects on pyloric ligation-induced gastric ulcer in rats. *Phytomedicine* **2014**, *21*, 1356–1363. [CrossRef]
18. Kohoutková, M.; Korimová, A.; Brázda, V.; Kohoutek, J. Early inflammatory profiling of schwannoma cells induced by lipopolysaccharide. *Histochem. Cell Biol.* **2017**, *148*, 607–615. [CrossRef]
19. Kai, K.; Zhou, X.; Wong, H.L.; Ng, C.F.; Fu, W.M.; Leung, P.C.; Peng, G.; Ko, C.H. In vivo and in vitro anti-inflammatory effects of Zao-Jiao-Ci (the spine of *Gleditsia sinensis* Lam.) aqueous extract and its mechanisms of action. *J. Ethnopharmacol.* **2016**, *192*, 192–200.
20. Liu, L.; Chen, L.; Jiang, C.; Xie, Y.; Cheng, Z. Berberine inhibits the LPS-induced proliferation and inflammatory response of stromal cells of adenomyosis tissues mediated by the LPS/TLR4 signalling pathway. *Exp. Ther. Med.* **2017**, *14*, 6125. [CrossRef]
21. Cuadrado, I.; Amesty, A.; Cedrón, J.C.; Oberti, J.C.; Estévez-Braun, A.; Hortelano, S.; Heras, B. Semisynthesis and Inhibitory Effects of Solidagenone Derivatives on TLR-Mediated Inflammatory Responses. *Molecules* **2018**, *23*, 3197. [CrossRef] [PubMed]
22. Oh, W.J.; Jung, U.; Eom, H.S.; Shin, H.J.; Park, H.R. Inhibition of Lipopolysaccharide-Induced Proinflammatory Responses by *Buddleja officinalis* Extract in BV-2 Microglial Cells via Negative Regulation of NF-κB and ERK1/2 Signalling. *Molecules* **2013**, *18*, 9195–9206. [CrossRef]
23. Kim, E.A.; Kim, S.Y.; Ye, B.R.; Kim, J.; Ko, S.C.; Lee, W.W.; Kim, K.N.; Choi, I.W.; Jung, W.K.; Heo, S.J. Anti-inflammatory effect of Apo-9′-fucoxanthinone via inhibition of MAPKs and NF-κB signalling pathway in LPS-stimulated RAW264.7 macrophages and zebrafish model. *Int. Immunopharmacol.* **2018**, *59*, 339–346. [CrossRef] [PubMed]
24. Lu, X.; Min, L.; Wei, J.; Gou, H.; Bao, Z.; Wang, Z.; Huang, Y.; An, B. Heliangin inhibited lipopolysaccharide-induced inflammation through signalling NF-κB pathway on LPS-induced RAW264.7 cells. *Biomed. Pharmacother.* **2017**, *88*, 102–108. [CrossRef] [PubMed]
25. Silva, D.F.; Alves, C.Q.; Brandão, H.N.; David, J.P.; Silva, R.L.; Franchin, M.; Cunha, T.M.; Martins, F.T.; Oliveirra, C.M. Poligalen, a new coumarin from *Polygala boliviensis*, reduces the release of TNF and IL-6 independent of NF-κB downregulation. *Fitoterapia* **2016**, *113*, 139–143. [CrossRef] [PubMed]
26. Bian, X.; Zhao, Y.; Guo, X.; Liu, J. Chiisanoside, a triterpenoid saponin, exhibits anti-tumor activity by promoting apoptosis and inhibiting angiogenesis. *RSC Adv.* **2017**, *7*, 41640–41650. [CrossRef]
27. Zhu, J.; Yang, H.; Li, Z.H.; Wang, G.K.; Feng, T.; Liu, J.K. Anti-inflammatory lupane triterpenoids from *Menyanthes trifoliata*. *J. Asian Nat. Prod. Res.* **2018**, 1–6. [CrossRef] [PubMed]
28. Mabhida, S.E.; Dludla, P.V.; Johnson, R.N.; Ndlovu, M.L.; Johan, O.; Andy, R.M.; Rebamang, A. Protective effect of triterpenes against diabetes-induced β-cell damage: An overview of in vitro and in vivo studies. *Pharmacol. Res.* **2018**, *137*, 179–192. [CrossRef] [PubMed]
29. Hotamisligil, G.S. Inflammation, metaflammation and immunometabolic disorders. *Nature* **2017**, *542*, 177–185. [CrossRef] [PubMed]
30. Afonina, I.S.; Zhang, Z.; Karin, M.; Beyaert, R. Limiting inflammation-the negative regulation of NF-κB and the NLRP3 inflammasome. *Nat. Immunol.* **2017**, *542*, 861–869. [CrossRef] [PubMed]
31. Moldogazieva, N.T.; Mokhosoev, I.M.; Feldman, N.B.; Lutsenko, S.V. ROS and RNS signalling: Adaptive redox switches through oxidative/nitrosative protein modifications. *Free Radic Res.* **2018**, *52*, 507–543. [CrossRef]
32. Kipanyula, M.J.; Etet, P.F.S.; Vecchio, L.; Farahna, M.; Nukenine, E.; Kamdje, A.H.N. Signalling pathways bridging microbial-triggered inflammation and cancer. *Cell. Signal.* **2013**, *25*, 403–416. [CrossRef]

33. Takano, K.; Ishida, N.; Kawabe, K.; Moriyama, M.; Hibino, S.; Choshi, T.; Hori, O.; Nakamura, Y. A dibenzoylmethane derivative inhibits lipopolysaccharide-induced NO production in mouse microglial cell line BV-2. *Neurochem. Int.* **2018**, *119*, 126–131. [CrossRef]
34. Zhang, S.; Li, Z.; Stadler, M.; Chen, H.P.; Huang, Y.; Gan, X.Q.; Feng, T.; Liu, J.K. Lanostane triterpenoids from *Tricholoma pardinum* with NO production inhibitory and cytotoxic activities. *Phytochemistry* **2018**, *152*, 105–112. [CrossRef]
35. Cao, T.; Tran, M.H.; Kim, J.A.; Tran, P.T.; Lee, J.H.; WOO, M.H.; Lee, H.K.; Min, B.S. Inhibitory effects of compounds from *Styrax obassia* on NO production. *Bioorg. Med. Chem. Lett.* **2015**, *25*, 5087–5091. [CrossRef]
36. Valilou, S.F.; Keshavarz-Fathi, M.; Silvestris, N.; Argentiero, A.; Rezaei, N. The role of inflammatory cytokines and tumor associated macrophages (TAMs) in microenvironment of pancreatic cancer. *Cytokine Growth Factor Rev.* **2018**, *39*, 46–61. [CrossRef]
37. Mao, R.; Zhang, C.; Chen, J.; Zhao, G. Different levels of pro- and anti-inflammatory cytokines in patients with unipolar and bipolar depression. *J. Affect. Disord.* **2018**, *237*, 65–72. [CrossRef]
38. Naseem, S.; Hussain, T.; Manzoor, S. Interleukin-6: A promising cytokine to support liver regeneration and adaptive immunity in liver pathologies. *Cytokine Growth Factor Rev.* **2018**, *39*, 39–45. [CrossRef]
39. Rahimifard, M.; Maqbool, F.; Moeini-Nodeh, S.; Niaz, K.; Abdollahi, M.; Braidy, N.; Nabavi, S.M.; Nabavi, S.F. Targeting the TLR4 signalling pathway by poly Anti-inflammatory potential of hentriacontane in LPS stimulated RAW264.7 cells and mice model phenols: A novel therapeutic strategy for neuroinflammation. *Ageing Res. Rev.* **2017**, *36*, 11–19. [CrossRef]
40. Chong, C.; Ai, N.; Ke, M.; Tan, Y.; Huang, Z.; Li, Y.; Lu, J.H.; Ge, W.; Su, H. Roles of Nitric Oxide Synthase Isoforms in Neurogenesis. *Mol. Neurobiol.* **2018**, *55*, 2645–2652. [CrossRef]
41. Genovese, S.; Taddeo, V.A.; Fiorito, S.; Epifano, F.; Marrelli, M.; Conforti, F. Inhibition of nitric oxide production by natural oxyprenylated coumarins and alkaloids in RAW264.7 cells. *Phytochem. Lett.* **2017**, *20*, 181–185. [CrossRef]
42. Khajuria, V.; Gupta, S.; Sharma, N.; Kumar, A.; Lone, N.A.; Khullar, M.; Dutt, P.; Sharma, P.R.; Bhagat, A.; Ahmed, Z. Anti-inflammatory potential of hentriacontane in LPS stimulated RAW264.7 cells and mice model. *Biomed. Pharmacother.* **2017**, *92*, 175–186. [CrossRef]
43. Han, H.; Shin, J.; Lee, S.; Park, J.C.; Lee, K.T. Cirsimarin, a flavone glucoside from the aerial part of *Cirsium japonicum* var. *ussuriense* (Regel) Kitam. ex Ohwi, suppresses the JAK/STAT and IRF-3 signalling pathway in LPS-stimulated RAW264.7 macrophages. *Chem. Biol. Interact.* **2018**, *293*, 38–47. [CrossRef]
44. Lee, W.S.; Shin, J.S.; Jang, D.S.; Lee, K.T. Cnidilide, an alkylphthalide isolated from the roots of *Cnidium officinale*, suppresses LPS-induced NO, PGE$_2$, IL-1β, IL-6 and TNF-α production by AP-1 and NF-κB inactivation in RAW264.7 macrophages. *Int. Immunopharmacol.* **2016**, *40*, 146–155. [CrossRef]
45. Lee, S.; Lee, W.S.; Shin, J.; Jang, D.S.; Lee, K.T. Xanthotoxin suppresses LPS-induced expression of iNOS, COX-2, TNF-α, and IL-6 via AP-1, NF-κB, and JAK-STAT inactivation in RAW264.7 macrophages. *Int. Immunopharmacol.* **2017**, *49*, 21–29. [CrossRef]
46. Chen, C.; Peng, W.; Tsai, K.D.; Hsu, S.L. Luteolin suppresses inflammation-associated gene expression by blocking NF-κB and AP-1 activation pathway in mouse alveolar macrophages. *Life Sci.* **2007**, *81*, 1602–1614. [CrossRef]
47. Jung, D.H.; Park, H.J.; Byun, H.E.; Park, Y.M.; Kim, T.W.; Kim, B.O.; Um, S.H.; Pyo, S. Diosgenin inhibits macrophage-derived inflammatory mediators through downregulation of CK2, JNK, NF-κB and AP-1 activation. *Int. Immunopharmacol.* **2010**, *10*, 1047–1054. [CrossRef]
48. Kwon, D.J.; Ju, S.M.; Youn, G.S.; Choi, S.Y.; Park, J. Suppression of iNOS and COX-2 expression by flavokawain A via blockade of NF-κB and AP-1 activation in RAW264.7 macrophages. *Food Chem. Toxicol.* **2013**, *58*, 479–486. [CrossRef]
49. Jeong, Y.J.; Shin, J.M.; Bae, Y.S.; Cho, H.J.; Park, K.K.; Choe, J.Y.; Han, S.M.; Moon, S.K.; Kim, W.J.; Choi, Y.H.; et al. Melittin has a chondroprotective effect by inhibiting MMP-1 and MMP-8 expressions via blocking NF-κB and AP-1 signalling pathway in chondrocytes. *Int. Immunopharmacol.* **2015**, *25*, 400–405. [CrossRef]
50. Paul, A.; Edwards, J.; Pepper, C.; Mackay, S. Inhibitory-κB Kinase (IKK) α and Nuclear Factor-κB (NF-κB)-Inducing Kinase (NIK) as anti-cancer drug targets. *Cells* **2018**, *7*, 176. [CrossRef]
51. Courtois, G.; Fauvarque, M.O. The many roles of ubiquitin in NF-κB signaling. *Biomedicines* **2018**, *6*, 43. [CrossRef]

52. Durham, W.J.; Li, Y.P.; Gerken, E.; Eric, G.; Farid, M.; Arbogast, S.; Wolfe, R.R.; Reid, M.B. Fatiguing exercise reduces DNA binding activity of NF-kappaB in skeletal muscle nuclei. *J. Appl. Physiol.* **2004**, *97*, 1740–1745. [CrossRef]
53. Covarrubias, A.J.; Aksoylar, H.I.; Horng, T. Control of macrophage metabolism and activation by mTOR and Akt signaling. *Semin. Immunol.* **2015**, *27*, 286–296. [CrossRef]
54. Yoo, S.; Kim, M.Y.; Cho, J.Y. Syk and Src-targeted anti-inflammatory activity of aripiprazole, an atypical antipsychotic. *Biochem. Pharmacol.* **2018**, *148*, 1–12. [CrossRef]
55. Kim, A.R.; Lee, M.S.; Shin, T.S.; Hua, H.; Jang, B.C.; Choi, J.S.; Byun, D.S.; Utstuki, T.; Ingram, D.; Kim, H.R. Phlorofucofuroeckol A inhibits the LPS-stimulated iNOS and COX-2 expressions in macrophages via inhibition of NF-κB, Akt, and p38 MAPK. *Toxicol. In Vitro* **2011**, *25*, 1789–1795. [CrossRef]
56. Kim, H.G.; Shrestha, B.; Lim, S.Y.; Yoon, D.H.; Chang, W.C.; Shin, D.J.; Han, S.K.; Park, J.H.; Park, H.I.; Sung, J.M.; et al. Cordycepin inhibits lipopolysaccharide-induced inflammation by the suppression of NF-κB through Akt and p38 inhibition in RAW 264.7 macrophage cells. *Eur. J. Clin. Pharmacol.* **2006**, *545*, 192–199. [CrossRef]
57. Ku, K.Y.; Huang, Y.L.; Huang, Y.J.; Chiou, W.F. Miyabenol A Inhibits LPS-Induced NO Production via IKK/IκB Inactivation in RAW 264.7 Macrophages: Possible Involvement of the p38 and PI3K Pathways. *J. Agric. Food Chem.* **2008**, *56*, 8911–8918. [CrossRef]
58. EL-Gamal, A. Cytotoxic lupane secolupane and oleanane type triterpenes from *Viburnum awabuki*. *Nat. Prod. Res.* **2008**, *22*, 191–197. [CrossRef]
59. Hu, W.; Wang, X.; Wu, L.; Shen, T.; Zhao, X.; Si, C.L.; Jiang, Y.; Wang, G. Apigenin-7-O-β-D-glucuronide inhibits LPS-induced inflammation through the inactivation of AP-1 and MAPK signalling pathways in RAW264.7 macrophages and protects mice against endotoxin shock. *Food Funct.* **2016**, *7*, 1002–1013. [CrossRef]
60. Bai, Y.; Jiang, Y.; Liu, T.; Li, F.; Zhang, J.; Luo, Y.; Zhang, L.; Yan, G.; Feng, Z.; Li, X.; et al. Xinjiang herbal tea exerts immunomodulatory activity via TLR2/4-mediated MAPK signalling pathways in RAW264.7 cells and prevents cyclophosphamide-induced immunosuppression in mice. *J. Ethnopharmacol.* **2019**, *228*, 179–187. [CrossRef]

Sample Availability: Samples of the compounds are available from the authors.

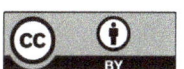

© 2019 by the authors. Licensee MDPI, Basel, Switzerland. This article is an open access article distributed under the terms and conditions of the Creative Commons Attribution (CC BY) license (http://creativecommons.org/licenses/by/4.0/).

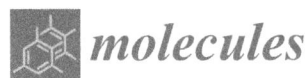

Article

Anti-Inflammatory and Anti-Oxidant Activity of *Portulaca oleracea* Extract on LPS-Induced Rat Lung Injury

Vafa Baradaran Rahimi [1,2,†], Hassan Rakhshandeh [1,†], Federica Raucci [3], Benedetta Buono [3], Reza Shirazinia [4], Alireza Samzadeh Kermani [5], Francesco Maione [3,*], Nicola Mascolo [3] and Vahid Reza Askari [1,6,*]

[1] Pharmacological Research Center of Medicinal Plants, Mashhad University of Medical Sciences, Mashhad 9177948564, Iran; baradaranv941@mums.ac.ir (V.B.R.); rakhshandehh@mums.ac.ir (H.R.)
[2] Department of Pharmacology, Faculty of Medicine, Mashhad University of Medical Sciences, Mashhad 9177948564, Iran
[3] Department of Pharmacy, School of Medicine and Surgery, University of Naples Federico II, Via Domenico Montesano 49, 80131 Naples, Italy; federicaraucci@gmail.com (F.R.); bened.buono@gmail.com (B.B.); nicola.mascolo@unina.it (N.M.)
[4] Department of Pharmacology, Faculty of Veterinary Medicine, University of Tehran, Tehran 1419963111, Iran; Rezashirazinia@ut.ac.ir
[5] Department of Chemistry, Faculty of Science, University of Zabol, Zabol 35856-98613, Iran; arsamzadeh@yahoo.com
[6] Neurogenic Inflammation Research Centre, Mashhad University of Medical Sciences, Mashhad 9177948564, Iran
* Correspondence: francesco.maione@unina.it (F.M.); askariv941@mums.ac.ir or Vahidrezaaskary@yahoo.com (V.R.A.); Tel.: +39-081678429 (F.M.); +98-513-8002-262 (V.R.A.); Fax: +98-513-8828564 (V.R.A.)
† These authors share first co-authorship.

Received: 16 December 2018; Accepted: 26 December 2018; Published: 1 January 2019

Abstract: Acute lung injury (ALI) and acute respiratory distress syndrome (ARDS) are classified as two lung complications arising from various conditions such as sepsis, trauma, and lung inflammation. Previous studies have shown that the extract of the leaves of *Portulaca oleracea* (PO) possesses anti-inflammatory and anti-oxidant activities. In the present study, the effects of PO (50–200 mg/kg) and dexamethasone (Dexa; 1.5 mg/kg) on lipopolysaccharide (LPS)-induced ALI were investigated. Subsequentially, the lung wet/dry ratio; white blood cells (WBC); levels of nitric oxide (NO); myeloperoxidase (MPO); malondialdehyde (MDA); thiol groups formation; super oxide dismutase (SOD) and catalase (CAT) activities; and levels of interleukin (IL)-1β, tumor necrosis factor (TNF)-α, IL-6, IL-10, prostaglandin E2 (PGE_2), and transforming growth factor (TGF)-β in the broncho alveolar lavage fluid (BALF) were evaluated in order to demonstrate the anti-oxidant and anti-inflammatory activity of PO. Our results show that PO suppresses lung inflammation by the reduction of IL-β, IL-6, TNF-α, PGE_2, and TGF-β, as well as by the increase of IL-10 levels. We also found that PO improves the level of WBC, MPO, and MDA, as well as thiol group formation and SOD and CAT activities, compared with the LPS group. The results of our investigation also show that PO significantly decreased the lung wet/dry ratio as an index of interstitial edema. Taken together, our findings reveal that PO extract dose-dependently displays anti-oxidant and anti-inflammatory activity against LPS-induced rat ALI, paving the way for rational use of PO as a protective agent against lung-related inflammatory disease.

Keywords: acute lung injury; *Portulaca oleracea*; inflammation

1. Introduction

Inflammation plays a dual protective and damaging role against cellular and tissue damages. Acute inflammation is usually considered a protective role to destroy and remove the noxious stimuli and injured tissues, thereby allowing the tissue repair. When this process becomes uncontrolled, another face of inflammation appears. In this regard, acute lung injury (ALI) and acute respiratory distress syndrome (ARDS) are known as two inflammatory lung complications with a high rate of morbidity and mortality [1,2]. These are characterized by severe pulmonary inflammation, massive recruitment of neutrophils and lymphocytes in interstitial tissue, edema, disruption of epithelial integrity, and the injury of lung parenchyma [3]. ALI and ARDS result from various diseases and pathological conditions such as trauma, pneumonia, sepsis, and endotoxemia [4,5].

Despite the great efforts to find new and/or most active pharmacological approaches for ALI/ARDS treatment and the discovery of the pathological factors, their mortality still presents a high rate (about of 40%) [6,7]. On this basis, the need for new therapeutic agents in the field of lung inflammatory-based diseases has prompted the investigation of several plant-based products for potential therapeutic application [8,9]. Portulaca oleracea (PO) belongs to the Portulacaceae family, commonly called qurfeh (Persia), purslane (the USA and Australia), pigweed (England), rigla (Egypt), pourpier (France), and Ma-Chi-Xian (China) [10]. This plant is commonly found in tropical and subtropical areas of the world, as well as in many regions of the United States, Mediterranean, and tropical Asian countries [11]. It has been used as a folk medicine in many countries for its febrifuge, antiseptic, and anthelmintic properties [12]. Congruently, it has been reported that PO exhibits great pharmacological properties including anti-oxidant [13], antibacterial [14], anti-ulcerogenic [15], anti-inflammatory [16], and wound-healing properties [17,18]. Indeed, recent studies have demonstrated that Oleracone, an alkaloid isolated from PO, attenuates inflammation induced by lipopolysaccharide (LPS) in RAW 264.7 macrophage cell lines [19] and that the extract of the leaves of PO possesses anti-inflammatory and immunomodulatory properties on Th1/Th2 lymphocytes profile [20]. It has also been reported that treatment of ovalbumin-sensitized rats with PO extract displays a modulation of lung inflammation and immune markers [21].

Lipopolysaccharide (LPS) is known as the predominant microbial inducer of inflammation processes accountable for the strong innate immune responses in ALI onset [5,22]. Alveolar epithelial cells (AECs) are the first cells faced by pathogenic microorganisms playing a central role in the beginning and progression of acute lung injury, followed by massive recruitment of neutrophils and lymphocytes [2,23]. Moreover, it has also been demonstrated that inflammation, due to inflammatory cyto-chemokines (in particular interleukin (IL)-6 and tumor necrosis factor (TNF)-α), plays an important role in lung injury onset [24,25] and the first innate immune response [26]. Therefore, in the present study, we aimed to investigate a new possible medication regarding the anti-inflammatory properties of PO for ALI using the LPS-induced animal model of ALI and lung inflammation. In the present study, we extended the previous observations about protective effects of PO, and shed new light on its anti-inflammatory and anti-oxidant mechanism of action.

2. Results

2.1. Effects of LPS and PO on Body and Absolute Organ Weights, and Lung Wet/Dry Ratio

LPS (5 mg/kg) significantly elevated the absolute organs weights (lung, $p \leq 0.001$; liver $p \leq 0.01$; and heart, $p \leq 0.001$) compared with the control group (Table 1). PO at doses of 50 mg/kg ($p \leq 0.01$), 100 mg/kg ($p \leq 0.001$), and 200 mg/kg ($p \leq 0.001$), as well as Dexa (1.5 mg/kg, $p \leq 0.001$) significantly attenuated the absolute lung weight compared with the LPS group (Table 1). Moreover, PO (200 mg/kg) and Dexa (1.5 mg/kg) notably decreased the increased absolute weights of liver ($p \leq 0.01$) and heart ($p \leq 0.001$) compared with the LPS group (Table 1). LPS at 5 mg/kg significantly increased lung wet/dry ratio compared with the control group (Figure 1, $p \leq 0.001$). PO at doses of 100 mg/kg

($p \leq 0.05$) and 200 mg/kg ($p \leq 0.001$) and Dexa ($p \leq 0.001$) at 1.5 mg/kg significantly reverted the lung wet/dry ratio increase compared with the LPS group (Figure 1).

Table 1. Body and absolute organs weights for different groups.

	C	LPS	Dexa	PO 50 mg/kg	PO 100 mg/kg	PO 200 mg/kg
Body weight (g)	220 ± 31	218 ± 22	208 ± 19	215 ± 21	223 ± 22	231 ± 19
Lung (g)	1.05 ± 0.08 ***	2.78 ± 0.15	1.28 ± 0.07 ***	1.87 ± 0.14 **	1.61 ± 0.09 ***	1.23 ± 0.11 ***
Liver (g)	5.41 ± 1.21 **	7.94 ± 1.24	5.77 ± 1.06 **	8.01 ± 1.28	7.23 ± 1.18	5.69 ± 1.13 **
Heart (g)	0.86 ± 0.08 ***	1.21 ± 0.09	0.89 ± 0.12 ***	1.17 ± 0.07	1.05 ± 0.17	0.83 ± 0.12 ***

Data are presented as means ± SD (n = 6). ** $p \leq 0.01$ and *** $p \leq 0.001$. PO—Portulaca oleracea.

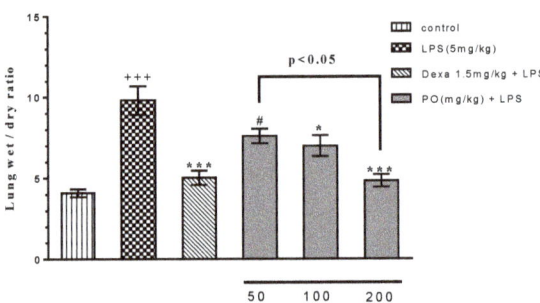

Figure 1. Effect of Portulaca oleracea (PO) extract on the lung wet/dry ratio in broncho alveolar lavage fluid (BALF). Data were presented as mean ± standard error of measurement (SEM) (n = 6). +++ $p \leq 0.001$ compared with the control group, * $p \leq 0.05$ and *** $p \leq 0.001$ compared with the lipopolysaccharide (LPS) group, and # $p \leq 0.05$ compared with the Dexa + LPS group.

2.2. Effects of LPS and PO on Bronchoalveolar Lavage Fluid (BALF) Hematologic Indices

Our results revealed that LPS treatment significantly modified hematologic indices of neutrophil, basophil, eosinophil, and monocyte/macrophage, as well as total white blood cells (Figure 2A–E, $p \leq 0.001$) and lymphocytes (Figure 2F, $p \leq 0.001$). Notably, PO extract (100 and 200 mg/kg) and Dexa (1.5 mg/kg) markedly reverted hematologic indices (Figure 2A–E, $p \leq 0.05$ to 0.001) and lymphocytes reduction (Figure 2F, $p \leq 0.001$).'

2.3. Effects of LPS and PO Extract on BALF Inflammatory Cytokines

LPS significantly increased the production of inflammatory cytokines including IL-1β (Figure 3A, $p \leq 0.001$), TNF-α (Figure 3B, $p \leq 0.001$), IL-6 (Figure 3C, $p \leq 0.001$), IL-10 (Figure 3D, $p \leq 0.05$), PGE$_2$ (Figure 3E, $p \leq 0.001$), and TGF-β (Figure 3F, $p \leq 0.001$) compared with the control group. Treatment with Dexa at 1.5mg/kg significantly decreased all measured parameters compared with the LPS group (Figure 3A–F, $p \leq 0.01$ to 0.001 for all cases). Interestingly, PO at doses of 100 and 200 mg/kg significantly modulated the expression of IL-1β, TNF-α, IL-6, PGE$_2$, and TGF-β, and the increase of increment in IL-10 level compared with the LPS group (Figure 3A–F, $p \leq 0.05$ to 0.001 for all cases).

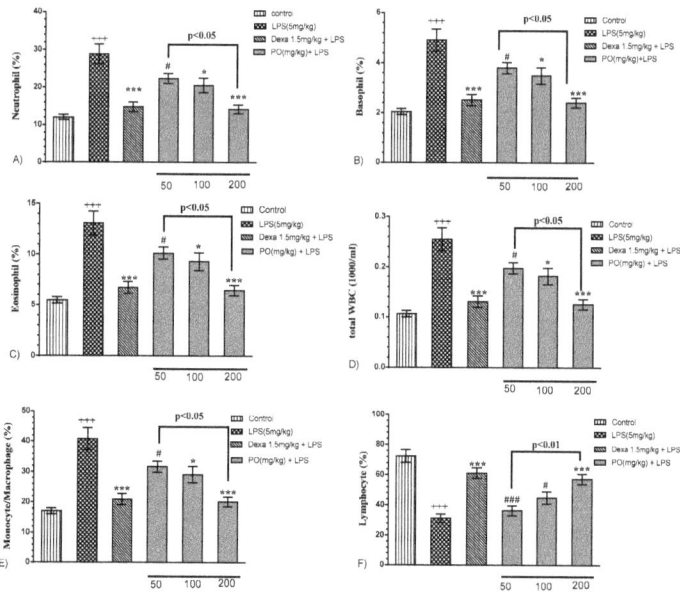

Figure 2. Effect of PO extract on hematologic indices (**A**) neutrophil, (**B**) basophil, (**C**) eosinophil, (**D**) total white blood cell, (**E**) monocyte/macrophage ratio, and (**F**) lymphocyte in BALF. Data were presented as mean ± SEM (n = 5). +++ $p \leq 0.001$ compared with the control group, * $p \leq 0.05$ and *** $p \leq 0.001$ compared with the LPS-induced group and # $p \leq 0.05$ and ### $p \leq 0.001$ compared with the Dexa + LPS group. WBC—white blood cells.

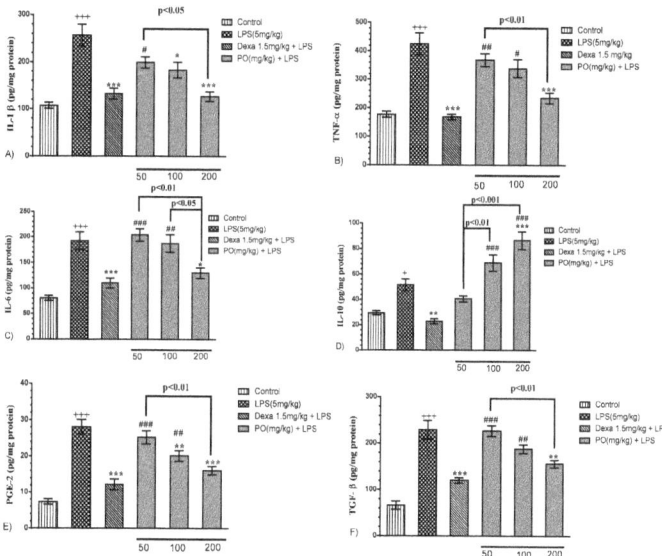

Figure 3. Effects of PO extract on inflammatory and anti-inflammatory biomarkers (**A**) interleukin (IL)-1β, (**B**) TNF-α, (**C**) IL-6, (**D**) IL-10, (**E**) PGE$_2$, and (**F**) TGF-β in BALF. Data were presented as mean ± SEM (n = 7). + $p \leq 0.05$ and +++ $p \leq 0.001$ compared with the control group; * $p \leq 0.05$, ** $p \leq 0.01$, and *** $p \leq 0.001$ compared with the LPS-induced group; and # $p \leq 0.05$, ## $p \leq 0.01$, and ### $p \leq 0.001$ compared with the Dexa + LPS group.

2.4. Impact of PO on the BALF Oxidant/Antioxidant Status

LPS notably increased malondialdehyde (MDA), myeloperoxidase (MPO), and nitric oxide (NO) levels, and contextually decreased super oxide dismutase SOD and catalase (CAT) activity, as well as thiol content, compared with the control group (Figure 4A–C, $p \leq 0.001$). However, PO (100 and 200 mg/kg) and Dexa (1.5 mg/kg) groups significantly decreased MDA, MPO, and NO levels (Figure 4A–C, $p \leq 0.05$ to 0.001) and reverted oxidant/anti-oxidant status that resulted in a significant increase in the levels of SOD ($p \leq 0.001$) and catalase ($p \leq 0.001$) activity, as well as total thiol content ($p \leq 0.001$) (Figure 5).

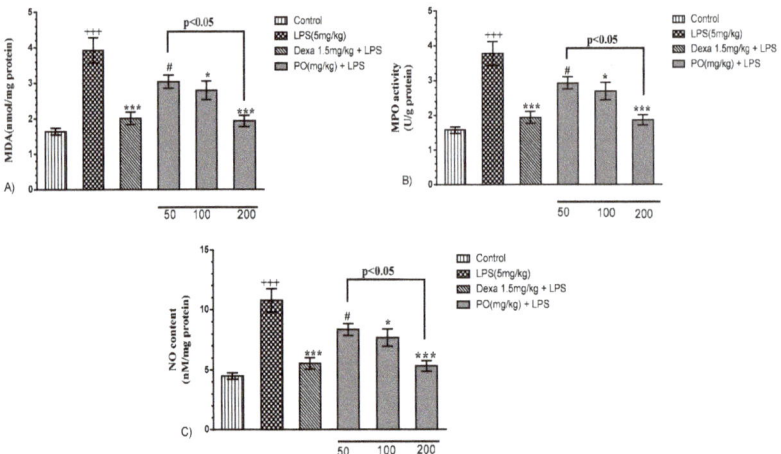

Figure 4. Effects of PO extract on oxidative indices: (**A**) malondialdehyde (MDA), (**B**) myeloperoxidase (MPO), and (**C**) NO in BALF and lung tissue. Data were presented as mean ± SEM ($n = 7$). $^{+++}$ $p \leq 0.001$ compared with the control group, * $p \leq 0.05$ and *** $p \leq 0.001$ compared with the LPS-induced group, and $^{\#}$ $p \leq 0.05$ compared with the Dexa + LPS group.

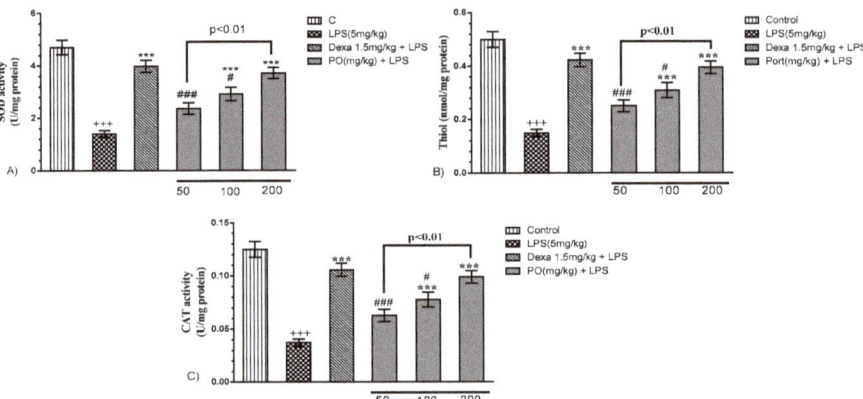

Figure 5. Effects of PO extract on anti-oxidative indices: (**A**) SOD, (**B**) thiol, and (**C**) catalase (CAT) in BALF and lung tissue. Data were presented as mean ± SEM ($n = 6$). $^{+++}$ $p \leq 0.001$ compared with the control group, *** $p \leq 0.001$ compared with the LPS-induced group, $^{\#}$ $p \leq 0.05$ and $^{\#\#\#}$ $p \leq 0.001$ compared with the Dexa + LPS group.

2.5. Characteristics of PO Hydro-Ethanolic Extract

HPLC peaks from PO extract chromatogram appeared at 320 nm (Figure 6B). Using the H-NMR method, we also detected the peaks at 220 and 320 nm between 8 and 12 min ascribed to kaempferol and apigenin derivatives, respectively (Figure 6A,B).

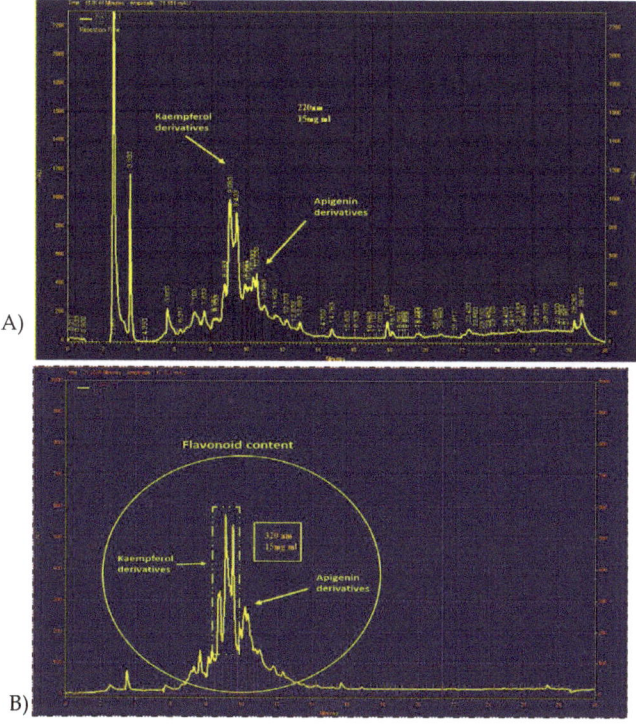

Figure 6. HPLC fingerprint of the hydro-ethanolic extract of *P. oleracea* at 220 nm (**A**) and 320 nm (**B**).

3. Discussion

LPS, as a gram-negative bacterial constituent, is a well-known and established cause of adventitious pneumonia from the community or hospital patients, and Toll-like receptor-4 (TLR4) activation by this stimuli is a reasonable way for activating the innate immunity against gram-negative pathogen/s [27,28]. It has been demonstrated that LPS leads to pulmonary inflammation such as ALI, which occurs after 4–48 h of pathogen exposure [29–31]. For this reason, previous studies have reported that LPS stimulation is a standard model for inducing experimental ALI and ARDS [32,33].

Inflammation is considered the major response to infections or injuries. However, uncontrolled prolongation of the inflammatory repertoire may lead to tissue damage and healing [24,28]. LPS activated macrophages produce inflammatory mediators such as TNF-α, PGE$_2$, IL-1β, and IL-6 [34–36], which play an important role in self-sustaining inflammatory conditions [37]. Therefore, suppressing the prolonged and/or chronic lung inflammation induced by LPS could represent a potential curative aspect for lung injury [38,39].

Portulaca oleracea is a medicinal plant widely used in traditional medicine [40]. Nowadays, many studies have revealed its valuable pharmacologic properties including anti-inflammatory, anti-oxidant, anti-microbial, and neuroprotective [41–48]. PGE$_2$ is a bioactive lipid associating with inflammation and cancer. Its synthesis is originated by phospholipases (PLAs) through liberating free fatty acids from membrane, including arachidonic acid (AA) [49]. There are several studies on the notion of the contribution of the dysregulation in the levels of arachidonic acid, and PGE$_2$ synthesis or degradation have been associated with a number of inflammatory diseases [49–51]. In the current study, we demonstrated that LPS significantly increases the levels of PGE$_2$ and other inflammatory cytokines in the BALF compared with the control group. Previous studies also described that an increase in the level of PGE$_2$ promotes the activation of both the innate and adaptive immunity including macrophage and Th$_{17}$ cells, a subset of CD4$^+$ helper T cells, by the production of interleukin-17 (IL-17) [49–51]. Our results showed that PO suppresses lung inflammation by the reduction of IL-1β, IL-6, TNF-α, PGE$_2$, and TGF-β, as well as by the increase of IL-10 levels. These results are in accordance with previous studies that reported anti-inflammatory effects of PO on RAW 264.7 macrophage cell line and human umbilical vein endothelial cells (HUVECs) treated with LPS [16,52]. In contrast, it has been reported that PO extract inhibits TNF-α-induced adhesion of HL-60 cells to HUVECs and mRNA expression of IL-8 and monocyte chemoattractant protein (MCP)-1 [12]. It has also been suggested that inhibition of inflammation by PO may be partly because of modulation of nuclear factor-kappa B (NF-κB) signaling pathway and decrement of p65 nuclear accumulation [53]. Indeed, all these pieces of evidence further support and validate the anti-inflammatory potential of *Portulaca oleracea* in other inflammatory-based illness such as colitis [54], peripheral pain [16], and liver injury [55]. Previous studies demonstrated that the levels of inflammatory (TNF-α and IL-1β) and anti-inflammatory (IL-10) cytokines are impressed by both transcription factors NF-κB and nuclear factor erythroid 2-related factor 2 (Nrf2), respectively [28,56,57]. As one of the current study's limitations, we did not evaluate changes in gene expression and/or activity of certain transcription factors related to the inflammatory and antioxidant response such as NFκB and Nrf2, respectively.

TLR-4, as the main receptor for LPS, possesses an essential role in the pathogenesis of ALI, also supported by its localization on airway vascular endothelial and epithelial cells [58]. Accordingly, Askari and coworkers [20] have shown that PO extract had modulatory effects on imbalanced lymphocytes through the reduction of inflammatory cytokines and increased expression of IL-10 may be correlated to TLR-4 modulation. LPS-induced lung injury is also characterized by neutrophils infiltration in lung tissues that occurs and is driven by the massive cytokines production [2,59,60]. Interestingly, we found that PO extract improves the level of WBC in BALF samples, as well as the level of MPO, compared with the LPS group as an index of a significative reduction of neutrophil recruitment and activity. Contextually, in ALI/ARDS onset, lung edema appears as a consequence of microvascular leakage associated with endothelial injury [61,62]. The results of our study showed that PO significantly decreased the lung wet/dry ratio as an index of interstitial edema. In addition, we observed that PO markedly prevented MDA and NO production as well as propagated thiol, catalase, and SOD in BALF. Lipid peroxidation is a condition under which free radicals attack lipids containing carbon–carbon double bonds leading to cell and organ damage [63–65]. The main bio-products produced in this process are MDA and SOD, widely used as lipid peroxidation index and as markers of lipid peroxidation in ALI/ARDS [66]. Furthermore, it has been suggested that NO and inducible nitric oxide synthase (iNOS) lead to oxidative stress and endothelial damage [63–65,67]. Therefore, inhibition of iNOS and reduction of NO content could be beneficial in these pathologies [68]. Free radicals are highly reactive species capable of destructing DNA, proteins, carbohydrates, and lipids, structurally leading to cell damage or apoptosis. Exogenous anti-oxidant enzymes such as catalase, SOD, and thiol groups protect cells against oxidative stress damages induced by free radicals [69–73]. It could be concluded that the significant modulation of SOD and catalase activities and of the level of thiol groups after PO treatments improve the lung antioxidant status in an LPS-induced rat lung injury.

The anti-oxidant and anti-inflammatory properties of this plant extract may be the result of the considerable amounts of anti-oxidant compounds including gallotannins, omega-3 fatty acids, ascorbic acid, α-tocopherols, kaempferol, quercetin, and apigenin [16,74,75], and because of the presence of flavonoids such as kaempferol and apigenin derivatives found in our chemical characterization. Accordingly, Chen et al. reported that aqueous extract of PO alleviated high fat diet-elicited oxidative stress including blood and liver anti-oxidant enzymatic systems by the modulation of leptin and liver peroxisome proliferator-activated receptor (PPAR)-γ [13,28]. Furthermore, it has been reported that aqueous extract of PO exhibits cytoprotective effects on 2,2′-azobis hydrochloride-induced hemolytic injuries of red blood cells (RBCs) [76].

4. Materials and Methods

4.1. Chemicals and Reagents

LPS (Escherichia coli 055: B5) was obtained from Sigma (St. Louis, MO, USA). Myeloperoxidase (MPO) assay kit, IL-1β, TNF-α, IL-6, IL-10, PGE_2, and TGF-β enzyme-linked immunosorbent assay (ELISA) kit were provided by eBioscience (San Diego, CA, USA). All other reagents were of analytical grade.

4.2. Preparation of PO Extract

PO extract was prepared according to our previously characterized and standardized method [20]. In brief, the hydroethanolic extract was made using the macerated method with 70% w/w ethanol for 72 h at room temperature (RT). The yield of the dried extract was 21% w/w in the ratio of dried powder, and kept in $-20\,^\circ$C until use. For the characterization of PO extract, we used a liquid chromatography system comprising of a 510 Waters pump (Waters Association, Milford, MA, U.S.A.), a variable wavelength (model 486 Waters UV detector), and a Waters sample injection system (U6K system). The mobile phase was formed by a mixture of methanol:acetonitrile/tetrahydrofuran/0.5% glacial acetic acid (5:3:18:74). This phase was filtered under vacuum, then degassed, and finally pumped through the Novapak C18 column (150 × 3.9 mm i.d.) at a flow rate of 1.0 mL/min. The chromatograms were recorded at 220 and 320 nm [62] and interpreted by Gloexir Pars ® Company, Mashhad, Iran. For total flavonoid content, we have followed the procedure previously adopted in our group [63,64]. Briefly, 5 mL of 2% aluminum trichloride ($AlCl_3$) in methanol was mixed with the same volume of PO extract, incubated for 15 min at RT, and then measured at 510 nm using a MultiSpec UV-vis spectrophotometer (Shimadzu, Tokyo, Japan). The total flavonoid content was measured based on the standard curve of different flavonoids at a range of 0–50 μg/mL.

4.3. Animals and Husbandry

Adult male Sprague–Dawley rats (weighing 220 ± 30 g) were provided by the animal laboratory of Faculty of Medicine, Mashhad University of Medical Sciences (Mashhad, Iran), and kept in an animal care facility under controlled temperature and humidity, and on a 12 h/12 h light/dark cycle, with ad libitum access to water and a standard laboratory chow diet. All experimental procedures were carried out in compliance with local and national law and policies (Grant No. 971254 of Ethical Committee of National Institute for Medical Research Development, Iran). All procedures were carried out to minimize the number of animals (n = 5–7 per group) and their suffering.

4.4. Experimental Protocol

Animals were randomly divided into six groups of 5–7 rats: (I) control group (saline); (II) LPS group (5 mg/kg); (III) LPS + Dexamethasone group (Dexa, 1.5 mg/kg); (IV) LPS + PO (50 mg/kg) group; (V) LPS + PO (100 mg/kg) group; and (VI) LPS + PO (200 mg/kg) group. LPS was administered using intraperitoneal (i.p.) injection to induce acute lung injury. PO and Dexa were administrated by oral gavage (po) 1 h before LPS injection. Dose adjustment was performed according to our preliminary study. Rats were sacrificed, and samples were collected at 4 h after LPS administration [61].

4.5. Absolute Organ Weight and Lung Wet/dry Weight Ratio

The whole body and absolute lung, heart, and liver weights were recorded. The measurement of water content of lungs was also carried out by assessing the wet/dry weight quantitative ratio of lung tissues. Briefly, the right lung inferior lobe was dissected and weighed to supply the 'wet' weight.

The lung was then dried at −80 °C for 72 h to get the 'dry' weight. Finally, the wet/dry ratio was calculated as wet/dry ratio = wet weight/dry weight.

4.6. Broncho-Alveolar Lavage Fluid (BALF) Preparation

As previously described [64], animals were anesthetized with urethane (50 mg/kg, i.p.) at the end of the experimental protocol. Successively, the chest was opened and lungs and trachea were dissected and washed with distilled water. Lungs were lavaged with 1 mL saline five times at controlled RT through the cannulated trachea. The collected BALF was centrifuged at 2500 g for 10 min and the obtained supernatant was stored at −80 °C for the subsequent analysis.

4.7. Measurement of Total and Differential White Blood Cells (WBC) in BALF

Briefly, 1 mL of BALF was stained with Turk solution (1 mL glacial acetic acid, 1 mL of gentian violet solution 1%, and 100 mL distilled water) and counted by Neubauer chamber. Differential cell analysis was carried out by the aim of a light microscope as previously described [77]. WBC and differential WBC were determined via light microscope according to morphological criteria and staining.

4.8. Oxidant-Antioxidant Assessment in BALF

For measurement of malondialdehyde (MDA) concentration, the sample was refluxed with a solution of HCl and TBA (thiobarbituric acid). Then, 2 mL of this solution was added to 1 mL of BALF and heated in a water bath at 50 °C for 40 min to dissolve TBA. After cooling and reaching RT, it was centrifuged at 1000 rpm for 10 min. Afterward, the absorbance was read at 535 nm and then the MDA concentration was calculated based on the following equation: $C (M) = A/1.65 \times 10^5$, where C indicated the concentration and A the absorbance [24,78]. To determine the thiol groups, the DTNB method (2, 2′-dinitro-5, 5′-dithiodibenzoic acid) was used. This reagent reacts with SH (thiol) groups and produces a yellow complex that has an absorbance peak at 412 nm and has a molar absorption coefficient of 13.6 mM^{-1}cm^{-1}. Then, 1 mL of Tris-EDTA buffer (pH 8.6) was added to 50 µL BALF and sample absorbance was read at 412 nm against Tris-EDTA buffer alone (A1). A total of 20 µL of DTNB reagents (10 nM in methanol) was added to the mixture and the samples were kept at RT for 15 min, after which the absorbance was read again (A2). The absorbance of DTNB reagent was also read as a blank (B) [78]. Total thiol concentration expressed as nmol/mg protein was calculated with the following equation: $(A2 - A1 - B) \times 1.07/0.05 \times 13.6$. Catalase (CAT) activity was measured based on its ability to decompose hydrogen peroxide (H_2O_2) by decreasing adsorption in a 240 nm absorption spectrum. For this purpose, 30 mM hydrogen peroxide was used as a substrate and 50 mM phosphate buffer with pH = 7 as substrate substitute in blank solution. The measuring solution contained a suitable volume of sample and a solution of hydrogen peroxide. The reaction was started by adding hydrogen peroxide and reduced absorption by spectrophotometer at 240 nm for 3 min. Each catalase activity unit was defined as the hydrogen peroxide µmol consumed per mg of protein [78]. Measurement of superoxide dismutase enzyme activity was performed based on previously described methods with slight modifications [63,64,79–81]. The method is based on the pyrogallol auto-oxidation and the inhibition of superoxide-dependent reduction of the tetrazolium dye, MTT (3-(4,5-dimethylthiazol-2-yl)-2,5-diphenyltetrazolium bromide) to its formazan. The reaction was stopped by adding dimethyl sulfoxide (DMSO), and then performed with a microtiter plate reader at 570 nm. A unit of SOD was defined as the amount of enzyme needed to control MTT reduction up to 50%.

4.9. Enzyme-Linked Immunosorbent Assay (ELISA) Assay

The levels of TNF-α, IL-6, IL-1β, IL-10, PGE$_2$, and TGF-β in the supernatants of obtained BALF were measured using commercially available enzyme-linked immunosorbent assay kit (ELISA kits, eBioscience Co., San Diego, CA, USA) according to the manufacturer instructions. Briefly, 100 µL of BALF supernatants, diluted standards, quality controls, and dilution buffer (blank) were applied on a pre-coated plate with the monoclonal antibody for 2 h. After washing, 100 µL of biotin-labeled antibody was added and incubation continued for 1 h. The plate was washed and 100 µL of the streptavidin–HRP conjugate was added and the plate was incubated for a further 30 min period in the dark. The addition of 100 µL of the substrate and stop solution represented the last steps before the reading of absorbance (measured at 450 nm) on a microplate reader [82].

4.10. Myeloperoxidase Assay

Leukocyte myeloperoxidase (MPO) activity was assessed by measuring the H_2O_2-dependent oxidation of 3,3′,5,5′-tetramethylbenzidine (TMB) as previously reported [82]. Aliquots of 20 µL of BALF were incubated with 160 µL of TMB and 20 µL of H_2O_2 (in 80 mM phosphate buffer, pH 5.4) in 96-well plates. Plates were incubated for 5 min at RT and optical density was read at 620 nm using a plate-reader (Biorad, Italy). The assay was performed in duplicates and normalized for protein content [82].

4.11. Statistical Analysis

The results obtained were expressed as the mean ± SEM. Normality test was carried out based on Kolmogorov–Smirnov. After passing the tests, statistical analysis was performed using one-way analysis of variance (ANOVA) followed by Bonferroni or Dunnett's post-test when comparing more than two groups. Student's t-test was used in cases where two groups were compared. Statistical analysis was performed using GraphPad Prism 6.0 software (San Diego, CA, USA). Data were considered statistically significant when a value of $p \leq 0.05$ was achieved. The data and statistical analysis comply with the recommendations on experimental design, analysis [83], and data sharing and presentation in preclinical pharmacology [84,85].

5. Conclusions

These studies are in accordance with our findings that demonstrate the protective effects of PO on LPS-induced acute rat lung injury, paving the way for rational use of this plant extract in lung-related inflammatory diseases, as well as in those characterized by an increase of free radicals and oxidative reactive products.

Author Contributions: V.B.R., H.R., F.R., B.B., R.S., and A.S.K. performed the experiments. F.M., N.M., and V.R.A. designed the study, and drafted and wrote the manuscript. F.R., F.M., and V.R.A. edited and revised the manuscript.

Funding: This study was financially supported by a grant from the National Institute for Medical Research Development Grant No. 971254.

Conflicts of Interest: The authors declare no conflict of interest. This Declaration acknowledges that this paper adheres to the principles for transparent reporting and scientific rigor of preclinical research recommended by funding agencies, publishers, and other organizations engaged with supporting research.

References

1. Villar, J.; Sulemanji, D.; Kacmarek, R.M. The acute respiratory distress syndrome: Incidence and mortality, has it changed? *Curr. Opin. Crit. Care* **2014**, *20*, 3–9. [CrossRef] [PubMed]
2. Matthay, M.A.; Zemans, R.L. The Acute Respiratory Distress Syndrome: Pathogenesis and Treatment. *Ann. Rev. Pathol. Mech. Dis.* **2011**, *6*, 147–163. [CrossRef] [PubMed]
3. Ware, L.B.; Matthay, M.A. The Acute Respiratory Distress Syndrome. *N. Engl. J. Med.* **2000**, *342*, 1334–1349. [CrossRef] [PubMed]
4. Mokra, D.; Kosutova, P. Biomarkers in acute lung injury. *Respir. Physiol. Neurobiol.* **2015**, *209*, 52–58. [CrossRef] [PubMed]

5. Arai, Y.; Watanabe, S.; Kimira, M.; Shimoi, K.; Mochizuki, R.; Kinae, N. Dietary intakes of flavonols, flavones and isoflavones by Japanese women and the inverse correlation between quercetin intake and plasma LDL cholesterol concentration. *J. Nutr.* **2000**, *130*, 2243–2250. [CrossRef] [PubMed]
6. Rubenfeld, G.D.; Caldwell, E.; Peabody, E.; Weaver, J.; Martin, D.P.; Neff, M.; Stern, E.J.; Hudson, L.D. Incidence and outcomes of acute lung injury. *N. Engl. J. Med.* **2005**, *353*, 1685–1693. [CrossRef] [PubMed]
7. Zambon, M.; Vincent, J.-L. Mortality rates for patients with acute lung injury/ARDS have decreased over time. *CHEST J.* **2008**, *133*, 1120–1127. [CrossRef]
8. Kim, H.P.; Lim, H.; Kwon, Y.S. Therapeutic Potential of Medicinal Plants and Their Constituents on Lung Inflammatory Disorders. *Biomol. Ther.* **2017**, *25*, 91–104. [CrossRef]
9. Maione, F.; Russo, R.; Khan, H.; Mascolo, N. Medicinal plants with anti-inflammatory activities. *Nat. Prod. Res.* **2016**, *30*, 1343–1352. [CrossRef]
10. Elkhayat, E.S.; Ibrahim, S.R.; Aziz, M.A. Portulene, a new diterpene from *Portulaca oleracea* L. *J. Asian Natl. Prod. Res.* **2008**, *10*, 1039–1043. [CrossRef]
11. Palaniswamy, U.R.; Bible, B.B.; McAvoy, R.J. Effect of nitrate: Ammonium nitrogen ratio on oxalate levels of purslane. *Trends New Crops New Uses* **2002**, *11*, 453–455.
12. Lee, A.S.; Kim, J.S.; Lee, Y.J.; Kang, D.G.; Lee, H.S. Anti-TNF-α activity of Portulaca oleracea in vascular endothelial cells. *Int. J. Mol. Sci.* **2012**, *13*, 5628–5644. [CrossRef] [PubMed]
13. Chen, B.; Zhou, H.; Zhao, W.; Zhou, W.; Yuan, Q.; Yang, G. Effects of aqueous extract of *Portulaca oleracea* L. on oxidative stress and liver, spleen leptin, PARα and FAS mRNA expression in high-fat diet induced mice. *Mol. Biol. Rep.* **2012**, *39*, 7981–7988. [CrossRef] [PubMed]
14. Zhang, X.; Ji, Y.; Qu, Z.; Xia, J.; Wang, L. Experimental studies on antibiotic functions of *Portulaca oleracea* L. in vitro. *Chin. J. Microecol.* **2002**, *14*, 277–280.
15. Karimi, G.; Hosseinzadeh, H.; Ettehad, N. Evaluation of the gastric antiulcerogenic effects of *Portulaca oleracea* L. extracts in mice. *Phytother. Res.* **2004**, *18*, 484–487. [CrossRef] [PubMed]
16. Chan, K.; Islam, M.; Kamil, M.; Radhakrishnan, R.; Zakaria, M.; Habibullah, M.; Attas, A. The analgesic and anti-inflammatory effects of *Portulaca oleracea* L. subsp. sativa (Haw.) Celak. *J. Ethnopharmacol.* **2000**, *73*, 445–451. [CrossRef]
17. Rashed, A.; Afifi, F.; Disi, A. Simple evaluation of the wound healing activity of a crude extract of *Portulaca oleracea* L.(growing in Jordan) in Mus musculus JVI-1. *J. Ethnopharmacol.* **2003**, *88*, 131–136. [CrossRef]
18. Xu, X.; Yu, L.; Chen, G. Determination of flavonoids in *Portulaca oleracea* L. by capillary electrophoresis with electrochemical detection. *J. Pharm. Biomed. Anal.* **2006**, *41*, 493–499. [CrossRef]
19. Meng, Y.; Ying, Z.; Xiang, Z.; Hao, D.; Zhang, W.; Zheng, Y.; Gao, Y.; Ying, X. The anti-inflammation and pharmacokinetics of a novel alkaloid from *Portulaca oleracea* L. *J. Pharm. Pharmacol.* **2016**, *68*, 397–405. [CrossRef]
20. Askari, V.R.; Rezaee, S.A.; Abnous, K.; Iranshahi, M.; Boskabady, M.H. The influence of hydro-ethanolic extract of *Portulaca oleracea* L. on Th1/Th2 balance in isolated human lymphocytes. *J. Ethnopharmacol.* **2016**, *194*, 1112–1121. [CrossRef]
21. Kaveh, M.; Eidi, A.; Nemati, A.; Boskabady, M.H. Modulation of lung inflammation and immune markers in asthmatic rats treated by Portulaca oleracea. *Avicenna J. Phytomed.* **2017**, *7*, 409–416. [PubMed]
22. Stearns-Kurosawa, D.J.; Osuchowski, M.F.; Valentine, C.; Kurosawa, S.; Remick, D.G. The Pathogenesis of Sepsis. *Ann. Rev. Pathol. Mech. Dis.* **2011**, *6*, 19–48. [CrossRef] [PubMed]
23. Lee, J.W.; Fang, X.; Dolganov, G.; Fremont, R.D.; Bastarache, J.A.; Ware, L.B.; Matthay, M.A. Acute lung injury edema fluid decreases net fluid transport across human alveolar epithelial type II cells. *J. Biol. Chem.* **2007**, *282*, 24109–24119. [CrossRef] [PubMed]
24. Rahimi, V.B.; Shirazinia, R.; Fereydouni, N.; Zamani, P.; Darroudi, S.; Sahebkar, A.H.; Askari, V.R. Comparison of honey and dextrose solution on post-operative peritoneal adhesion in rat model. *Biomed. Pharmacother.* **2017**, *92*, 849–855. [CrossRef] [PubMed]
25. Hu, J.; Zhang, Y.; Dong, L.; Wang, Z.; Chen, L.; Liang, D.; Shi, D.; Shan, X.; Liang, G. Design, Synthesis, and Biological Evaluation of Novel Quinazoline Derivatives as Anti-inflammatory Agents against Lipopolysaccharide-induced Acute Lung Injury in Rats. *Chem. Biol. Drug Des.* **2015**, *85*, 672–684. [CrossRef] [PubMed]

26. Meduri, G.U.; Kohler, G.; Headley, S.; Tolley, E.; Stentz, F.; Postlethwaite, A. Inflammatory Cytokines in the BAL of Patients With ARDS: Persistent Elevation Over Time Predicts Poor Outcome. *Chest* **1995**, *108*, 1303–1314. [CrossRef] [PubMed]
27. Schurr, J.R.; Young, E.; Byrne, P.; Steele, C.; Shellito, J.E.; Kolls, J.K. Central role of toll-like receptor 4 signaling and host defense in experimental pneumonia caused by Gram-negative bacteria. *Infect. Immunity* **2005**, *73*, 532–545. [CrossRef]
28. Askari, V.R.; Shafiee-Nick, R. Promising neuroprotective effects of β-caryophyllene against LPS-induced oligodendrocyte toxicity: A mechanistic study. *Biochem. Pharmacol.* **2018**, *159*, 154–171. [CrossRef]
29. Szarka, R.J.; Wang, N.; Gordon, L.; Nation, P.; Smith, R.H. A murine model of pulmonary damage induced by lipopolysaccharide via intranasal instillation. *J. Immunol. Methods* **1997**, *202*, 49–57. [CrossRef]
30. Thangavel, J.; Samanta, S.; Rajasingh, S.; Barani, B.; Xuan, Y.T.; Dawn, B.; Rajasingh, J. Epigenetic modifiers reduce inflammation and modulate macrophage phenotype during endotoxemia-induced acute lung injury. *J. Cell Sci.* **2015**, *128*, 3094–3105. [CrossRef]
31. Sarma, J.V.; Ward, P.A. Oxidants and redox signaling in acute lung injury. *Compr. Physiol.* **2011**, *1*, 1365–1381. [CrossRef] [PubMed]
32. Brigham, K.L.; Meyrick, B. Endotoxin and lung injury. *Am. Respir. Dis.* **1986**, *133*, 913–927.
33. Martin, M.A.; Silverman, H.J. Gram-negative sepsis and the adult respiratory distress syndrome. *Clin. Infect. Dis.* **1992**, *14*, 1213–1228. [CrossRef] [PubMed]
34. Morrison, D.C.; Ryan, J.L. Endotoxins and disease mechanisms. *Ann. Rev. Med.* **1987**, *38*, 417–432. [CrossRef] [PubMed]
35. Adams, D.O. Molecular biology of macrophage activation: A pathway whereby psychosocial factors can potentially affect health. *Psychosom. Med.* **1994**, *56*, 316–327. [CrossRef] [PubMed]
36. Cheung, D.W.; Koon, C.M.; Wat, E.; Ko, C.H.; Chan, J.Y.; Yew, D.T.; Leung, P.C.; Chan, W.Y.; Lau, C.B.; Fung, K.P. A herbal formula containing roots of Salvia miltiorrhiza (Danshen) and Pueraria lobata (Gegen) inhibits inflammatory mediators in LPS-stimulated RAW 264.7 macrophages through inhibition of nuclear factor kappaB (NFkappaB) pathway. *J. Ethnopharmacol.* **2013**, *145*, 776–783. [CrossRef] [PubMed]
37. Xie, X.; Sun, S.; Zhong, W.; Soromou, L.W.; Zhou, X.; Wei, M.; Ren, Y.; Ding, Y. Zingerone attenuates lipopolysaccharide-induced acute lung injury in mice. *Int. Immunopharmacol.* **2014**, *19*, 103–109. [CrossRef] [PubMed]
38. Do-Umehara, H.C.; Chen, C.; Urich, D.; Zhou, L.; Qiu, J.; Jang, S.; Zander, A.; Baker, M.A.; Eilers, M.; Sporn, P.H.S.; et al. Suppression of inflammation and acute lung injury by the transcription factor Miz1 via repression of C/EBP-δ. *Nat. Immunol.* **2013**, *14*, 461–469. [CrossRef]
39. Kim, K.H.; Kwun, M.J.; Han, C.W.; Ha, K.-T.; Choi, J.-Y.; Joo, M. Suppression of lung inflammation in an LPS-induced acute lung injury model by the fruit hull of Gleditsia sinensis. *BMC Complement. Altern. Med.* **2014**, *14*, 402. [CrossRef]
40. Iranshahy, M.; Javadi, B.; Iranshahi, M.; Jahanbakhsh, S.P.; Mahyari, S.; Hassani, F.V.; Karimi, G. A review of traditional uses, phytochemistry and pharmacology of *Portulaca oleracea* L. *J. Ethnopharmacol.* **2017**, *205*, 158–172. [CrossRef]
41. Dan, Z. Study on Antimicrobial Effect of Flavonoids from *Portulace oleracea* L. *J. Anhui Agric. Sci.* **2006**, *34*, 7.
42. Malek, F.; Boskabady, M.; Borushaki, M.; Tohidi, M. Bronchodilatory effect of Portulaca oleracea in airways of asthmatic patients. *J. Ethnopharmacol.* **2004**, *93*, 57–62. [CrossRef] [PubMed]
43. Hozayen, W.; Bastawy, M.; Elshafeey, H. Effects of aqueous purslane (portulaca oleracea) extract and fish oil on gentamicin nephrotoxicity in albino rats. *Nat. Sci.* **2011**, *9*, 47–62.
44. Wang, W.-Y.; Gu, L.-M.; Dong, L.-W.; Wang, X.-L.; Ling, C.-Q.; Li, M. Protective effect of Portulaca oleracea extracts on hypoxic nerve tissue and its mechanism. *Asia Pac. J. Clin. Nutr.* **2007**, *16*, 227–233. [PubMed]
45. Parry, O.; Marks, J.; Okwuasaba, F. The skeletal muscle relaxant action of Portulaca oleracea: Role of potassium ions. *J. Ethnopharmacol.* **1993**, *40*, 187–194. [CrossRef]
46. Eidi, A.; Mortazavi, P.; Moghadam, J.Z.; Mardani, P.M. Hepatoprotective effects of Portulaca oleracea extract against CCl4-induced damage in rats. *Pharm. Biol.* **2015**, *53*, 1042–1051. [CrossRef] [PubMed]
47. Kumar, A.; Sharma, A.; Vijayakumar, M.; Rao Ch, V. Antiulcerogenic Effect Of Ethanolic Extract Of Portulaca oleracea Experimental Study. *Pharmacol. Online* **2010**, *1*, 417–432.
48. Hanumantappa, B.N.; Ramesh, L.; Umesh, M. Evaluation of Potential Antifertility activity of Total Flavonoids, Isolated from Portulaca oleracea L on female albino rats. *Int. J. PharmTech Res.* **2014**, *6*, 783–793.

49. Ricciotti, E.; FitzGerald, G.A. Prostaglandins and inflammation. *Arterioscler. Thromb. Vasc. Biol.* **2011**, *31*, 986–1000. [CrossRef]
50. Askari, V.R.; Alavinezhad, A.; Boskabady, M.H. The impact of "Ramadan fasting period" on total and differential white blood cells, haematological indices, inflammatory biomarker, respiratory symptoms and pulmonary function tests of healthy and asthmatic patients. *Allergol. Immunopathol.* **2016**, *44*, 359–367. [CrossRef]
51. Askari, V.R.; Baradaran Rahimi, V.; Rezaee, S.A.; Boskabady, M.H. Auraptene regulates Th1/Th2/TReg balances, NF-κB nuclear localization and nitric oxide production in normal and Th2 provoked situations in human isolated lymphocytes. *Phytomedicine* **2018**, *43*, 1–10. [CrossRef] [PubMed]
52. Azab, A.; Nassar, A.; Azab, A.N. Anti-Inflammatory activity of natural products. *Molecules* **2016**, *21*, 1321. [CrossRef] [PubMed]
53. Chuang, K.-H.; Peng, Y.-C.; Chien, H.-Y.; Lu, M.-L.; Du, H.-I.; Wu, Y.-L. Attenuation of LPS-Induced Lung Inflammation by Glucosamine in Rats. *Am. J. Respir. Cell Mol. Biol.* **2013**, *49*, 1110–1119. [CrossRef] [PubMed]
54. Kong, R.; Luo, H.; Wang, N.; Li, J.; Xu, S.; Chen, K.; Feng, J.; Wu, L.; Li, S.; Liu, T.; et al. Portulaca Extract Attenuates Development of Dextran Sulfate Sodium Induced Colitis in Mice through Activation of PPARγ. *PPAR Res.* **2018**, *2018*, 11. [CrossRef] [PubMed]
55. Shi, H.; Liu, X.; Tang, G.; Liu, H.; Zhang, Y.; Zhang, B.; Zhao, X.; Wang, W. Ethanol extract of *Portulaca oleracea* L. reduced the carbon tetrachloride induced liver injury in mice involving enhancement of NF-kappaB activity. *Am. J. Transl. Res.* **2014**, *6*, 746–755. [PubMed]
56. Valenzuela, R.; Illesca, P.; Echeverria, F.; Espinosa, A.; Rincon-Cervera, M.A.; Ortiz, M.; Hernandez-Rodas, M.C.; Valenzuela, A.; Videla, L.A. Molecular adaptations underlying the beneficial effects of hydroxytyrosol in the pathogenic alterations induced by a high-fat diet in mouse liver: PPAR-alpha and Nrf2 activation, and NF-kappaB down-regulation. *Food Funct.* **2017**, *8*, 1526–1537. [CrossRef] [PubMed]
57. Hernandez-Rodas, M.C.; Valenzuela, R.; Echeverria, F.; Rincon-Cervera, M.A.; Espinosa, A.; Illesca, P.; Munoz, P.; Corbari, A.; Romero, N.; Gonzalez-Manan, D.; et al. Supplementation with Docosahexaenoic Acid and Extra Virgin Olive Oil Prevents Liver Steatosis Induced by a High-Fat Diet in Mice through PPAR-alpha and Nrf2 Upregulation with Concomitant SREBP-1c and NF-kB Downregulation. *Mol. Nutr. Food Res.* **2017**, *61*. [CrossRef] [PubMed]
58. Martin, T.R.; Wurfel, M.M. A TRIFfic Perspective on Acute Lung Injury. *Cell* **2008**, *133*, 208–210. [CrossRef]
59. Reutershan, J.; Morris, M.A.; Burcin, T.L.; Smith, D.F.; Chang, D.; Saprito, M.S.; Ley, K. Critical role of endothelial CXCR2 in LPS-induced neutrophil migration into the lung. *J. Clin. Investig.* **2006**, *116*, 695–702. [CrossRef] [PubMed]
60. Lucas, R.; Verin, A.D.; Black, S.M.; Catravas, J.D. Regulators of endothelial and epithelial barrier integrity and function in acute lung injury. *Biochem. Pharmacol.* **2009**, *77*, 1763–1772. [CrossRef]
61. Feng, G.; Sun, B.; Li, T.Z. Daidzein attenuates lipopolysaccharide-induced acute lung injury via toll-like receptor 4/NF-kappaB pathway. *Int. Immunopharmacol.* **2015**, *26*, 392–400. [CrossRef] [PubMed]
62. Han, S.; Mallampalli, R.K. The acute respiratory distress syndrome: From mechanism to translation. *J. Immunol.* **2015**, *194*, 855–860. [CrossRef] [PubMed]
63. Rahimi, V.B.; Askari, V.R.; Shirazinia, R.; Soheili-Far, S.; Askari, N.; Rahmanian-Devin, P.; Sanei-Far, Z.; Mousavi, S.H.; Ghodsi, R. Protective effects of hydro-ethanolic extract of Terminalia chebula on primary microglia cells and their polarization (M1/M2 balance). *Mult. Scler. Relat. Disord.* **2018**, *25*, 5–13. [CrossRef] [PubMed]
64. Askari, V.R.; Rahimi, V.B.; Zamani, P.; Fereydouni, N.; Rahmanian-Devin, P.; Sahebkar, A.H.; Rakhshandeh, H. Evaluation of the effects of Iranian propolis on the severity of post operational-induced peritoneal adhesion in rats. *Biomed. Pharmacother.* **2018**, *99*, 346–353. [CrossRef] [PubMed]
65. Askari, V.R.; Fereydouni, N.; Baradaran Rahimi, V.; Askari, N.; Sahebkar, A.H.; Rahmanian-Devin, P.; Samzadeh-Kermani, A. β-Amyrin, the cannabinoid receptors agonist, abrogates mice brain microglial cells inflammation induced by lipopolysaccharide/interferon-γ and regulates Mφ1/Mφ2 balances. *Biomed. Pharmacother.* **2018**, *101*, 438–446. [CrossRef] [PubMed]
66. Till, G.O.; Hatherill, J.R.; Tourtellotte, W.W.; Lutz, M.J.; Ward, P.A. Lipid peroxidation and acute lung injury after thermal trauma to skin. Evidence of a role for hydroxyl radical. *Am. J. Pathol.* **1985**, *119*, 376–384. [PubMed]

67. Ayala, A.; Muñoz, M.F.; Argüelles, S. Lipid Peroxidation: Production, Metabolism, and Signaling Mechanisms of Malondialdehyde and 4-Hydroxy-2-Nonenal. *Oxid. Med. Cell. Longev.* **2014**, *2014*, 31. [CrossRef]
68. Kristof, A.S.; Goldberg, P.; Laubach, V.; Hussain, S.N.A. Role of Inducible Nitric Oxide Synthase in Endotoxin-induced Acute Lung Injury. *Am. J. Respir. Crit. Care Med.* **1998**, *158*, 1883–1889. [CrossRef]
69. Sheng, Y.; Abreu, I.A.; Cabelli, D.E.; Maroney, M.J.; Miller, A.-F.; Teixeira, M.; Valentine, J.S. Superoxide Dismutases and Superoxide Reductases. *Chem. Rev.* **2014**, *114*, 3854–3918. [CrossRef]
70. Lobo, V.; Patil, A.; Phatak, A.; Chandra, N. Free radicals, antioxidants and functional foods: Impact on human health. *Pharmacogn. Rev.* **2010**, *4*, 118–126. [CrossRef]
71. Brigham, K.L. Role of Free Radicals in Lung Injury. *Chest* **1986**, *89*, 859–863. [CrossRef]
72. He, G.; Dong, C.; Luan, Z.; McAllan, B.M.; Xu, T.; Zhao, L.; Qiao, J. Oxygen free radical involvement in acute lung injury induced by H5N1 virus in mice. *Influ. Other Respir. Viruses* **2013**, *7*, 945–953. [CrossRef] [PubMed]
73. Junod, A.F. Oxygen free radicals and lungs. *Intensiv. Care Med.* **1989**, *15* (Suppl. 1), S21–S23. [CrossRef]
74. Zhu, H.; Wang, Y.; Liu, Y.; Xia, Y.; Tang, T. Analysis of Flavonoids in *Portulaca oleracea* L. by UV-Vis Spectrophotometry with Comparative Study on Different Extraction Technologies. *Food Anal. Methods* **2010**, *3*, 90–97. [CrossRef]
75. Hwang, J.; Hwang, H.; Lee, H.W.; Suk, K. Microglia signaling as a target of donepezil. *Neuropharmacology* **2010**, *58*. [CrossRef] [PubMed]
76. Karimi, G.; Aghasizadeh, M.; Razavi, M.; Taghiabadi, E. Protective effects of aqueous and ethanolic extracts of *Nigella sativa* L. and *Portulaca oleracea* L. on free radical induced hemolysis of RBCs. *Daru* **2011**, *19*, 295–300. [PubMed]
77. Feizpour, A.; Boskabady, M.H.; Ghorbani, A. Adipose-Derived Stromal Cell Therapy Affects Lung Inflammation and Tracheal Responsiveness in Guinea Pig Model of COPD. *PLoS ONE* **2014**, *9*, e108974. [CrossRef]
78. Kaveh, M.; Eidi, A.; Nemati, A.; Boskabady, M.H. The Extract of Portulaca oleracea and its Constituent, Alpha Linolenic Acid Affects Serum Oxidant Levels and Inflammatory Cells in Sensitized Rats. *Iran. J. Allergy Asthma Immunol.* **2017**, *16*, 256–270. [PubMed]
79. Bahramsoltani, R.; Farzaei, M.H.; Abdolghaffari, A.H.; Rahimi, R.; Samadi, N.; Heidari, M.; Esfandyari, M.; Baeeri, M.; Hassanzadeh, G.; Abdollahi, M.; et al. Evaluation of phytochemicals, antioxidant and burn wound healing activities of Cucurbita moschata Duchesne fruit peel. *Iran. J. Basic Med. Sci.* **2017**, *20*, 798–805. [CrossRef]
80. Rahimi, V.B.; Askari, V.R.; Emami, S.A.; Tayarani-Najaran, Z. Anti-melanogenic activity of Viola odorata different extracts on B16F10 murine melanoma cells. *Iran. J. Basic Med. Sci.* **2017**, *20*, 242–249. [CrossRef]
81. Rahimi, V.B.; Askari, V.R.; Mehrdad, A.; Sadeghnia, H.R. Boswellia serrata has promising impact on glutamate and quinolinic acid-induced toxicity on oligodendroglia cells: In vitro study. *Acta Pol. Pharm.* **2017**, *74*, 1803–1811.
82. Maione, F.; Paschalidis, N.; Mascolo, N.; Dufton, N.; Perretti, M.; D'Acquisto, F. Interleukin 17 sustains rather than induces inflammation. *Biochem. Pharmacol.* **2009**, *77*, 878–887. [CrossRef] [PubMed]
83. Curtis, M.J.; Bond, R.A.; Spina, D.; Ahluwalia, A.; Alexander, S.P.; Giembycz, M.A.; Gilchrist, A.; Hoyer, D.; Insel, P.A.; Izzo, A.A.; et al. Experimental design and analysis and their reporting: New guidance for publication in BJP. *Br. J. Pharmacol.* **2015**, *172*, 3461–3471. [CrossRef] [PubMed]
84. George, C.H.; Stanford, S.C.; Alexander, S.; Cirino, G.; Docherty, J.R.; Giembycz, M.A.; Hoyer, D.; Insel, P.A.; Izzo, A.A.; Ji, Y.; et al. Updating the guidelines for data transparency in the British Journal of Pharmacology—Data sharing and the use of scatter plots instead of bar charts. *Br. J. Pharmacol.* **2017**, *174*, 2801–2804. [CrossRef]
85. Alexander, S.P.H.; Roberts, R.E.; Broughton, B.R.S.; Sobey, C.G.; George, C.H.; Stanford, S.C.; Cirino, G.; Docherty, J.R.; Giembycz, M.A.; Hoyer, D.; et al. Goals and practicalities of immunoblotting and immunohistochemistry: A guide for submission to the British Journal of Pharmacology. *Br. J. Pharmacol.* **2018**, *175*, 407–411. [CrossRef] [PubMed]

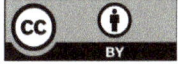

© 2019 by the authors. Licensee MDPI, Basel, Switzerland. This article is an open access article distributed under the terms and conditions of the Creative Commons Attribution (CC BY) license (http://creativecommons.org/licenses/by/4.0/).

Article

Iso-α-Acids, the Bitter Components of Beer, Suppress Microglial Inflammation in rTg4510 Tauopathy

Yasuhisa Ano [1,2,*], Yuta Takaichi [1], Kazuyuki Uchida [1], Keiji Kondo [2], Hiroyuki Nakayama [1] and Akihiko Takashima [3,4]

1. Graduate School of Agricultural and Life Sciences, The University of Tokyo, Tokyo 113-8657, Japan; takaichi.yuta.5110@gmail.com (Y.T.); auchidak@mail.ecc.u-tokyo.ac.jp (K.U.); anakaya@mail.ecc.u-tokyo.ac.jp (H.N.)
2. Research Laboratories for Health Science & Food Technologies, Kirin Company Ltd., Kanagawa 236-0004, Japan; kondok@kirin.co.jp
3. Department of Aging Neurobiology, National Center for Geriatrics and Gerontology, Obu 474-8511, Japan; 20160021@gakushuin.ac.jp
4. Faculty of Science, Gakushuin University, Tokyo 171-8588, Japan
* Correspondence: Yasuhisa_Ano@kirin.co.jp; Tel.: +81-45-330-9007

Academic Editor: Francesco Maione
Received: 15 November 2018; Accepted: 27 November 2018; Published: 29 November 2018

Abstract: Due to the growth in aging populations, prevention for cognitive decline and dementia are in great demand. We previously demonstrated that the consumption of iso-α-acids (IAA), the hop-derived bitter compounds in beer, prevents inflammation and Alzheimer's disease pathology in model mice. However, the effects of iso-α-acids on inflammation induced by other agents aside from amyloid β have not been investigated. In this study, we demonstrated that the consumption of iso-α-acids suppressed microglial inflammation in the frontal cortex of rTg4510 tauopathy mice. In addition, the levels of inflammatory cytokines and chemokines, including IL-1β and MIP-1β, in the frontal cortex of rTg4510 mice were greater than those of wild-type mice, and were reduced in rTg4510 mice fed with iso-α-acids. Flow cytometry analysis demonstrated that the expression of cells producing CD86, CD68, TSPO, MIP-1α, TNF-α, and IL-1β in microglia was increased in rTg4510 mice compared with wild-type mice. Furthermore, the expression of CD86- and MIP-1α-producing cells was reduced in rTg4510 mice administered with iso-α-acids. Moreover, the consumption of iso-α-acids reduced the levels of phosphorylated tau in the frontal cortex. Collectively, these results suggest that the consumption of iso-α-acids prevents the inflammation induced in tauopathy mice. Thus, iso-α-acids may help in preventing inflammation-related brain disorders.

Keywords: inflammation; iso-α-acids; microglia; tau; tauopathy

1. Introduction

Dementia and cognitive impairment are becoming an increasing burden not only on patients and their families, but also on national healthcare systems worldwide, concomitant with the rapid growth in aging populations. Owing to the lack of disease-modifying therapies for dementia, preventive approaches, including diet, exercise, and learning are garnering increased attention. Etiological studies of lifestyle have demonstrated that low-to-moderate consumption of alcohol, such as wine and beer, may reduce the risk of cognitive decline and the development of dementia. Indeed, individuals who consume low-to-moderate levels of alcoholic beverages on a daily basis were shown to have a significantly lower risk of developing a neurodegenerative disease, as compared with individuals who abstained from alcohol beverages or drank heavily [1–3]. Apart from the effects of alcohol itself, resveratrol, a polyphenolic compound present in red wine, has been shown to be neuroprotective [4–7]. We previously demonstrated that the consumption of iso-α-acids, the bitter components present in beer, prevents Alzheimer's pathology in 5 × FAD transgenic model mice. In addition, iso-α-acids suppress the microglial inflammation induced by amyloid β deposition in the brain, resulting in protection against cognitive decline. Iso-α-acids activate the peroxisome proliferator-activated receptor-γ (PPAR-γ) and regulate microglial phagocytosis and inflammation [8]. However, the effects of iso-α-acids on inflammation induced by other agents aside from amyloid β have not been investigated. In Alzheimer's disease, neurofibrillary tangles (NFTs) composed of hyperphosphorylated tau are observed in each brain region with aging, as well as senile plaques composed of amyloid β [9]. Tauopathy is characterized by fibrillar tau accumulation in neurons and glial cells, which is associated with neuronal dysfunction [10]. Proliferation and activation of microglia in the brain around NFTs and senile plaques are prominent features of Alzheimer's disease. Inflammation caused by activated microglia is associated with the disease progressions [11]. rTg4510 tauopathy model mice overexpress human P301L mutant tau and show neuroinflammation in the brain, accompanied by disease progression [12]. On the other hand, there is no report evaluating the preventive effects of nutritional components with anti-inflammatory activity in rTg4510 mice. Therefore, in the present study, the effects of iso-α-acids on inflammation in rTg4510 tauopathy mice were investigated.

2. Results

2.1. Effects of Iso-α-Acids on Inflammation in the Brain with Tauopathy

To evaluate the effects of iso-α-acids on inflammation in the brain of rTg4510 tauopathy mice, the levels of proinflammatory cytokines and chemokines in the frontal cortex of tauopathy mice fed with iso-α-acids were measured. The levels of IL-1β, TNF-α, MIP-1β, and IL-12p40 in the frontal cortex of rTg4510 mice were higher than those of wild-type mice (Figure 1a–d). The administration of iso-α-acids reduced the levels of IL-1β and MIP-1β in rTg4510 mice (Figure 1a,c), but did not change those in wild-type mice. These results indicate that proinflammatory cytokines and chemokines are increased in the frontal cortex in rTg4510 mice, and the consumption of iso-α-acids reduce the inflammation induced in tauopathy mice.

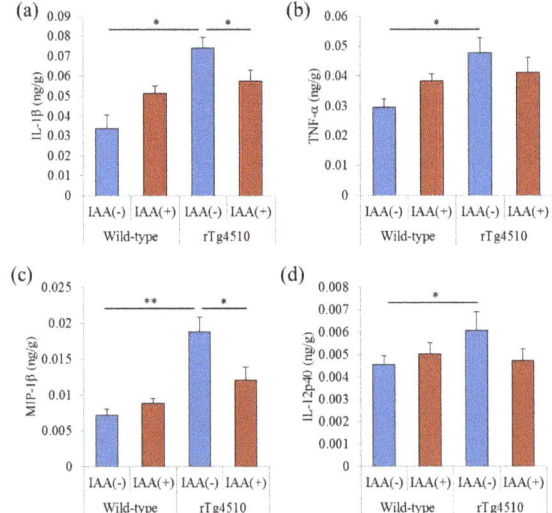

Figure 1. Effects of iso-α-acids on rTg4510 mice. Three-month-old rTg4510 mice and wild-type mice were fed 0% or 0.05% (w/w) iso-α-acids (IAA) for three months. (**a–d**), the levels of IL-1β, TNF-α, MIP-1α, and IL-12p40 in the frontal cortex, respectively. Data are the means ± SEM of 12 (wild-type mice without IAA), 6 (wild-type mice with IAA), 12 (rTg4510 mice without IAA), and 10 (rTg4510 mice with IAA) mice. p-values shown in the graph were calculated by one-way ANOVA, followed by the Tukey-Kramer test. * $p < 0.05$ and ** $p < 0.01$.

2.2. Effects of Iso-α-Acids on Microglial Phenotype in the Brain of Tauopathy

To evaluate the effects of iso-α-acids on microglia in rTg4510 tauopathy mice, CD11b-positive microglia were isolated and analyzed using flow cytometry. The expression of CD86, a costimulatory molecule, on CD11b-positive cells in the brain was increased in rTg4510 mice compared with wild-type mice and reduced in rTg4510 mice fed with iso-α-acids (Figure 2a). The expressions of CD68 and TSPO in CD11b-positive microglia were increased in rTg4510 mice compared with wild-type, but did not change in rTg4510 mice fed with iso-α-acids (Figure 2b,c). MIP-1α-, TNF-α-, and IL-1β-producing cells were also increased in rTg4510 mice, and MIP-1α-producing cells were decreased by iso-α-acids (Figure 2d–f). These results indicate that the microglia phenotype was induced into the proinflammatory type in rTg4510 mice, and some of these inflammatory inductions were suppressed by the consumption of iso-α-acids.

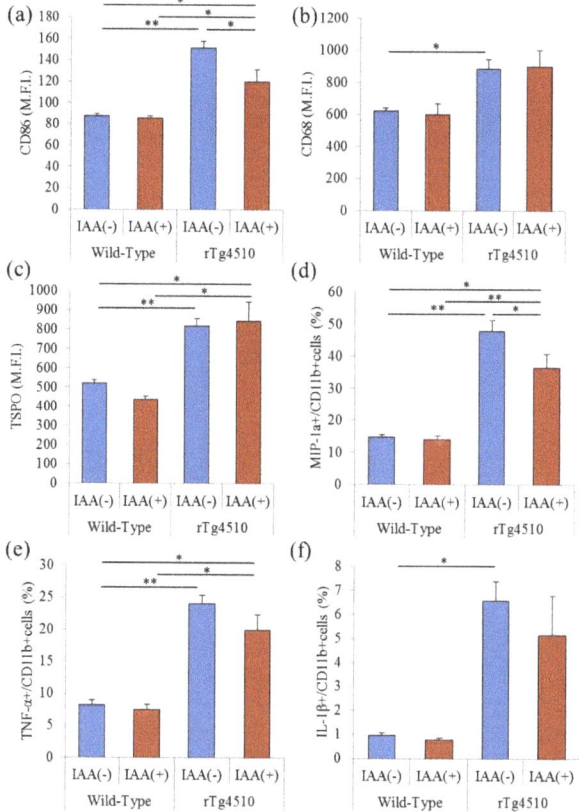

Figure 2. Analysis of microglia in rTg4510 mice. Microglia in the brains of rTg4510 mice were isolated using magnetic cell sorting and analyzed using a flow cytometer. (**a–c**), the expression of CD86, CD68, and TSPO in CD11b-positive microglia of rTg4510 or wild-type mice, respectively. (**d–f**), the percentages of intracellular MIP-1α-, TNF-α-, and IL-1β-producing cells in CD11b-positive cells, respectively. Data are the means ± SEM of five mice in each group. p-values shown in the graph were calculated by one-way ANOVA, followed by the Tukey-Kramer test. * $p < 0.05$ and ** $p < 0.01$.

2.3. Effects of Iso-α-Acids on Tau Phosphorylation in Tauopathy Mice

To evaluate the effects of iso-α-acids on the phosphorylation of tau, the levels of total tau and phosphorylated tau in the hippocampus and frontal cortex were measured. The levels of total tau were not changed by the consumption of iso-α-acids (Figure 3a). However, the levels of phosphorylated tau (pS199) soluble in TBS buffer in the frontal cortex were significantly decreased with the consumption of iso-α-acids (Figure 3b). The levels of phosphorylated tau (pS396 and pT231) in rTg4510 mice fed with iso-α-acids were lower, but this change was not significantly different from control rTg4510 mice (Figure 3c,d). pTau soluble in lauric acid and formic acid was not changed by the administration of iso-α-acids. The levels of phosphorylated tau in the hippocampus of rTg4510 mice and the levels of total tau and phosphorylated tau (pS199) in the frontal cortex of wild-type mice were not changed by the consumption of iso-α-acids. These results indicate that the consumption of iso-α-acids reduces the phosphorylation of tau in rTg4510 mice.

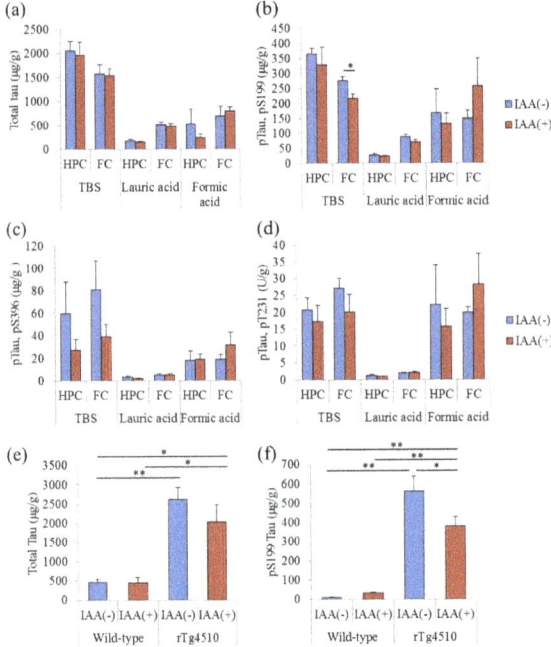

Figure 3. Effects of iso-α-acids on the phosphorylation of tau in rTg4510 mice. Three-month-old rTg4510 mice and wild-type mice were fed 0% or 0.05% (w/w) iso-α-acids (IAA) for three months. (**a–d**), the levels of total tau and phosphorylated tau (pS199, pS396, and pT231) soluble in tris-buffered saline (TBS) buffer, lauric acid, and formic acid of rTg4510 were measured. p-values shown in the graph were calculated by Student's t-test. * $p < 0.05$. (**e,f**), the levels of total tau and phosphorylated tau (pS199) soluble in TBS buffer of rTg4510 and wild-type mice fed with 0% or 0.05% (w/w) IAA, respectively. p-values shown in the graph were calculated by one-way ANOVA, followed by the Tukey-Kramer test. * $p < 0.05$ and ** $p < 0.01$.

3. Discussion

In the present study, we demonstrated that the consumption of iso-α-acids mitigated microglial inflammation and the phosphorylation of tau in the frontal cortex of tauopathy rTg4510 mice. To evaluate the effects of iso-α-acids on tauopathy, rTg4510 tauopathy mice were fed with iso-α-acids, and the levels of proinflammatory cytokines and pTau were measured. The consumption of iso-α-acids suppressed the levels of cytokines and chemokines in the frontal cortex and induced microglia into the anti-inflammatory type in rTg4510 mice. We previously reported that iso-α-acids activate PPAR-γ [13], and PPAR-γ activation by iso-α-acids is involved in the suppression of microglial inflammation using primary microglia [8]. It has also been reported that PPAR-γ activation induces microglia into the M2 anti-inflammatory type [14,15]. Pioglitazone, an agonist of PPAR-γ, induced microglia into the M2 type and showed anti-inflammatory effects in vivo [16]. These results suggest that iso-α-acids also suppress tau-induced microglial inflammation.

Inflammation in the brain has increasingly become a focus for studies of preventive and therapeutic approaches for Alzheimer's disease [17]. Epidemiological investigations have suggested that the intake of non-steroidal anti-inflammatory drugs (NSAIDs) has a preventive effect on Alzheimer's disease [18,19]. In addition, the potential of pioglitazone for medical treatments related to Alzheimer's disease has been suggested. Microglia play a crucial role in inflammation in the brain. In general, microglia remove the old synapses and waste products in the brain to maintain the environment [20]. On the other hand, massively activated microglia produce neurotoxic substances, including reactive oxygen spices and inflammatory cytokines [21]. It has been suggested that the polarization of microglia between the M1 inflammatory type and the M2 anti-inflammatory type is important for improving the neurological pathology and cognitive decline observed in Alzheimer's disease [22]. CD86 and MIP-1 proinflammatory markers of microglia are increased in rTg4510 mice [23,24], and consumption of iso-α-acids suppressed the expression of CD86 in rTg4510 mice. Therefore, it is suggested that iso-α-acids suppress the induction of microglia into the M1 proinflammatory type in rTg4510 mice.

We next evaluated the effects of iso-α-acids on the phosphorylation of tau, and the concentrations of tau and pTau were measured. pTau (Ser199), soluble in TBS, in rTg4510 mice fed with iso-α-acids was significantly lower than that of control rTg4510 mice. It has been reported that inflammation in the brain accelerates the phosphorylation of tau [25,26]. Intraventricular injection with lipopolysaccharide (LPS) in rTg4510 mice induces microglia into the proinflammatory type and increases the phosphorylation of tau (Ser199) in the frontal cortex and hippocampus [25]. These reports suggest that the suppression of inflammation in the frontal cortex of rTg4510 mice reduces the phosphorylation of tau. However, in the present study, we did not evaluate the direct effects of iso-α-acids on the phosphorylation of tau. Thus, further study is needed to further evaluate the relationship between inflammation and phosphorylation of tau.

In summary, in the present study, we analyzed the microglial inflammatory phenotype in rTg4510 mice; induced microglial inflammation in rTg4510 was suppressed by the consumption of iso-α-acids. Iso-α-acids are considered a safe food material because they are generated from α-acids in hops, and hops have been used as a material for brewing beer for more than 1000 years. The consumption of iso-α-acids suppresses the inflammation induced by various agents, including amyloid β [8], a high-fat diet [27], and pTau; therefore, it may help in preventing inflammatory-related brain disorders. Further study as part of a clinical trial is needed to evaluate the effects of iso-α-acids on cognitive function.

4. Materials and Methods

4.1. Animals

rTg4510 mice [28], a transgenic mouse model for human tauopathy, and control FVB/N-C57BL/6J mice (wild-type mice) were used in this study. Animals were maintained in an experimental facility at the University of Tokyo. rTg4510 mice overexpress human tau that contains the frontotemporal dementia-associated P301L mutation, and tau expression can be suppressed with doxycycline treatment [28]. For the expression of mutant tau in rTg4510 mice, the mutated gene, located downstream of a tetracycline-operon-responsive element, must be co-expressed with an activator transgene consisting of a tet-off open reading frame located downstream of the Ca^{2+}-calmodulin kinase II promoter elements [28]. Wild-type control mice lack both the tau responder and the activator transgene. Mice under 3 months of age were housed in cages, with free access to a standard purified rodent growth diet (AIN-93G, Oriental Yeast, Tokyo, Japan); mice over 3 months of age were housed with free access to a maintenance diet (AIN-93M, Oriental Yeast). Three-month-old mice were fed 0% or 0.05% (w/w) iso-α-acids for 3 months. The number of mice were 12 (wild-type mice without iso-α-acids), 6 (wild-type mice with iso-α-acids), 12 (rTg4510 mice without iso-α-acids), and 10 (rTg4510 mice with iso-α-acids). The Institutional Animal Care and Use Committee of the Graduate School of Agricultural and Life Science at the University of Tokyo approved all experiments in 2017 (Approval No. P17-020). All efforts were made to minimize suffering.

4.2. Preparation of Iso-α-Acids

Iso-α-Acids consist predominantly of three congeners: Cohumulone, humulone, and adhumulone. During the brewing process, they are each isomerized into two epimeric isomers, namely, *cis*- and *trans*-iso-α-acids (Figure 4). A purchased isomerized hop extract (IHE; Hopsteiner, Mainburg, Germany) with 30.5% (w/v) iso-α-acids, comprising *cis*-isocohumulone (7.61% w/v), *cis*-isohumulone

(14.0% *w/v*), and *cis*-isoadhumulone (3.37% *w/v*), *trans*-isocohumulone (1.74% *w/v*), *trans*-isohumulone (3.05% *w/v*), and *trans*-isoadhumulone (0.737% *w/v*) was used in this study.

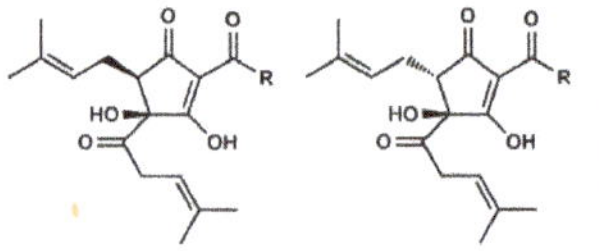

Figure 4. Chemical structures of iso-α-acids. Structures of *cis*-iso-α-acids: *Cis*-isocohumulone (**1a**), *cis*-isohumulone (**1b**), and *cis*-isoadhumulone (**1c**). Structures of *trans*-iso-α-acids: *Trans*-isocohumulone (**2a**), *trans*-isohumulone (**2b**), and *trans*-isoadhumulone (**2c**).

4.3. Microglia Analysis

Primary microglial cells were isolated from the brain via magnetic cell sorting after conjugation with anti-CD11b antibodies (Miltenyi Biotec, Bergisch Gladbach, Germany), as previously described [29]. Isolated CD11b-positive cells (>90% pure as evaluated by flow cytometry) were stained with anti-CD86-FITC (eBioscience, CA, USA), anti-CD68-APC (BioLegend, CA, USA), anti-TSPO-PE (PBR, Abcam, Cambridge, UK), and anti-CD11b-APC-Cy7 (BD Biosciences, CA, USA) antibodies after treatment with the BD Cytofix/Cytoperm Fixation/Permeabilization kit (BD Biosciences). To measure intracellular cytokines, microglia were plated in poly-D-lysine (PDL)-coated 96-well plates (BD Biosciences) and cultured in DMEM/F-12 (Gibco, CA, USA) medium supplemented with 10% fetal calf serum (Gibco) and 100 U/mL penicillium/streptomycin (Sigma-Aldrich, MO, USA) containing a leukocyte activation-cocktail with BD GolgiPlug^{TM} (BD Biosciences) for 12 h. Microglia cells were treated with the BD Cytofix/Cytoperm Fixation/Permeabilization kit (BD Biosciences) and then stained with anti-IL-1β-FITC (eBiosciences), anti-MIP-1α-PE (eBiosciences), anti-TNF-α-APC (BD Pharmingen, CA, USA), and anti-CD11b-APC-Cy7 (BD Biosciences) antibodies. Stained cells were analyzed using a flow cytometer (FACSCanto II; BD Biosciences).

4.4. Cytokines and Tau Measurement in Transgenic Mice

To measure cytokines and tau in the brain, the hippocampus and frontal cortex were homogenized in TBS buffer (Wako, Monza, Monza and Brianza, Lombardy, Italy) containing protease inhibitor cocktail (Biovision, CA, USA) and phosphatase inhibitor cocktail l and II (Wako) with a multi-bead shocker (Yasui Kikai, Osaka, Japan). After centrifugation at $50,000 \times g$ for 20 min (MX-107, Tommy, Tokyo, Japan), the supernatant was collected. The pellets were sonicated in sarkosyl solution (1% *N*-lauroylsarcosine (Sarkosyl) in 1 mM Tris, 1 mM EGTA, 1 mM DTT, and 10% sucrose, pH 7.5), and the supernatant was collected after centrifugation at $386,000 \times g$ for 20 min at 4 °C. The pellets were treated with formic acid and dried. The samples were dissolved in an assay buffer (0.2 g/L KCl, 0.2 g/L KH_2PO_4, 8.0 g/L NaCl, 1.150 g/L Na_2HPO_4, 5% BSA, 0.03% Tween 20, and 1× protease inhibitor cocktail (Calbiochem) in ultrapure water, pH 7.4). The total protein concentration of each supernatant was measured using a BCA protein assay kit (ThermoScientific, Yokohama, Japan). Each supernatant was assayed for quantifying total tau and phosphorylated tau (pTau) of pS199, pS396, and pT231 (Thermo Scientific, Waltham, MA, USA) by ELISA. For quantifying cytokines and chemokines, the first supernatant was evaluated by a Bio-Plex assay system (Bio-Rad, Hercules, CA, USA).

4.5. Statistical Analysis

The data represent the mean ± SEM. Data were analyzed by one-way ANOVA, followed by the Tukey-Kramer test or Student's *t*-test, as described in the figure legends. All statistical analyses were performed using the Ekuseru-Toukei 2012 software program (Social Survey Research Information, Tokyo, Japan). A value of $p < 0.05$ was considered statistically significant.

Author Contributions: Y.A. conducted most of biochemical analysis and wrote the majority of the paper. A.T., Y.T., K.U. and H.N. conducted the experiments using rTg4510 model mice, while K.K., A.T. and H.N. wrote the manuscript.

Funding: There is no funding in the present study.

Acknowledgments: We appreciate the technical support for Yuka Yoshino.

Conflicts of Interest: Ano, Y. and Kondo, K. are employed by Kirin Company Ltd. All other authors declare no competing interests.

References

1. Horvat, P.; Richards, M.; Kubinova, R.; Pajak, A.; Malyutina, S.; Shishkin, S.; Pikhart, H.; Peasey, A.; Marmot, M.G.; Singh-Manoux, A.; et al. Alcohol consumption, drinking patterns, and cognitive function in older Eastern European adults. *Neurology* **2015**, *84*, 287–295. [CrossRef] [PubMed]
2. Matsui, T.; Yoshimura, A.; Toyama, T.; Matsushita, S.; Higuchi, S. Preventive effect of moderation in drinking on dementia. *Nihon Rinsho. Jpn. J. Clin. Med.* **2011**, *69*, 217–222.
3. Neafsey, E.J.; Collins, M.A. Moderate alcohol consumption and cognitive risk. *Neuropsych. Dis. Treat.* **2011**, *7*, 465–484. [CrossRef] [PubMed]
4. Porquet, D.; Grinan-Ferre, C.; Ferrer, I.; Camins, A.; Sanfeliu, C.; Del Valle, J.; Pallas, M. Neuroprotective role of trans-resveratrol in a murine model of familial Alzheimer's disease. *J. Alzheimers Dis.* **2014**, *42*, 1209–1220. [CrossRef] [PubMed]
5. Arntzen, K.A.; Schirmer, H.; Wilsgaard, T.; Mathiesen, E.B. Moderate wine consumption is associated with better cognitive test results: A 7 year follow up of 5033 subjects in the Tromso Study. *Acta Neurol. Scand.* **2010**, *122*, 23–29. [CrossRef] [PubMed]
6. Vidavalur, R.; Otani, H.; Singal, P.K.; Maulik, N. Significance of wine and resveratrol in cardiovascular disease: French paradox revisited. *Exp. Clin. Cardiol.* **2006**, *11*, 217–225. [PubMed]
7. Witte, A.V.; Kerti, L.; Margulies, D.S.; Floel, A. Effects of resveratrol on memory performance, hippocampal functional connectivity, and glucose metabolism in healthy older adults. *J. Neurosci.* **2014**, *34*, 7862–7870. [CrossRef] [PubMed]
8. Ano, Y.; Dohata, A.; Taniguchi, Y.; Hoshi, A.; Uchida, K.; Takashima, A.; Nakayama, H. Iso-α-acids, Bitter Components of Beer, Prevent Inflammation and Cognitive Decline Induced in a Mouse Model of Alzheimer's Disease. *J. Biol. Chem.* **2017**, *292*, 3720–3728. [CrossRef] [PubMed]
9. Binder, L.I.; Guillozet-Bongaarts, A.L.; Garcia-Sierra, F.; Berry, R.W. Tau, tangles, and Alzheimer's disease. *Biochim. Biophys. Acta* **2005**, *1739*, 216–223. [CrossRef] [PubMed]
10. Leyns, C.E.G.; Holtzman, D.M. Glial contributions to neurodegeneration in tauopathies. *Mol. Neurodegener.* **2017**, *12*, 50. [CrossRef] [PubMed]
11. Hansen, D.V.; Hanson, J.E.; Sheng, M. Microglia in Alzheimer's disease. *J. Cell Biol.* **2018**, *217*, 459–472. [CrossRef] [PubMed]
12. Sahara, N.; Maeda, J.; Ishikawa, A.; Tokunaga, M.; Suhara, T.; Higuchi, M. Microglial Activation during Pathogenesis of Tauopathy in rTg4510 Mice: Implications for the Early Diagnosis of Tauopathy. *J. Alzheimers Dis.* **2018**, *64*, 1–7. [CrossRef] [PubMed]
13. Yajima, H.; Ikeshima, E.; Shiraki, M.; Kanaya, T.; Fujiwara, D.; Odai, H.; Tsuboyama-Kasaoka, N.; Ezaki, O.; Oikawa, S.; Kondo, K. Isohumulones, bitter acids derived from hops, activate both peroxisome proliferator-activated receptor α and γ and reduce insulin resistance. *J. Biol. Chem.* **2004**, *279*, 33456–33462. [CrossRef] [PubMed]
14. Pan, J.; Jin, J.L.; Ge, H.M.; Yin, K.L.; Chen, X.; Han, L.J.; Chen, Y.; Qian, L.; Li, X.X.; Xu, Y. Malibatol A regulates microglia M1/M2 polarization in experimental stroke in a PPARγ-dependent manner. *J. Neuroinflamm.* **2015**, *12*, 51. [CrossRef] [PubMed]
15. Wen, L.; You, W.; Wang, H.; Meng, Y.; Feng, J.; Yang, X. Polarization of Microglia to the M2 Phenotype in a Peroxisome Proliferator-Activated Receptor Gamma-Dependent Manner Attenuates Axonal Injury Induced by Traumatic Brain Injury in Mice. *J. Neurotraum.* **2018**. [CrossRef] [PubMed]
16. Mandrekar-Colucci, S.; Karlo, J.C.; Landreth, G.E. Mechanisms underlying the rapid peroxisome proliferator-activated receptor-γ-mediated amyloid clearance and reversal of cognitive deficits in a murine model of Alzheimer's disease. *J. Neurotraum.* **2012**, *32*, 10117–10128. [CrossRef] [PubMed]

17. Fernandez, P.L.; Britton, G.B.; Rao, K.S. Potential immunotargets for Alzheimer's disease treatment strategies. *J. Alzheimers Dis.* **2013**, *33*, 297–312. [CrossRef] [PubMed]
18. Stewart, W.F.; Kawas, C.; Corrada, M.; Metter, E.J. Risk of Alzheimer's disease and duration of NSAID use. *Neurology* **1997**, *48*, 626–632. [CrossRef] [PubMed]
19. Breitner, J.C.; Welsh, K.A.; Helms, M.J.; Gaskell, P.C.; Gau, B.A.; Roses, A.D.; Pericak-Vance, M.A.; Saunders, A.M. Delayed onset of Alzheimer's disease with nonsteroidal anti-inflammatory and histamine H2 blocking drugs. *Neurobiol. Aging* **1995**, *16*, 523–530. [CrossRef]
20. Kettenmann, H.; Kirchhoff, F.; Verkhratsky, A. Microglia: New roles for the synaptic stripper. *Neuron* **2013**, *77*, 10–18. [CrossRef] [PubMed]
21. Lull, M.E.; Block, M.L. Microglial activation and chronic neurodegeneration. *Neurotherapeutics* **2010**, *7*, 354–365. [CrossRef] [PubMed]
22. Sarlus, H.; Heneka, M.T. Microglia in Alzheimer's disease. *J. Clin. Investig.* **2017**, *127*, 3240–3249. [CrossRef] [PubMed]
23. Saqib, U.; Sarkar, S.; Suk, K.; Mohammad, O.; Baig, M.S.; Savai, R. Phytochemicals as modulators of M1-M2 macrophages in inflammation. *Oncotarget* **2018**, *9*, 17937–17950. [CrossRef] [PubMed]
24. Zhou, T.; Huang, Z.; Sun, X.; Zhu, X.; Zhou, L.; Li, M.; Cheng, B.; Liu, X.; He, C. Microglia Polarization with M1/M2 Phenotype Changes in rd1 Mouse Model of Retinal Degeneration. *Front. Neuroanat.* **2017**, *11*, 77. [CrossRef] [PubMed]
25. Lee, D.C.; Rizer, J.; Selenica, M.L.; Reid, P.; Kraft, C.; Johnson, A.; Blair, L.; Gordon, M.N.; Dickey, C.A.; Morgan, D. LPS-induced inflammation exacerbates phospho-tau pathology in rTg4510 mice. *J. Neuroinflamm.* **2010**, *7*, 56. [CrossRef] [PubMed]
26. Metcalfe, M.J.; Figueiredo-Pereira, M.E. Relationship between tau pathology and neuroinflammation in Alzheimer's disease. *Mt. Sinai J. Med.* **2010**, *77*, 50–58. [CrossRef] [PubMed]
27. Ayabe, T.; Ohya, R.; Kondo, K.; Ano, Y. Iso-α-acids, bitter components of beer, prevent obesity-induced cognitive decline. *Sci. Rep.* **2018**, *8*, 4760. [CrossRef] [PubMed]
28. Spires, T.L.; Orne, J.D.; SantaCruz, K.; Pitstick, R.; Carlson, G.A.; Ashe, K.H.; Hyman, B.T. Region-specific dissociation of neuronal loss and neurofibrillary pathology in a mouse model of tauopathy. *Am. J. Pathol.* **2006**, *168*, 1598–1607. [CrossRef] [PubMed]
29. Ano, Y.; Ozawa, M.; Kutsukake, T.; Sugiyama, S.; Uchida, K.; Yoshida, A.; Nakayama, H. Preventive effects of a fermented dairy product against Alzheimer's disease and identification of a novel oleamide with enhanced microglial phagocytosis and anti-inflammatory activity. *PLoS ONE* **2015**, *10*, e0118512. [CrossRef] [PubMed]

Sample Availability: Samples of the compounds of isomerized hop extracts are available from the authors only for the academic science.

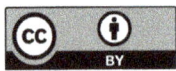

© 2018 by the authors. Licensee MDPI, Basel, Switzerland. This article is an open access article distributed under the terms and conditions of the Creative Commons Attribution (CC BY) license (http://creativecommons.org/licenses/by/4.0/).

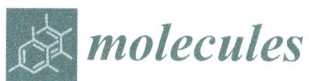

Article

Nuciferine Inhibits Proinflammatory Cytokines via the PPARs in LPS-Induced RAW264.7 Cells

Chao Zhang [1,2,†], Jianjun Deng [3,†], Dan Liu [1], Xingxia Tuo [1], Yan Yu [1], Haixia Yang [1,*] and Nanping Wang [2,4,*]

1. Department of Nutrition and Food Safety, College of Public Health, Xi'an Jiaotong University, Xi'an 710061, China; zhangchao9277@163.com (C.Z.); liudan940305@163.com (D.L.); yyyyyy_214@163.com (X.T.); yuyan@mail.xjtu.edu.cn (Y.Y.)
2. Cardiovascular Research Center, Xi'an Jiaotong University, Xi'an 710061, China
3. Shaanxi Key Laboratory of Degradable Biomedical Materials, School of Chemical Engineering, Northwest University, Xi'an 710069, China; dengjianjun@nwu.edu.cn
4. The Advanced Institute for Medical Sciences, Dalian Medical University, Dalian 116044, China
* Correspondence: yanghx@xjtu.edu.cn (H.Y.); nanpingwang2003@yahoo.com (N.W.); Tel.: +86-029-8265-5107 (H.Y.)
† These authors contributed equally to this work.

Academic Editor: Francesco Maione
Received: 29 September 2018; Accepted: 21 October 2018; Published: 22 October 2018

Abstract: Inflammation is important and has been found to be an underlying cause in many acute and chronic human diseases. Nuciferine, a natural alkaloid containing an aromatic ring, is found in the *nelumbo nucifera* leaves. It has been shown to have potential anti-inflammatory activities, but the molecular mechanism has remained unclear. In this study, we found that nuciferine (10 µM) significantly inhibited the lipopolysaccharide (LPS)-induced inflammatory cytokine IL-6 and TNF-α production in RAW 264.7 cells. In addition, the luciferase reporter assay results of different subtypes of the peroxisome proliferator-activated receptor (PPAR) showed that nuciferine dose-dependently activated all the PPAR activities. Specific inhibitors of PPARα and PPARγ significantly abolished the production of inflammatory cytokines as well as IκBα degradation. However, PPARδ inhibitor did not show this effect. Our results suggested a potential molecular mechanism of the anti-inflammatory effects of nuciferine in LPS-induced inflammation, at least in part, by activating PPARα and PPARγ in RAW 264.7 cells.

Keywords: nuciferine; inflammation; PPARs; IL-6; TNF-α

---

1. Introduction

Inflammatory responses are widely implicated in vast kinds of acute and chronic human diseases, including cancer, atherosclerosis, and diabetes [1]. Macrophages play a critical role and are involved in the self-regulating cycle of inflammation, as macrophages produce multiple pro-inflammatory cytokines and mediators that are involved in inflammation, such as the TNFα and the IL-6 [2]. Interference therapy that target macrophages and related cytokines may be some new approaches for controlling inflammatory diseases.

Regulation of the inflammatory response depends on a variety of potential mechanisms, including peroxisome proliferator-activated receptors (PPARs) actions [3]. PPARs are activated by their synthetic or natural ligands/modulators, which lead to the PPARs to bind to their specific DNA response elements, as heterodimers, with the retinoid X receptor (RXR) [4]. PPARs have been found to have three subtypes, which are named PPARα, PPARβ/δ, and PPAR. They play crucial roles in the regulation of lipid and glucose metabolism. In addition, accumulating evidence reveals that activation of the PPARs are involved in the various types of inflammatory processes, due to the inhibition of pro-inflammatory genes expression and negative regulation of pro-inflammatory transcription factor signaling pathways, in inflammatory cells [5]. Furthermore, activation of PPARs shows the anti-inflammatory effect by inhibiting the activation of nuclear factor-κB (NF-κB), leading to a decrease of pro-inflammatory cytokines and mediators [6]. Therefore, PPARs have been shown to be the drug targets to treat various related inflammatory diseases, such as vascular diseases, cancer, and neurodegenerative diseases [7]. Searching for the effective ligands or modulators of PPARs, for the prevention and clinical therapeutic options, is of great interest.

The natural product nuciferine ((R)-1,2-dimethoxyaporphine; Nuci) is an alkaloid found within the leaves of *Nymphaea caerulea* and *Nelumbo nucifera*, which is widely planted in Asia, the Middle East, and some countries in Africa [8]. Especially in China, lotus leaves are usually commercially available for tea due to its pharmacologic effects, such as losing weight, heat-clearing, and detoxifying, according to the traditional theory of Chinese medicine [9]. Recent studies showed that nuciferine, an important component of lotus leave extracts, can improve hepatic lipid metabolism [10], increase the glucose consumption, and stimulate insulin secretion [11]. Anti-inflammation activity of nuciferine was also reported in potassium oxonate-induced kidney inflammation [12], as well as Fructose-induced inflammatory responses [13], in vivo. However, the underlying molecular mechanisms of its anti-inflammatory effects are not fully understood. Based on the inflammatory-related functions of PPARs and the differences of the distinct tissue-specific expression, physiology, and ligand specificity of the PPARα, PPARβ/δ, and the PPARγ, the aim of this study was to investigate the effect of nuciferine on inflammation in lipopolysaccharide (LPS)-induced RAW264.7 cells and to observe if this effect is mediated by the three PPAR subtypes.

2. Results

2.1. Cytotoxicity of Nuciferine on RAW264.7 Cells

To test the effect of nuciferine on the cell viabilities of RAW264.7 cells, 3-(4,5-dimethyl-2-thiazolyl)-2,5-diphenyltetrazolium bromide (MTT) assay was performed in RAW264.7 cells, using different concentrations of nuciferine, ranging from 1 to 50 μM. After treatment for 24 h, cell viabilities were measured, and the results are shown in Figure 1. Compared with the control group (without nuciferine), no significant difference ($p > 0.05$) were found between control and all the treatment groups, indicating that nuciferine had no direct cytotoxicity, in this cell line. To avoid using a concentration of nuciferine higher than the normal physiological concentration, 10 μM was used in all of the following experiments.

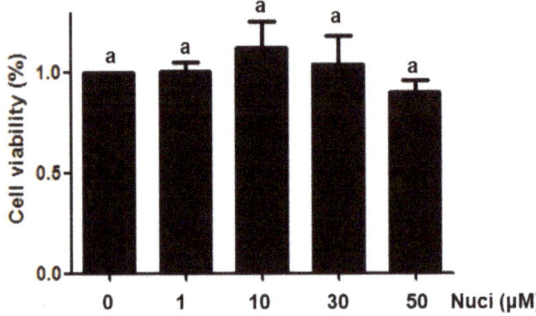

Figure 1. Cytotoxicity of Nuciferine on macrophage RAW264.7 cells. Cell viabilities of RAW264.7 cells treated with Nuciferine (0, 1, 3, 10 or 50 μM), for 24 h, were measured by MTT assay.

2.2. Nuciferine Inhibited IL-6 and TNFα Production in LPS-Induced RAW264.7 Cells

In order to evaluate whether the nuciferine has potential anti-inflammatory activity in RAW264.7 cells, the cells were pretreated with nuciferine (1~50 μM), for 24 h, before exposure to LPS, and the pro-inflammatory cytokines IL-6 and TNFα were examined (Figure 2). Without the LPS stimulation, the concentrations of TNFα and IL-6, in the cell medium, by ELISA were 380.5 ± 51.3 pg/mL and 352.1 ± 60.1 pg/mL, respectively (Figure 2A,B). The LPS treatment significantly increased ($p < 0.05$) both TNFα and IL-6 levels by 679.2% and 472.6%, respectively. Importantly, the nuciferine decreased both these cytokine levels induced by the LPS, in a dose-dependent manner. Meanwhile, gene expression of these cytokines, by RT-qPCR, showed the same trends as the ELISA results (Figure 2C,D). Pearson correlation analysis of both the protein and the mRNA levels of TNFα and IL-6, with the nuciferine concentrations, are shown in Table 1. With the LPS treatment, it showed significant negative correlation of the ratio of nuciferine concentration versus IL-6 protein level (Pearson $r = -0.62$, $p = 0.004$, $n = 20$) or mRNA level (Pearson $r = -0.50$, $p = 0.02$, $n = 20$). Similarly, significant negative correlations were found between nuciferine concentration and TNFα protein level (Pearson $r = -0.58$, $p = 0.02$, $n = 20$) or mRNA level (Pearson $r = -0.69$, $p = 0.01$, $n = 20$). All these results indicated that nuciferine had a potential anti-inflammatory effect, by reducing inflammatory cytokines production.

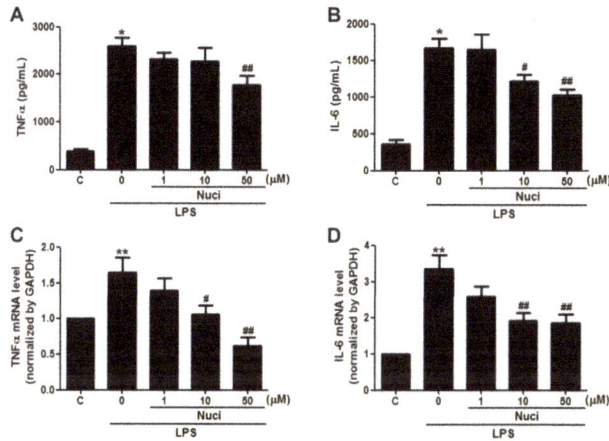

Figure 2. Nuciferine inhibits the LPS-induced TNFα and IL-6 production in RAW264.7 cells. RAW 264.7 cells were pretreated with nuciferine (0, 1, 10 or 50 μM for 24 h) and then stimulated with the LPS (500 ng/mL for 12 h), with a nuciferine withdrawal. (**A,B**) TNFα and IL-6 releases and (**C,D**) mRNA level of TNFα and IL-6, respectively. * $p < 0.05$ ** $p < 0.01$ vs. control, # $p < 0.05$ ## $p < 0.01$ vs. LPS treatment.

Table 1. Nuciferine inhibits the LPS-induced TNFα and IL-6 production in RAW264.7 cells.

Nuciferine (μM)	LPS (ng/mL)	TNFα		IL-6	
		Protein (pg/mL)	mRNA	Protein (pg/mL)	mRNA
0	0	380.51 ± 51.27	0.99 ± 0.01	352.01 ± 60.02	1.01 ± 0.01
0	500	2584.46 ± 179.60 *	1.64 ± 0.21 **	1663.71 ± 137.20 *	3.34 ± 0.39 **
1	500	2315.98 ± 146.64	1.39 ± 0.17	1643.94 ± 209.69	2.59 ± 0.28
10	500	2139.87 ± 275.53	1.05 ± 0.13 #	1216.91 ± 88.18 #	1.92 ± 0.20 ##
50	500	1772.82 ± 203.58 ##	0.61 ± 0.11 ##	1028.78 ± 74.61 ##	1.85 ± 0.21 ##

Quantitative data are presented as mean ± SEM. * $p < 0.05$ ** $p < 0.01$ vs. control, # $p < 0.05$ ## $p < 0.01$ vs. LPS treatment.

2.3. Nuciferine Increased the PPARs Activity

PPARs are involved in the various types of inflammatory processes [5]. To study the potential molecular mechanism of nuciferine on the LPS-induced inflammation, we examined the effects of nuciferine on PPARs activity by a luciferase reporter assay. The cells were transfected with PPARs isoforms (PPARα/PPARδ/PPARγ) plasmid and reporter plasmid, followed by the treatment of nuciferine (1 or 10 µM) or PPARs agonists, for 24 h. All the selective agonists WY14643 for PPARα, GW501516 for PPARβ/δ, and rosiglitazone (Rosi) for PPARγ, significantly increased the fluorescence signal in the both the RAW264.7 cells and HEK 293 cells, confirming that the systems for detecting PPARs transactivation activity were correct. In the RAW 264.7 cells, nuciferine significantly increased the transcriptional activities of PPARα and PPARγ, in a dose-dependent manner, compared to control group. However, it did not affect PPARβ/δ activity (Figure 3A–C). Pearson correlation analysis (Table 2) shows a significant positive correlation of the ratio of nuciferine concentration, versus the PPARα activity (Pearson $r = 0.70$; $p = 0.004$, $n = 15$) and a significant positive correlation of the ratio of nuciferine concentration versus the PPARγ activity (Pearson $r = 0.51$; $p = 0.05$, $n = 15$). However, there was no significant correlation of the ratio of nuciferine concentration versus the PPARβ/δ activity (Pearson $r = 0.29$; $p = 0.11$, $n = 15$). Meanwhile, the luciferase reporter assay was carried out using the HEK 293 cells (Supplementary Figure S1) to verify the results. All the results showed that nuciferine increased the activities of the three PPARs but only significantly increased the PPARα and PPARγ activity. The mRNA levels of the targets genes of PPARs, such as carnitine palmitoyltransferase 1A (CPT-1A) for PPARα [14], adipose differentiation related protein (ADRP) for PPARβ/δ [15], CD36 for PPARγ [16], were further investigated (Figure 3D). All these target genes expressions were up-regulated by nuciferine, at 10 µM, in the RAW264.7 cells. Together, these results indicated that nuciferine could enhance PPARs transcriptional activity in mononuclear macrophages.

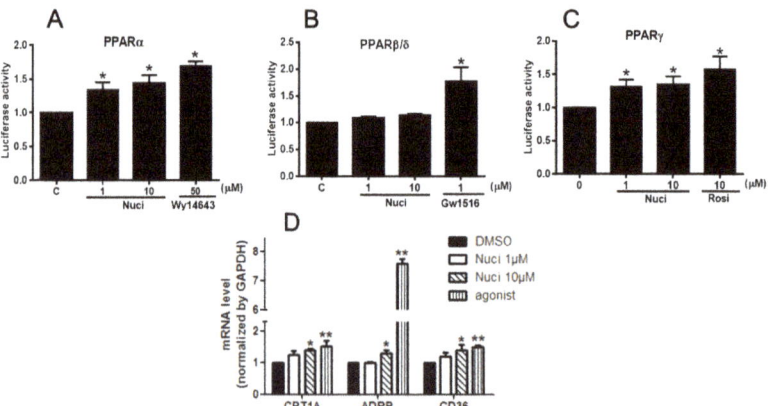

Figure 3. Effect of Nuciferine on PPARs transcription activities. (**A**–**C**) Luciferase reporter assay in RAW264.7 cells. (**D**) The relative mRNA expression of PPARs target genes. * $p < 0.05$ ** $p < 0.01$ vs. control.

Table 2. Effect of Nuciferine on PPARs transcription activities in RAW264.7 cells.

Nuci (µM)	PPARα	PPARβ/δ	PPARγ
0	1.03 ± 0.04	0.99 ± 0.01	1.02 ± 0.01
1	1.34 ± 0.11 *	1.03 ± 0.19	1.31 ± 0.09 *
10	1.44 ± 0.11 *	1.13 ± 0.27	1.35 ± 0.12 *
agonist	1.69 ± 0.06 *	1.17 ± 0.22 *	1.57 ± 0.13 *

Quantitative data are presented as mean ± SEM. * $p < 0.05$ vs. control.

2.4. Antagonists of PPARα and PPARγ Abolished the Anti-Inflammatory Effects of Nuciferine

To further clarify whether the anti-inflammatory effect of nuciferine are mediated by PPARs, antagonists GW5417 for PPARα, GSK0660 for PPARβ/δ, GW9662 for PPARγ were co-administered with nuciferine, for 24 h, in the LPS-induced RAW264.7 cells, respectively (Figure 4). As the results before, when stimulated with the LPS, the content of IL-6 and TNFα were increased. All these antagonists increased the pro-inflammatory cytokines, compared with the group treated with the LPS only. However, the effect of nuciferine was abolished in the presence of the PPARα and PPARγ antagonists, indicating that the anti-inflammatory effect of nuciferine, at least partially, went through the PPARs activation.

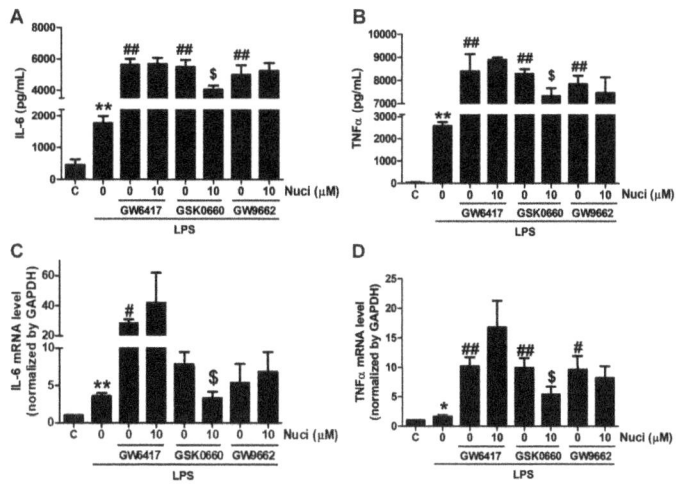

Figure 4. Antagonist of PPARα and PPARγ abolished the effects of nuciferine on the LPS-induced TNFα and IL-6 production. RAW264.7 cells were pretreated with GW6417/GSK0660/GW9662, for 12 h, followed by the nuciferine incubation, for 24 h, and then stimulated with LPS for 12 h. (**A,B**) production of the IL-6 and the TNFα in a cell medium supernatant. (**C,D**) mRNA expression of IL-6 and TNFα. * $p < 0.05$ ** $p < 0.01$ vs. control. # $p < 0.05$, ## $p < 0.01$ vs. LPS treatment. $ $p < 0.05$ vs. antagonist pretreatment followed by the LPS stimulation.

2.5. Nuciferine Decreased LPS Induced IκB-α Degradation through PPARs Activation

PPARs exert anti-inflammatory effects by regulating the NF-κB signal pathway. To further investigate the mechanisms of nuciferine on anti-inflammatory effect, the degradation of IκB-α protein levels were determined with exposure to the nuciferine in the LPS-treated RAW 264.7 cells (Figure 5, original results see Figure S2). When stimulated only with LPS, the cytosolic IκB-α protein was markedly degraded, consistent with the THP-1 treatment results [17]. However, nuciferine treatment attenuated the pro-inflammatory effect of the LPS. Furthermore, the effects of nuciferine were abolished by a co-incubation with PPARs antagonists. The results suggested that nuciferine dramatically inhibited the LPS-induced NF-κB activation and its effect was PPARs-dependent.

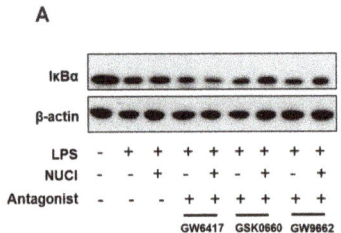
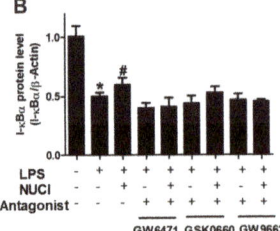

Figure 5. Anti-inflammatory effects of nuciferine on the LPS-induced inflammatory response, are PPARs dependent. RAW264.7 cells were pretreated with GW6417/GSK0660/GW9662, for 12 h, followed by the Nuciferine incubation and then stimulated by the LPS with a nuciferine withdrawal. Levels of the expression of IκBα were detected by Western blotting. * $p < 0.05$ vs. control group; # $p < 0.05$ vs. LPS group.

3. Discussion

Our present study has shown that treatment with nuciferine ameliorates the LPS-induced inflammation in RAW264.7 cells. Importantly, it was found that the protective effect of nuciferine is mediated by PPARs activation. These results highlight the potential use of nuciferine for preventing inflammation.

Overexpression of the inflammatory mediators is closely associated with systemic injury. There is evidence that anti-inflammatory treatment has become an important component of inflammatory diseases [18]. Inflammatory mediator inhibitors can be shown to have beneficial effects in improving the severity of inflammation-related diseases. A wide variety of phytochemicals derived from natural plant have anti-inflammatory effects, such as phenolics, terpenolids, and alkaloids [19]. Nuciferine, an alkaloid found in the lotus leaves, exerted a protective effect against inflammation, in vivo [20] and in vitro [21]. Our results showed that nuciferine decreased the expression of inflammatory cytokines IL-6 and TNFα, in both protein and gene levels, dose dependently, in the LPS-treated RAW264.7 cells, indicating that nuciferine had potential anti-inflammatory effects.

Nuciferine, a natural alkaloid from the lotus leaves, have been reported to exert multiple beneficial effects, in vivo and in vitro, such as anti-tumor [22] and insulin stimulatory effects [23]. Our recent results showed that nuciferine improved the hepatic steatosis in high-fat diet/streptozocin-induced diabetic mice [24]. Some studies reported that nuciferine suppressed the inflammation by regulating inflammatory signaling through different signal pathways. For example, in hyperuricemia mouse model, nuciferine inhibited renal inflammation through suppression of Toll-like receptor 4/myeloid differentiation factor 88/NF-κB signaling and a NOD-like receptor family, pyrin domain containing 3 (NLRP3) inflammasome [12]. Similarly, in vitro studies, nuciferine exerted the anti-inflammatory and antilipemic effects, as well as the siRNA Per-Arnt-Sim kinase treatment group in oleic acid-induced hepatic steatosis, in HepG$_2$ cells, indicating a potential molecular pathway of the anti-inflammation effect of nuciferine [21]. As we know, the three subtypes of PPARs exert anti-inflammatory effects in vivo and in vitro by several different molecular mechanisms [25–27]. PPARα [28] and PPARγ [29] were shown to repress some other transcription factors, such as NF-κB signal pathway, to reduce the release of inflammatory cytokines including IL-6 and TNFα, when they were activated by their ligands. The anti-inflammatory effects of PPARβ are mediated by ligand-independent repression [30]. Owing to the anti-inflammatory effect of PPARs, we used the luciferase reporter assay and the target gene transcription of PPARα/PPARγ/PPARδ to test if the PPAR family is involved in the anti-inflammatory effect of nuciferine. The results showed that nuciferine activated the PPAR family, especially the PPARα and the PPARγ. Moreover, the antagonists of the PPAR family GW6417/GSK0660/GW9662 were treated in the cells to block the PPARs activities, before the nuciferine treatment. What's interesting is that all the antagonist treatment increased the inflammation markers. The protective effect of nuciferine was remarkably diminished by the inhibition of PPARα and PPARγ, indicating that the anti-inflammatory effect of nuciferine, at least in part, went through the PPARs receptor activation. To confirm these results, the protein expression of the activated PPARs and the total PPARs should also be tested, using immunoblotting, in the further studies. Our recent in vivo results also clarified that nuciferine-activated PPARα in the liver tissues, in a diabetic mouse model [24]. Nuciferine is hydrophobic, consistent with the structures of most PPAR agonists. It could interact with the ligand-binding domain of PPARs, in theory, leading to the stabilization of the configuration of the hydrophobic core and subsequently the activation of PPARs to regulate the gene transcription [31]. However, more binding mechanisms between the nuciferine and the PPARs should be further studied.

It is well known that NF-κB is an important target for inflammatory therapeutic strategy [32]. PPARs have recently been shown to exert the anti-inflammatory activity by reducing the DNA-binding activity of NF-κB and suppressing its nucleus translocation, which attenuates the cytokine production and reduces tissue injury [32–34]. NF-κB is a crucial factor to activate the inflammatory genes transcription, including pro-inflammatory cytokines, such as TNFα and IL-6 [35]. In addition, IκBα expression was accompanied by a decrease in NF-κB DNA binding activity [36]. Our results showed that nuciferine treatment alters the IκBα cellular content in LPS stimulation. Moreover, the specific inhibitors for PPARs reversed the effect of nuciferine, partially or completely, indicating that nuciferine could prevent IκBα degradation via PPARs activation, under the LPS stimulated conditions.

Overall, our studies demonstrated that nuciferine, with a concentration of 10 μM, attenuated the LPS-induced inflammation through activation of PPARs, especially PPAR-α and -γ, in RAW264.7 cells. These findings suggest that nuciferine may be a potentially important candidate for inflammatory diseases.

4. Materials and Methods

4.1. Reagents

Nuciferine (purity by HPLC > 98.0%) was purchased from APP-CHEM (YHI-039, Xi'an, Shanxi, China). Dulbecco's modified Eagle's medium-high glucose (DMEM), fetal bovine serum (FBS), 3-(4,5-dimethylthiazol-2-yl)-2,5-diphenyltetrazolium bromide (MTT), and Lipofectamine 2000 reagent were purchased from Invitrogen (Carlsbad, CA, USA). Lipopolysaccharide (LPS), PPARs agonists WY14643, GW501516, rosiglitazone (Rosi) were purchased from Sigma (St. Louis, MO, USA). TRIzol reagent was purchased from Invitrogen (Carlsbad, CA, USA). IL-6 and TNF-α Mouse ELISA Kit was obtained from Elabscience Biotechnology Co. Ltd. (Wuhan, Hubei, China). Super Script II Rnase H Reverse Transcriptase kit was purchased from Invitrogen (Carlsbad, CA, USA).

4.2. Cell Culture

Murine macrophage RAW264.7 cells (ATCC, Rockville, MD, USA) and human embryonic kidney cells (HEK293 cells, ATCC, Rockville, MD, USA) were cultured with DMEM containing 10% FBS, 100 U/mL penicillin, and 100 U/mL streptomycin. Cells were maintained at 37 °C, in a humidified atmosphere of 5% CO_2 and 95% air. RAW264.7 cells were seeded into plates and treated at approximately 80% confluence.

4.3. Cytotoxicity

RAW264.7 cells were seeded at a density of 1.5×10^3 cells/well in 96-well plates. After 24 h, cells were treated with different concentrations of nuciferine (0–50 μM), for 24 h, followed by an addition 20 μL MTT solution (5 g/L), to each well, for 4 h. The insoluble formazan product was dissolved in 150 μL/well dimethyl sulfoxide (DMSO), after washing out the supernatant [37]. Then, the absorbance at 490 nm was measured using a microplate reader (Olympus America Inc., New York, NY, USA). The percentage of cytotoxicity was calculated by the equation: Cytotoxicity (%) = (1 − A_{490} of sample)/A_{490} of control well.

4.4. IL-6 and TNFα Levels Determination

RAW264.7 cells were grown into 12-well plates, treated with different concentrations of nuciferine (0, 1, 10 or 50 µM) and stimulated with LPS (500 ng/mL). Cell-free supernatants were collected and the levels of pro-inflammatory cytokines, TNFα and IL-6 were measured using ELISA kits, by a determination of the absorbance at 450 nm, according to the manufacturer's instructions. Standard curves were used to calculate the concentration of TNFα and IL-6 in each sample.

4.5. PPARs Luciferase Reporter Assay

HEK293T cells and RAW264.7 cells were plated into 12-well plates at 4×10^5 cells/well without antibiotics. After 24 h at 60% confluence, cells were transfected according to the manufacturer's instructions. Briefly, PPARs isoforms (PPARα/PPARδ/PPARγ) plasmid (0.9 µg), reporter plasmid PPRE×3-TK-LUC (0.3 µg) and β-gal (0.1 µg) were transfected into the cells, using Lipofectamine 2000 reagents (1:1), for 4 h. Since transfection efficiency is typically low in RAW264.7 cells, more Lipofectamine 2000 was needed (1:2.5) and the transfection time was extended to 24 h. The medium was replaced with a complete media containing DMSO, nuciferine, or PPARs agonists, for 24 h. The cells were harvested and lysed to measure the luciferase activities using a luciferase assay kit, according to the manufacturer's instructions. The β-gal was transfected to normalize the transfection efficiency [38].

4.6. RNA Isolation and Analysis

Cells were cultured into 12-well plate with a density of 4×10^5 cells/well. Total RNA was isolated using TRIzol reagent and reverse transcribed into cDNA. Real-time quantitative polymerase chain reaction (RT-qPCR) was performed as described by Yang et al. [39]. Glyceraldehyde-3-phosphate dehydrogenase (*Gapdh*) was used as an internal control. Ct values of the sample were calculated, and the mRNA levels were analyzed by $2^{-\Delta\Delta Ct}$ method and normalized to *Gapdh* [40]. The primer sequences were listed in Supplemental Table S1.

4.7. Immunoblotting

RAW264.7 Cell lysates were prepared using a lysis buffer containing 0.1% Triton X-100 and proteinase inhibitors (Roche, Nutley, NJ, USA). Protein concentrations were determined using the BCA protein assay kit (Thermo Scientific, PA, USA). Western blot was performed as described by Yang et al. [39]. After blocking the membranes, primary rabbit antibody against IκBα (Santa Cruz Biotechnology, Dallas, TX, USA) was incubated with a ratio of 1:1000 overnight. β-actin (1:5000, Santa Cruz Biotechnology, Dallas, TX, USA) was used as a loading control. Membranes were then washed with TBST and incubated with the secondary antibodies conjugated to anti-rabbit or anti-mouse HRP-conjugated secondary antibodies (1:3000, Santa Cruz Biotechnology, Dallas, TX, USA) for 1 h. Bands were detected by enhanced chemiluminescence using ECL (Amersham Biosciences, Picataway, NJ, USA) and then visualized by X-ray films.

4.8. Data Statistics

Quantitative data are expressed as mean ± SEM using SPSS 18.0 (IBM Corporation, Chicago, IL, USA). Student *t* test and ANOVA followed by Tukey's post hoc test were used to analyze the significant difference between two or more groups, respectively. The rank-based test methods were employed when data were not in a normal distribution or the variances were not homogeneous. All the results were representative of at least three independent experiments.

Supplementary Materials: The following are available online, Figure S1: Effect of Nuciferine on PPARs transcription activities in HEK 293 cells. Figure S2: Original western blot films of Figure 5A. Table S1: Sequences of primers for qRT-PCR.

Author Contributions: C.Z., J.D., N.W. and H.Y. conceived and designed the experiments and wrote the paper; C.Z. performed the experiments; D.L., X.T., and Y.Y. analyzed the data and check the manuscript. All authors read and approved the final manuscript.

Funding: This project was supported by the National Natural Science Foundation of China (21676212), China Postdoctoral Science Foundation (2016M602833), Shaanxi Postdoctoral Science Foundation (2017BSHTDZZ14), and Shaanxi Provincial Scientific Technology Research and Development Program (2018KJXX-017).

Conflicts of Interest: The authors declare no conflict of interest.

References

1. Boteanu, R.M.; Suica, V.I.; Uyy, E.; Ivan, L.; Dima, S.O.; Popescu, I.; Simionescu, M.; Antohe, F. Alarmins in chronic noncommunicable diseases: Atherosclerosis, diabetes and cancer. *J. Proteomics* **2017**, *153*, 21–29. [CrossRef] [PubMed]
2. Laskin, D.L.; Pendino, K.J. Macrophages and inflammatory mediators in tissue injury. *Annu. Rev. Pharmacol. Toxicol.* **1995**, *35*, 655–677. [CrossRef] [PubMed]
3. Moraes, L.A.; Piqueras, L.; Bishop-Bailey, D. Peroxisome proliferator-activated receptors and inflammation. *Pharmacol. Ther.* **2006**, *110*, 371–385. [CrossRef] [PubMed]
4. Fan, W.; Evans, R. PPARs and ERRs: Molecular mediators of mitochondrial metabolism. *Curr. Opin. Cell Biol.* **2015**, *33*, 49–54. [CrossRef] [PubMed]
5. Daynes, R.A.; Jones, D.C. Emerging roles of PPARs in inflammation and immunity. *Nat. Rev. Immunol.* **2002**, *2*, 748–759. [CrossRef] [PubMed]
6. He, X.; Liu, W.; Shi, M.; Yang, Z.; Zhang, X.; Gong, P. Docosahexaenoic acid attenuates LPS-stimulated inflammatory response by regulating the PPARgamma/NF-κB pathways in primary bovine mammary epithelial cells. *Res. Vet. Sci.* **2017**, *112*, 7–12. [CrossRef] [PubMed]
7. Flores-Bastías, O.; Karahanian, E. Neuroinflammation produced by heavy alcohol intake is due to loops of interactions between Toll-like 4 and TNF receptors, peroxisome proliferator-activated receptors and the central melanocortin system: A novel hypothesis and new therapeutic avenues. *Neuropharmacology* **2018**, *128*, 401–407. [CrossRef] [PubMed]
8. Sharma, B.R.; Gautam, L.N.; Adhikari, D.; Karki, R. A Comprehensive Review on Chemical Profiling of Nelumbo Nucifera: Potential for Drug Development. *Phytother. Res.* **2017**, *31*, 3–26. [CrossRef] [PubMed]
9. Li, Z.; Liu, J.; Zhang, D.; Du, X.; Han, L.; Lv, C.; Li, Y.; Wang, R.; Wang, B.; Huang, Y. Nuciferine and paeoniflorin can be quality markers of Tangzhiqing tablet, a Chinese traditional patent medicine, based on the qualitative, quantitative and dose-exposure-response analysis. *Phytomedicine* **2018**, *44*, 155–163. [CrossRef] [PubMed]
10. Ma, C.; Li, G.; He, Y.; Xu, B.; Mi, X.; Wang, H.; Wang, Z. Pronuciferine and nuciferine inhibit lipogenesis in 3T3-L1 adipocytes by activating the AMPK signaling pathway. *Life Sci.* **2015**, *136*, 120–125. [CrossRef] [PubMed]
11. Nguyen, K.H.; Ta, T.N.; Pham, T.H.; Nguyen, Q.T.; Pham, H.D.; Mishra, S.; Nyomba, B.L. Nuciferine stimulates insulin secretion from beta cells-an in vitro comparison with glibenclamide. *J. Ethnopharmacol.* **2012**, *142*, 488–495. [CrossRef] [PubMed]
12. Wang, M.X.; Liu, Y.L.; Yang, Y.; Zhang, D.M.; Kong, L.D. Nuciferine restores potassium oxonate-induced hyperuricemia and kidney inflammation in mice. *Eur. J. Pharmacol.* **2015**, *747*, 59–70. [CrossRef] [PubMed]
13. Wang, M.X.; Zhao, X.J.; Chen, T.Y.; Liu, Y.L.; Jiao, R.Q.; Zhang, J.H.; Ma, C.; Liu, J.H.; Pan, Y.; Kong, L.D. Nuciferine Alleviates Renal Injury by Inhibiting Inflammatory Responses in Fructose-Fed Rats. *J. Agric. Food Chem.* **2016**. [CrossRef] [PubMed]
14. Ohashi, K.; Munetsuna, E.; Yamada, H.; Ando, Y.; Yamazaki, M.; Taromaru, N.; Nagura, A.; Ishikawa, H.; Suzuki, K.; Teradaira, R.; et al. High fructose consumption induces DNA methylation at PPARalpha and CPT1A promoter regions in the rat liver. *Biochem. Biophys. Res. Commun.* **2015**, *468*, 185–189. [CrossRef] [PubMed]
15. Zhao, S.; Kanno, Y.; Li, W.; Wakatabi, H.; Sasaki, T.; Koike, K.; Nemoto, K.; Li, H. Picrasidine N Is a Subtype-Selective PPARβ/δ Agonist. *J. Nat. Prod.* **2016**, *79*, 879–885. [CrossRef] [PubMed]
16. Zhong, Q.; Zhao, S.; Yu, B.; Wang, X.; Matyal, R.; Li, Y.; Jiang, Z. High-density lipoprotein increases the uptake of oxidized low density lipoprotein via PPARgamma/CD36 pathway in inflammatory adipocytes. *Int. J. Biol. Sci.* **2015**, *11*, 256–265. [CrossRef] [PubMed]

17. Bao, W.; Luo, Y.; Wang, D.; Li, J.; Wu, X.; Mei, W. Sodium salicylate modulates inflammatory responses through AMP-activated protein kinase activation in LPS-stimulated THP-1 cells. *J. Cell. Biochem.* **2018**, *119*, 850–860. [CrossRef] [PubMed]
18. Wu, Y.; Xie, G.; Xu, Y.; Ma, L.; Tong, C.; Fan, D.; Du, F.; Yu, H. PEP-1-MsrA ameliorates inflammation and reduces atherosclerosis in apolipoprotein E deficient mice. *J. Transl. Med.* **2015**, *13*, 316. [CrossRef] [PubMed]
19. Zhu, F.; Du, B.; Xu, B. Anti-inflammatory effects of phytochemicals from fruits, vegetables, and food legumes: A review. *Crit. Rev. Food Sci. Nutr.* **2018**, *58*, 1260–1270. [CrossRef] [PubMed]
20. Wu, H.; Yang, Y.; Guo, S.; Yang, J.; Jiang, K.; Zhao, G.; Qiu, C.; Deng, G. Nuciferine Ameliorates Inflammatory Responses by Inhibiting the TLR4-Mediated Pathway in Lipopolysaccharide-Induced Acute Lung Injury. *Front. Pharmacol.* **2017**, *8*, 939. [CrossRef] [PubMed]
21. Zhang, D.D.; Zhang, J.G.; Wu, X.; Liu, Y.; Gu, S.Y.; Zhu, G.H.; Wang, Y.Z.; Liu, G.L.; Li, X.Y. Nuciferine downregulates Per-Arnt-Sim kinase expression during its alleviation of lipogenesis and inflammation on oleic acid-induced hepatic steatosis in HepG2 cells. *Front. Pharmacol.* **2015**, *6*, 238. [CrossRef] [PubMed]
22. Liu, W.; Yi, D.D.; Guo, J.L.; Xiang, Z.X.; Deng, L.F.; He, L. Nuciferine, extracted from Nelumbo nucifera Gaertn, inhibits tumor-promoting effect of nicotine involving Wnt/β-catenin signaling in non-small cell lung cancer. *J. Ethnopharmacol.* **2015**, *165*, 83–93. [CrossRef] [PubMed]
23. Ma, C.; Wang, J.; Chu, H.; Zhang, X.; Wang, Z.; Wang, H. Purification and characterization of aporphine alkaloids from leaves of Nelumbo nucifera Gaertn and their effects on glucose consumption in 3T3-L1 adipocytes. *Int. J. Mol. Sci.* **2014**, *15*, 3481–3494. [CrossRef] [PubMed]
24. Zhang, C.; Deng, J.; Liu, D.; Tuo, X.; Xiao, L.; Lai, B.; Yao, Q.; Liu, J.; Yang, H.; Wang, N. Nuciferine ameliorates hepatic steatosis in high-fat diet/streptozocin-induced diabetic mice through a PPARalpha/PPARgamma coactivator-1alpha pathway. *Br. J. Pharmacol.* **2018**. [CrossRef] [PubMed]
25. Adhikary, T.; Wortmann, A.; Schumann, T.; Finkernagel, F.; Lieber, S.; Roth, K.; Toth, P.M.; Diederich, W.E.; Nist, A.; Stiewe, T.; et al. The transcriptional PPARβ/δ network in human macrophages defines a unique agonist-induced activation state. *Nucleic Acids Res.* **2015**, *43*, 5033–5051. [CrossRef] [PubMed]
26. Yang, W.; Rachez, C.; Freedman, L.P. Discrete roles for peroxisome proliferator-activated receptor gamma and retinoid X receptor in recruiting nuclear receptor coactivators. *Mol. Cell. Biol.* **2000**, *20*, 8008–8017. [CrossRef] [PubMed]
27. Bougarne, N.; Paumelle, R.; Caron, S.; Hennuyer, N.; Mansouri, R.; Gervois, P.; Staels, B.; Haegeman, G.; De Bosscher, K. PPARα blocks glucocorticoid receptor α-mediated transactivation but cooperates with the activated glucocorticoid receptor α for transrepression on NF-κB. *Proc. Natl. Acad. Sci. USA* **2009**, *106*, 7397–7402. [CrossRef] [PubMed]
28. Azuma, Y.T.; Nishiyama, K.; Matsuo, Y.; Kuwamura, M.; Morioka, A.; Nakajima, H.; Takeuchi, T. PPARalpha contributes to colonic protection in mice with DSS-induced colitis. *Int. Immunopharmacol.* **2010**, *10*, 1261–1267. [CrossRef] [PubMed]
29. Barish, G.D.; Atkins, A.R.; Downes, M.; Olson, P.; Chong, L.W.; Nelson, M.; Zou, Y.; Hwang, H.; Kang, H.; Curtiss, L.; et al. PPARδ regulates multiple proinflammatory pathways to suppress atherosclerosis. *Proc. Natl. Acad. Sci. USA* **2008**, *105*, 4271–4276. [CrossRef] [PubMed]
30. Yang, H.; Xiao, L.; Wang, N. Peroxisome proliferator-activated receptor α ligands and modulators from dietary compounds: Types, screening methods and functions. *J. Diabetes* **2017**, *9*, 341–352. [CrossRef] [PubMed]
31. Tak, P.P.; Firestein, G.S. NF-κB: A key role in inflammatory diseases. *J. Clin. Investig.* **2001**, *107*, 7–11. [CrossRef] [PubMed]
32. Hernandez-Rodas, M.C.; Valenzuela, R.; Echeverria, F.; Rincon-Cervera, M.A.; Espinosa, A.; Illesca, P.; Munoz, P.; Corbari, A.; Romero, N.; Gonzalez-Manan, D.; et al. Supplementation with Docosahexaenoic Acid and Extra Virgin Olive Oil Prevents Liver Steatosis Induced by a High-Fat Diet in Mice through PPAR-alpha and Nrf2 Upregulation with Concomitant SREBP-1c and NF-kB Downregulation. *Mol. Nutr. Food Res.* **2017**, *61*. [CrossRef] [PubMed]
33. Silva-Veiga, F.M.; Rachid, T.L.; de Oliveira, L.; Graus-Nunes, F.; Mandarim-de-Lacerda, C.A.; Souza-Mello, V. GW0742 (PPAR-β agonist) attenuates hepatic endoplasmic reticulum stress by improving hepatic energy metabolism in high-fat diet fed mice. *Mol. Cell. Endocrinol.* **2018**, *474*, 227–237. [CrossRef] [PubMed]

34. Sharma, S.; Sharma, P.; Kulurkar, P.; Singh, D.; Kumar, D.; Patial, V. Iridoid glycosides fraction from Picrorhiza kurroa attenuates cyclophosphamide-induced renal toxicity and peripheral neuropathy via PPAR-gamma mediated inhibition of inflammation and apoptosis. *Phytomedicine* **2017**, *36*, 108–117. [CrossRef] [PubMed]
35. Imanifooladi, A.A.; Yazdani, S.; Nourani, M.R. The role of nuclear factor-κB in inflammatory lung disease. *Inflamm. Allergy-Drug Targets* **2010**, *9*, 197–205. [CrossRef] [PubMed]
36. Delerive, P.; Gervois, P.; Fruchart, J.C.; Staels, B. Induction of IkappaBalpha expression as a mechanism contributing to the anti-inflammatory activities of peroxisome proliferator-activated receptor-alpha activators. *J. Biol. Chem.* **2000**, *275*, 36703–36707. [CrossRef] [PubMed]
37. Tolosa, L.; Donato, M.T.; Gomez-Lechon, M.J. General Cytotoxicity Assessment by Means of the MTT Assay. *Methods Mol. Biol.* **2015**, *1250*, 333–348. [CrossRef] [PubMed]
38. Cheung, S.T.; Shakibakho, S.; So, E.Y.; Mui, A.L.F. Transfecting RAW264.7 Cells with a Luciferase Reporter Gene. *J. Visualized Exp.* **2015**, *100*. [CrossRef] [PubMed]
39. Yang, H.; Xiao, L.; Yuan, Y.; Luo, X.; Jiang, M.; Ni, J.; Wang, N. Procyanidin B2 inhibits NLRP3 inflammasome activation in human vascular endothelial cells. *Biochem. Pharmacol.* **2014**, *92*, 599–606. [CrossRef] [PubMed]
40. Livak, K.J.; Schmittgen, T.D. Analysis of relative gene expression data using real-time quantitative PCR and the $2^{-\Delta\Delta CT}$ Method. *Methods* **2001**, *25*, 402–408. [CrossRef] [PubMed]

Sample Availability: Not available.

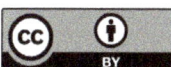

© 2018 by the authors. Licensee MDPI, Basel, Switzerland. This article is an open access article distributed under the terms and conditions of the Creative Commons Attribution (CC BY) license (http://creativecommons.org/licenses/by/4.0/).

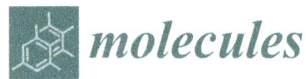

Review

Therapeutic Approaches of Resveratrol on Endometriosis via Anti-Inflammatory and Anti-Angiogenic Pathways

Ana-Maria Dull, Marius Alexandru Moga, Oana Gabriela Dimienescu *, Gabriela Sechel *, Victoria Burtea and Costin Vlad Anastasiu

Department of Medical and Surgical Specialties, Faculty of Medicine, Transilvania University of Brasov, 500019 Brasov, Romania; dullana2005@yahoo.com (A.-M.D.); moga.og@gmail.com (M.A.M.); victoriaburtea@yahoo.com (V.B.); canastasiu@gmail.com (C.V.A.)
* Correspondence: dimienescu.oana@gmail.com (O.G.D.); gabisechel@yahoo.com (G.S.);
  Tel.: +40-268-412-185 (O.G.D.); +40-268-412-185 (G.S.)

Academic Editor: Francesco Maione
Received: 2 January 2019; Accepted: 11 February 2019; Published: 13 February 2019

Abstract: Endometriosis represents a severe gynecological pathology, defined by implantation of endometrial glands and stroma outside the uterine cavity. This pathology affects almost 15% of women during reproductive age and has a wide range of consequences. In affected women, infertility has a 30% rate of prevalence and endometriosis implants increase the risk of ovarian cancer. Despite long periods of studies and investigations, the etiology and pathogenesis of this disease still remain not fully understood. Initially, endometriosis was related to retrograde menstruation, but new theories have been launched, suggesting that chronic inflammation can influence the development of endometriosis because inflammatory mediators have been identified elevated in patients with endometriosis, specifically in the peritoneal fluid. The importance of dietary phytochemicals and their effect on different inflammatory diseases have been highlighted, and nowadays more and more studies are focused on the analysis of nutraceuticals. Resveratrol is a phytoestrogen, a natural polyphenolic compound with antiproliferative and anti-inflammatory actions, found in many dietary sources such as grapes, wine, peanuts, soy, berries, and stilbenes. Resveratrol possesses a significant anti-inflammatory effect via inhibition of prostaglandin synthesis and it has been proved that resveratrol can exhibit apoptosis-inducing activities. From the studies reviewed in this paper, it is clear that the anti-inflammatory effect of this natural compound can contribute to the prevention of endometriosis, this phenolic compound now being considered a new innovative drug in the prevention and treatment of this disease.

Keywords: cytokines; resveratrol; endometriosis; anti-inflammatory; inflammatory disease

1. Introduction

Endometriosis represents a severe gynecological disease that affects almost 15% of women in reproductive age, described by the implantation of endometrial tissue outside the uterus [1]. In endometriosis, endometrial tissue fragments are present mainly on the ovaries, on the pelvic peritoneum, in the pouch of Douglas, and the rectovaginal septum [2]. Frequently, this dissemination of the endometrial cells is explained by the theory of retrograde menstruation, consisting of the presence of menstrual blood in the abdominal cavity, due to reflux through the Fallopian tubes, an approach first described by Sampson in 1927 [3]. The favorable hormonal environment and some immunological factors are involved in the implantation of endometrial cells in abnormal sites outside the uterus and in the failure to eliminate these cells from the inappropriate places [4].

There are three types of endometriosis, according to its localization in the pelvis: peritoneal, ovarian, and rectovaginal, presented in the first stage of implantations as red lesions similar to the eutopic endometrium. In time, these red lesions become black by an inflammatory reaction that provokes a process of scarification [2].

The clinical presentation of endometriosis is variable and includes some severe symptoms: dyspareunia, chronic pelvic pain, dysmenorrhea, and subfertility or infertility [5]. The severity of symptoms increases with age [6].

Even the pathogenesis and the mechanisms of initial development and subsequent progression of endometriosis are still unclear. There are proofs that this disorder is a pelvic inflammatory process and chronic inflammation has a significant role in the development and progression of the pathology [7].

Based on this pro-inflammatory hypothesis, various studies report that in the peritoneal fluid of patients with endometriosis increased numbers of activated macrophages, cytokines, angiogenic factors, and growth factors have been identified, [8] produced through the alteration of the regular activity of peritoneal cells [9].

A study conducted by Kobayashi et al. [10] highlights that endometriosis may be stimulated through the activation of the inflammatory cells. Also, subsequent inflammation and microbial infections of the upper genital tract are also involved in the initial development and progression of the lesions [10]. Peritoneal oxidative stress is also considered a significant component of endometriosis-related inflammation, and it can regulate genes that encode immunoregulators, cytokines, and cell adhesion molecules [11].

In the literature, there have been several studies conducted to highlight the importance of diet and its impact on the prevention and treatment of a wide range of diseases, raising more and more interest in the analysis of dietary polyphenols [12]. Polyphenols are micronutrients found in dietary sources and proof of their impact on the prevention of diseases is emerging [13]. The most common coccurrences of polyphenols are in herbs, fruits, beverages, vegetables and spices, several of these polyphenols have been proven to exhibit anti-inflammatory actions. Besides, several studies maintain that the consumption of food abundant in polyphenols can reduce the incidence of chronic inflammatory pathologies [14].

Resveratrol is a natural phytoalexin (trans-3,5,40-trihydroxystilbene), synthesized by plants due to ultraviolet radiation and fungal infections [15,16]. High levels were identified in grapes, wine, berries, Itadori tea, nuts, and stilbenes. Analysis of peanuts, raisins, and Itadori tea confirm the predominance of trans-resveratrol glucoside and, in counterpoint, the study of red wine shows that it contains mainly the aglycones cis- and trans-resveratrol forms [17].

Several studies indicate that resveratrol possesses various beneficial actions, including anti-neoplastic, anti-inflammatory, anti-oxidative, anti-microbial, anti-atherogenic, and anti-angiogenic properties [16,18]. It is also useful because it may provide cardiovascular protection [19].

Regarding the mechanism of action of resveratrol, numerous studies have shown that it includes multiple cellular targets affecting signal transduction pathways. AKT (protein kinase B) represents these pathways, Signal transducer and activator of transcription 3 (STAT3), ribosomal protein S6 kinase beta-2 (RPS6KB2), mitogen-activated protein kinase 1/3 (MAPK1/3; ERK1/2), Mitogen-Activated Protein Kinase 14 (MAPK14 (p38)), protein kinase C, and peroxisome proliferator-activated receptors (PPAR) gamma [20–22]. Some of the pathways are relevant for the mechanisms of endometriosis-related development on the impact of resveratrol as an anti-inflammatory agent [23,24]. This hypothesis supports that resveratrol seems to be a possible innovative alternative agent in the prevention and treatment of severe disease, but further studies are necessary to elucidate the useful potential of this phytochemical and also the potential adverse effects that may appear.

Bruner-Tran et al. [25] pointed out the inhibition of endometriotic lesions by resveratrol in a study published in 2011. Their study concluded that the oral gavage of resveratrol could reduce the quantity and dimensions of endometriotic lesions. The in vivo study was performed on nude mice and consisted of transplantation of induced human endometrial tissue into the peritoneal cavity of these mice. This effect of resveratrol was linked to reduced proliferative action and up-regulation of apoptotic cell death into the lesions.

The essential mechanism of resveratrol in the prevention of endometriosis is considered anti-inflammatory activity. It has been demonstrated to be manifested through the inhibition of prostaglandin synthesis via the inhibition of COX enzyme synthesis, inhibition of activated immune cells, and inhibition of pro-inflammatory cytokines [26].

Endometriosis, a chronic inflammatory disease is a frequent gynecological pathology, which has a severe impact on women worldwide, therefore by understanding the pathophysiology, and the mechanism of action of resveratrol we may improve the development of this disorder and the treatment strategies, using natural products. With low toxicity, high accessibility, and low price, resveratrol may become an alternative therapeutical agent for the prevention and treatment of endometriosis.

2. Biochemistry of Resveratrol

Resveratrol is a phytochemical found in high concentration in grapes, wine, tea, peanuts, and berries also called a "miracle molecule" because it exhibits many beneficial properties [27,28]. This molecule was discovered and described for the first time in the year 1939 [29,30] when it was isolated from the roots of *Veratrum grandifloorum* and in the year 1963, it was isolated from a plant used in complementary medicine in China, *Polygonum cuspidatum*. Since the first discovery of the compound, numerous scientific researches have been conducted to study the activity of resveratrol. In 2002, Burns et al. [31] reported 92 new resveratrol compounds from the *Dipterocarpaceae*, *Vitaceae*, *Paeoniaceae*, *Gnetaceae*, *Leguminosae*, *Polygonaceae*, *Gramineae*, *Cyperaceae*, and *Poaceae* families. According to Sobolev et al., two new dimers of resveratrol were isolated from peanut seeds [32], and this phytochemical has also been separated from baking chocolate, cocoa powder, and dark chocolate (0.35–1.85 mg/kg in commonly consumed quantities) [33]

Resveratrol is part of the large chemical class of stilbenes and as well as the resveratrol molecule and its analogs, a stilbene is considered a monomer, a primary building block that leads to subsequent polymerization. In the last five years, over 60 naturally occurring stilbenes have been isolated, and it is a fact that stilbenes exhibit a large wide of oligomeric constructions and polymerization [34].

The universal skeleton of stilbenes is a C6–C2–C6 unit, namely, a 1,2-diphenylethylene moiety [34]. Resveratrol is a polyphenolic phytoalexin that possesses two aromatic rings linked to each other by a double ethylene bridge [35]. The chemical structure of resveratrol (trans-3,5,4'-trihydroxystilbene) is responsible for the two isomeric forms, *cis*-resveratrol, and respectively *trans*-resveratrol [36]. In plants, wine, and in natural food, resveratrol is found as both *cis*- and *trans*-isomers, although the significant and more stable form of resveratrol is *trans*-resveratrol, which is useful as a preventive agent in cancer, vascular diseases, infections, etc. [37]. Figure 1 illustrates the two isomers of resveratrol.

The synthesis of resveratrol is a condensation reaction including three molecules of malonyl-CoA and one molecule of 4-coumaroyl CoA. From this reaction, out of resveratrol, also result four molecules of CO_2 [38]. The synthesis of resveratrol is shown in Figure 2.

The conversion of *cis*-isoform into *trans*-isoform is called cis-isomerization, and this phenomenon is possible when a *trans*-isoform is exposed to UV radiation or sunlight [39,40]. Therefore, because the *cis*-form is less stable [39], many studies use *trans*-resveratrol for administration, to highlight the biological effects of this phytoalexin.

As with any others polyphenols, resveratrol can undergo an auto-oxidation process and O_2 and H_2O_2 are produced. This can also result in a mixture of quinines and semiquinones that may be cytotoxic [41]. Regarding the metabolism of resveratrol, studies revealed that it is metabolized into glucuronide and sulfate conjugates. Regarding the crystalline resveratrol and its glucoside, a study of Jensen et al. [42] maintains that both of these forms are stable for more than three months, a low degree of degradation may occur in various conditions such as air exposure, fluorescent light, UV light, high temperature, etc.

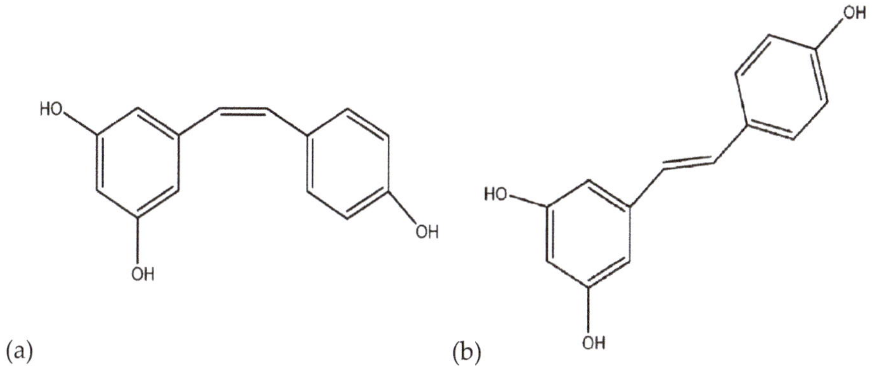

(a) (b)

Figure 1. The two isomers of resveratrol; (**a**) cis-resveratrol and (**b**) trans-resveratrol [37].

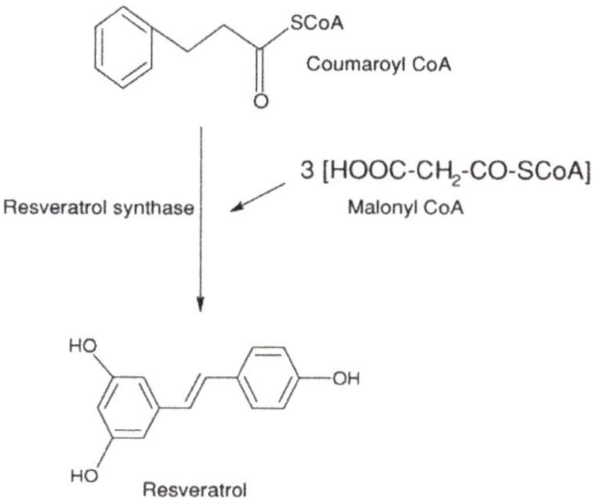

Figure 2. Resveratrol synthesis from malonyl-CoA and 4-coumaroyl CoA [43].

Recently, five tetramers of resveratrol were separated from the roots of *Vitis amurensis*: amurensins I–M, together with five resveratrol tetramers, named isohopeaphenol, (+)-vitisifuran A, heyneanol A, (+)-hopeaphenol, vitisin A, From all of these tetramers, vitisin A, (+)-hopeaphenol, isohopeaphenol, heyneanol A, and (+)-vitisifuran A showed a potent anti-inflammatory activity and also presented strong inhibition of the biogenesis of leukotriene B4 (LTB4) [44].

3. Development of the Endometriosis-Role of Inflammation

Endometriosis is characterized by functional endometrial stroma and gland implants outside of the uterine cavity. The main symptoms of this gynecological disease are chronic abdominal pain, dysmenorrhea, infertility [45,46], and anxiety or depression related to the severity of the pelvic-abdominal pain [47].

Regarding the pathophysiology of endometriosis and the biological mechanism of endometriosis-associated pain, these still remain controversial and unclear. Endometriosis is considered a multi-factorial condition with immunological, genetic, and hormonal environment contribution, characterized by an abnormal expression of inflammatory factors [48]. An essential step in the progression of endometriosis is represented by the link between inflammation and activation of the aromatase gene in the endometrium, followed by the local production of estrogens [49]. In healthy patients, the aromatase gene is inhibited, but in affected women, the promoter of this gene is activated by exposure to pro-inflammatory prostaglandins (PGE2). A malicious cycle between estrogen production and chronic inflammation is created, and through this cycle, the survival of heterotopic endometrial cells is maintained [50]. NF-kB is the link between aromatase expression and inflammation in endometriosis, the activation and translocation of NF-kB from the cytoplasm to cell nuclei being the first step to induce the inflammation process [51].

In patients with endometriosis and adenomyosis, the nuclear factor-kB subunit bound to a cell has been observed more often than in control cases [52,53]. The inflammatory environment in endometriosis points out an increased production of estrogens, which also increases prostaglandin production through NF-kB and COX-2 activation [54]. Recent studies also suggest that an essential cause of endometriosis development is neurovascular formation, or angiogenesis [55]. Angiogenesis is a complex process of new blood vessels formation that involves the extravasation of growth factors, degradation of the extracellular matrix, and new tube formation by endothelial cells. Endometriosis is dependent on the development of new blood vessels [56,57] that also associate a wide range of angiogenesis-related factors, such as VEGFR, VEGF, Delta-like 4 (Dll4)-Notch signal pathways, and angiopoietin [58].

VEGF and VEGFR are angiogenesis-related factors that affect the proliferation, migration, and permeability of the cells. A study of Gagne et al. [59] showed that the level of vascular endothelial growth factor in the peritoneal fluid of type IV endometriosis patients is significantly higher compared to type I/II endometriosis. VEGFC is an angiogenesis factor that acts on endothelial cells and promotes angiogenic responses through VEGFR2-mediated pathways, to improve endothelial function and vascular permeability in endometriosis [60].

Other constituents implicated in the development and progression of this chronic disease, are matrix metalloproteinases (MMPs), cyclo-oxygenase (COX), tumor necrosis factor (TNF-α), and hypoxia-inducible factor 1α (HIF-1) [48]. MMPs are involved in endometrial adhesion and angiogenesis, TNF-α promotes angiogenesis, and COX promotes the implantation of heterotopic endometrial cells [61,62]. Ectopic implants of the endometrial cell have shown increased expression of cyclo-oxygenase-2, while cyclo-oxygenase-2 inhibitors have been largely studied in the treatment of endometriosis-related abdominal pain [63]. The activity of MMP-2 in endothelial cells is significantly increased by PGE2 and is suppressed by the inhibition of COX-2 and all those factors, either directly or indirectly, are able to affect endometriosis-associated angiogenesis [64].

In the inflammatory panel of endometriosis, NF-kB has a crucial role in the progression of the disease. This factor is activated by several cytokines pro-inflammatory: tumor necrosis factor - α, interleukin 1β, and NF-kB activates multiple inflammatory mediators like IL-8 [65]. Activated macrophages are the key in the defense against infections because they can secrete cytokines pro-inflammatory: interleukin -1, interleukin -6, interleukin -12 and tumor necrosis factor-α and uncontrolled activation of these factors results in persistent inflammation. In the context of chronic inflammation, high levels of these cytokines have been identified in the peritoneal fluid of patients with endometriotic lesions [66]. TNF-α promotes inflammation in the Fallopian tubes, and this results in tissue repair and fibrosis in the tubes, which impairs reproduction, leading to poor quality of oocytes. IL-1 can promote angiogenesis in endometrial lesions and interfere with peritoneal immune surveillance. IL-8 has been identified in high levels in the peritoneal fluid of the patients with endometriosis and promotes cell attachment and cell growth [67].

So, the basis of endometriosis pathophysiology is represented by the pro-inflammatory cytokines axis, which was named by Soares et al. [68] "the crossroads of the molecular pathways." This process involves cytokines (tumor necrosis factor-α, interleukin-6, interleukin-8, monocyte chemoattractant protein, macrophage inhibitory factor, and granulocyte macrophage colony-stimulating factor) [69]. Matrix metalloproteinase-1, matrix metalloproteinase-2, matrix metalloproteinase-3, matrix metalloproteinase-7, matrix metalloproteinase-9 [70], nitric oxide (NO), and VEGF are involved in neoangiogenesis [71]. Figure 3 illustrates the pattern of the most relevant molecular pathways implicated in the pathophysiology of this pathology.

The purpose of the management of this chronic inflammatory disease is to improve chronic abdominal pain and successfully achieve a pregnancy in infertile women while the treatment is both medical and surgical. Regarding medical treatment, this involves a wide range of therapeutic agents including cyclo-oxygenase-2 inhibitors, TNF-α blockers, nuclear factor-kB inhibitors, statins, mitogen-activated protein kinase inhibitors, immunomodulators, MMP inhibitors, Metformin, antiangiogenic agents, and antioxidants [68].

Recent studies have shown the importance of natural therapy assessment for endometriosis treatment. Nowadays, natural compounds from food and various plants, named phytochemicals, are considered useful for the treatment of several diseases, including endometriosis. These new agents promise a new and revolutionary perspective in the treatment of endometriosis.

Resveratrol, the miraculous phytoalexin contained in grapes and red wine is an agent with multiple beneficial activities, and its role in endometriosis development and progression has been studied to demonstrate its effectiveness as a therapeutic agent. This study focuses on complementary medicines for the treatment of endometriosis, especially on the effect of resveratrol and examines its therapeutic efficacy and mechanism of action.

4. Anti-Inflammatory Molecular Mechanisms of Resveratrol

Resveratrol exerts different effects on various molecular pathways involved in inflammation, such as arachidonic acid, Nf-kB, Ah receptor or AP-1. We summarize in this subchapter how this natural compound affects these signaling pathways.

4.1. Arachidonic Acid Pathway

Various stimuli, such as hormones, cytokines, and stress signals activate the arachidonic acid (AA) pathway, under the action of phospholipase A2, the results being the release of this acid from the cell membranes [72]. Through the activity of lipoxygenase and COX, arachidonic acid is converted to several eicosanoids. Cyclo-oxygenase plays an essential role in inflammation because it catalyzes the formation of prostaglandin H2 (PGH2). The primary mechanism, namely the conversion of AA to PGH2 involves two steps: bisdioxygenation of arachidonic acid to PGG2 and peroxidative cleavage of PGG2 to PGH2, releasing the active biological prostanoids (PGE2, PGF2α, PGI2, and thromboxane A2) [72].

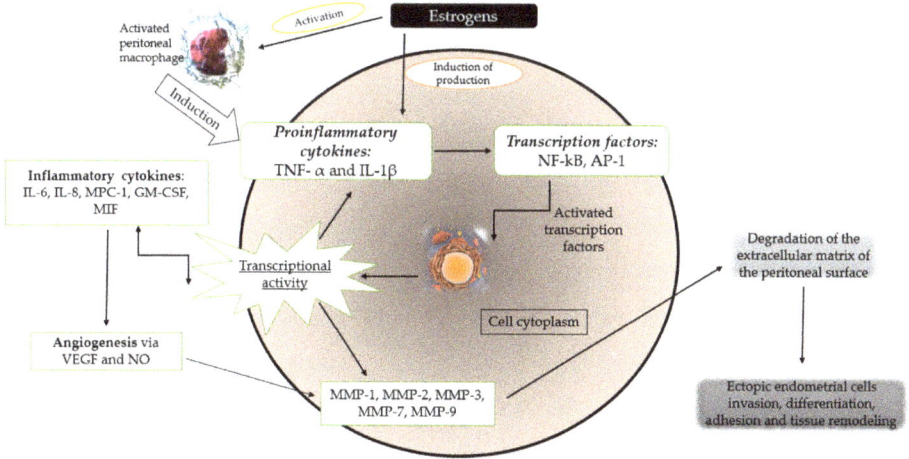

Figure 3. Illustration of molecular pathways in the development of endometriosis [7,68,73–75].

Regarding resveratrol, several types of research have pointed out that this compound interacts with the arachidonic acid pathway suppressing COX-2 effects on various levels. Subbaramaiah K et al. concluded in their study that the mechanism through which resveratrol inhibits inflammation is represented by suppression of PMA induced cyclooxygenase transcription in mammary epithelial cells, mainly through inhibition of the protein kinase C pathway [76]. This compound also prevents the induction of cyclooxygenase 2 promoter activity (known to be mediated by ERK-1 and c-Jun). Camp responses element (CRE) is also an essential element in the inflammatory process. When interfering with resveratrol, it suppresses COX-2 expression. Xie et al. [77] reported in their study that C-Jun (a component of activator protein 1) activates cyclooxygenase promoter through the camp responses element.

4.2. Aryl Hydrocarbon Receptor (AhR)

AhR has an essential role in the immune system, being a mediator of dioxin toxicity [78]. Furthermore, Esser et al. demonstrated in their study that aryl hydrocarbon receptor could bind different factors (estrogen receptors, NF- κB, E2F1) [79]. Because dioxin induces immunosuppression, agonists for AhR have been studied during the last years, aiming to identify natural products that interfere with this unique molecular pathway of inflammation. Resveratrol is one of the natural compounds that was identified to have antagonist effects on AhR [80,81]. It has been pointed out that essential roles in the regulation of the immune system are played by FoxP3+ Tregs and effector Th17 subset [82]. The research results of Bettelli E et al. showed that resveratrol inhibited the development of Th17 cells and FoxP3+ Treg [83]. Another in vitro study highlighted that resveratrol could block Th17 development [84]. These findings reflect the beneficial activity of resveratrol on inflammation, through inhibition of Th17.

4.3. Activator Protein 1 Pathway

In the inflammatory process the activator protein 1 is also involved, along with NF-κB, NFAT, and STATs, playing an essential role in the initiation of the process, by promoting the transcription of various biomolecules and pro-inflammatory cytokines. AP-1 factor includes multiple members of JUN, FOS, ATF, and MAF protein families [85]. Activation of AP-1 is induced by various cytokines (especially through JNK and MAPK signaling), hormones, growth factors (through extracellular-signal-regulated-kinase), and cellular stress. Cytokines activate this pathway especially through JNK and MAPK signaling. The cytokines (IL-2, IL-3, IL-4, IL-5, IL-13, IFN-γ, TNF-α) influenced by AP-1 are regulated by a transcription factor complex that involves NFAT. The activated AP-1 proteins have an essential role in the differentiation of T cells, it being known that several inflammatory diseases are characterized by this type of T-cell response [86,87]. Some studies suggested that resveratrol interferes with the inflammation process through AP-1 pathways, inhibiting COX-2 activity indirectly, after inhibition of AP-1. So, the AP-1 pathway is indispensable when discussing the anti-inflammatory effects of this natural compound [88,89].

4.4. NF-κB Pathway

The proteins of the NF-κB family proteins contain a Rel homology domain that serves as their dimerization, DNA-binding, and a primary regulatory domain, according to Ghosh et al. [90]. NF-κB proteins activation is dependent on the phosphorylation of IκB proteins. After the activation of IκB proteins, the released NF-κB proteins activate various target genes associated with cell proliferation, and inflammatory responses [91]. Manna et al. suggested that resveratrol modulates NF-κB through suppressing its activation in several cell types, blocking TNF-α and inducing activation of NF-κB [92]. Other researchers showed that this natural compound could prevent NF-κB activation by different stimuli besides TNF-α, such as other pro-inflammatory cytokines (IL-1β) or LPS, H2O2, okadaic acid, and ceramide [93].

5. Studies of Resveratrol as Anti-Inflammatory Agent in Endometriosis

Resveratrol, a natural non-flavonoid antioxidant, is a phytoalexin found in high levels in red wine, approximately 1.52 mg/L and in grapes skin, 50–100 µg/g [94]. Resveratrol has been shown to possess significant activity as anti-inflammatory, antioxidant, antiangiogenic agent and it also has immunomodulatory properties [95]. In demonstrating the anti-inflammatory effect of resveratrol several studies shown that this natural compound suppresses the production of ROS and inhibits COX-2 expression and prostaglandin synthesis [96]. In Tables 1 and 2, we summarized the most representative preclinical and clinical studies conducted to demonstrate the efficiency of resveratrol in the management of endometriosis.

5.1. Preclinical Studies

In the initiation and progression of this disease, activation of peritoneal macrophages is a crucial step [97]. This mechanism is responsible for the increased lipid peroxidation. Several authors concluded that the increased production of free oxygen radicals, elevates oxidized lipoproteins in the peritoneal fluid and lower levels of SOD and GSH-Px are often identified in patients with endometriosis. Another marker of lipoprotein peroxidation is lysophosphatidylcholine, which was found elevated in patients with this pathology, according to Murphy et al. [98,99]. The imbalance oxidation–antioxidation appears to be responsible for the pathophysiology of endometriosis. The authors of this study identified increased levels of MDA (increased lipid peroxidation in peritoneal plasma and implants), but after supplementing with resveratrol in a dose-dependent manner, the increased levels were suppressed, speculating that this natural compound can have beneficial effects as a potent antioxidant [98–102].

As we described in Section 4, resveratrol possesses anti-inflammatory effects through various pathways. Chen et al. [103] concluded in their study that resveratrol acts through inhibition of the expression of two enzymes induced by dioxin (CYP1A1 and CYP 1B1) via the AhR pathway. Another possible mechanism involving this natural compound is described by Casper et al., who found that resveratrol, in the presence of TCCD competes with AhR and inhibits CYP1A1 expression, resulting in anti-inflammatory activity [80].

Research of Yavuz S. et al. [104] was carried out to demonstrate the efficiency of resveratrol as a therapeutical agent in the treatment of endometriosis. The study included surgically induced lesions of endometriosis in 24 female rats. Four weeks after the procedure, the injuries were measured in three groups of study: control group, low resveratrol dose (1 mg/kg/day), and high resveratrol dose (10 mg/kg/day). Resveratrol was administered intraperitoneal over seven days, and at the end of the period, a laparotomy was completed for the purpose of observing the volume of endometriotic lesions and serum/tissue levels of antioxidant enzymes also detected. Their study indicated that resveratrol significantly reduced the volume of endometriotic lesions. Histological scores were also decreased in the treated groups compared. Therefore, resveratrol is a phytochemical with potential ameliorative effects in endometriosis, probably due to its anti-oxidative potency.

Another experimental endometriosis model was used in a prospective study of Tekin et al. [105]. The authors aimed to compare the biological activity of resveratrol in patients affected by endometriosis with the effects of leuprolide acetate. Endometriosis experimental pattern was surgically induced in thirty-three female rats, the cohort was divided into the following groups: group 1 (30 mg/kg resveratrol i.m. for 14 days), group 2 (1 mg/kg leuprolide acetate s.c. single dose), group 3 (resveratrol and leuprolide acetate), and group 4 was the control group, with no medication. The treatment was carried out for two weeks, and after administration, the lesions size, histopathology, immunoreactivity to matrix metalloproteinase-2, matrix metalloproteinase-9, and the vascular endothelial growth factor were evaluated. Peritoneal fluid levels of interleukin-6, interleukin-8, and TNF-α were also studied.

Authors concluded that resveratrol alone might be an efficient alternative to leuprolide acetate in the treatment of this pathology. Moreover, their combination decreased the activity of each therapeutical agent, mostly the anti-inflammatory and anti-angiogenic effects. Plasmatic and peritoneal levels of interleukin-6, interleukin-8, and TNF-α were reduced in the group that received only one therapeutical agent (1 and 2), and the volume of implant lesions was also significantly reduced. The study of Amaya et al. summarized these effects of resveratrol, pointing out that low concentrations of resveratrol associated to E2 possess a high estrogenic activity, suggesting that this compound can be considered as a new approach in the treatment of this disease [106].

Sex steroids are used in the treatment of endometriosis and resveratrol, at high doses, has been demonstrated to decrease the proliferation of human endometrial cells through estrogen receptor 1 (ESR 1) [80]. Another study used ovariectomized immunodeficient RAG-2-γ(c) mice with implanted human endometrial cells. Amaya S. et al. administered a one-month treatment with subcutaneous pellets of estradiol, estradiol and progesterone, and estradiol and resveratrol (6, 30, or 60 mg). They concluded that resveratrol functions in low doses as an estrogen agonist and in high doses as an estrogen antagonist.

Another study of Cenksoy et al. investigated the effect of resveratrol as an anti-angiogenic and anti-inflammatory agent in in vivo research on mice with induced endometriosis [26]. They surgically induced endometrial implants in 24 female rats and after the endometriosis foci had been confirmed, they divided the rats into the following groups: a first group that received resveratrol, the second group that received leuprolide acetate, and the control group. The treatment was administered for 21 days, and at the end of the administration, the authors evaluated the volume and histopathology of lesions. Vascular endothelial growth factor and monocyte chemoattractant protein one measurement in peritoneal samples and blood samples were performed.

The mean areas and volumes of the implants decreased after treatment with both resveratrol and leuprolide acetate. Serum and peritoneal levels of MCP-1 and VEGF also appeared to be significantly lower in both groups, so the effectiveness of resveratrol is comparable with that of leuprolide acetate, a well-known therapeutical agent used for endometriosis regression.

A study in vivo and in vitro from 2011 regarding the effects of resveratrol on endometriosis [25] reported that this compound increases cell death and decreases the proliferation of endometriosis lesions, inhibiting the development of this disease. Another in vivo research on rats demonstrated that after experimentally inducing endometriosis in the subjects, and after treatment with resveratrol, the implant sizes decreased, and also the levels of VEGF and MCP-1 from peritoneal fluid. VEGF expression was also suppressed in the endometriosis tissues after treatment [107]. By inhibiting VEGF expression and synthesis, resveratrol acts as an anti-angiogenic compound while the inhibition of synthesis, receptor activity secretion, and chemotactic activity of MCP-1 have anti-inflammatory effects. The same results were identified by Cenksoy et al., who continued their research with the administration of GnRHa, pointing out that resveratrol had the same impact as leuprolide acetate. Resveratrol acts like synthetic estrogens, binding and activating the estrogen receptors [108].

A study of Taguchi et al. [109] demonstrated that resveratrol alone could reduce significantly surviving mRNA expression, but did not induce apoptosis in human endometriotic stromal cells. Also, pre-treatment with resveratrol in the case of endometriosis significantly enhanced TNF-α-related-apoptosis-inducing ligand (TRAIL), known as a pro-apoptotic molecule.

5.2. Clinical Studies

Over time, the use of complementary and alternative medicine have been widely studied for the treatment of endometriosis [110] and many plant-based products, including resveratrol, have been reported to exhibit efficacy against this disease. Although the results of preclinical studies have been favorable and have revealed the effectiveness of resveratrol in the treatment of this disease, clinical trials using resveratrol have been limited. The hypothesis of most of the clinical trials involving resveratrol administration was that the combination of oral contraceptives with naturally occurring aromatase inhibitors might show promise for the treatment of endometriosis.

Resveratrol can potentiate the actions of oral contraceptives in the treatment of endometriosis-related symptoms (such as dysmenorrhea). The mechanism of action, in this case, consists of decreasing the expression of cyclooxygenase-2 and aromatase expression [81].

The suppression of aromatase and Cox-2 expression in the endometrium is a necessary premise for the control of chronic pelvic pain. Besides the suppression of aromatase, resveratrol possesses the ability to block SIRT 1 and transform growth factor-beta genes. Synthetic aromatase inhibitors do not share this characteristic [111]. Although the real mechanism of the anti-inflammatory effect of resveratrol is not fully known, it seems to include the inhibition of NF-kB activation and its translocation to cell nuclei. There, it stimulates the transcription of several genes connected to the inflammatory cascade [112].

Because the excess of estrogen in endometriosis takes place in lesions as a consequence of the expression of the aromatase p450 enzyme, progesterone resistance may develop as a consequence of this hyperestrogenic milieu. Therefore aromatase expression may persist into the endometrium of patients using oral contraceptives during the first months of treatment and pelvic pain and bleeding may continue despite the treatment. [113]. The breakthrough that bleeding in oral contraceptive users was associated with Cox-2 and nuclear factor kappa beta activation, thereby suggested that the recommencement of inflammation plays a significant role in the resumption of uterine bleeding and pain.

In this respect, the anti-inflammatory effect of resveratrol will contribute towards decreasing the pain associated with endometriosis, potentiating the therapeutic impact of drospirenone and rendering the patients pain-free [114,115].

Maia H. Jr et al. [116] investigated 12 patients with endometriosis-associated dysmenorrhea, who failed positive results after administration of oral contraceptive, containing drospirenone + ethinylestradiol. They added 30 mg of resveratrol to the standard hormone therapy and concluded that the pain scores significantly reduced after two months of treatment. A separate study of the same authors included 42 women with endometriosis submitted to laparoscopy and hysteroscopy, where they investigated aromatase and cyclooxygenase-2 expression from endometrial tissue of these patients. Sixteen patients used before hospital admission oral contraceptives alone and 26 received oral contraceptives and resveratrol combined. The authors concluded that the inhibition of aromatase and COX-2 was increased in the group with combined therapy.

Mendes da Silva et al. [117] also conducted a randomized clinical trial to observe the effectiveness of resveratrol in the management of endometriosis, associated with monophasic contraceptive pills. They included in the study 44 women aged 20 to 50, who randomly received two pills for 42 days: one tablet was an oral contraceptive and the other 40 mg of resveratrol or placebo pills. After the end of the study, the authors concluded that resveratrol did not prove any additional effects to placebo for the treatment of endometriosis-related symptoms because the differences between median pain scores in the two groups were insignificant.

NF-kB is one of the significant transcription agents involved in the inflammatory pathway of this disease. Another factor that seems to play an essential role in inflammation is an NAD^+ dependent histone deacetylase, SIRT1. It was discovered that this factor is also involved in carcinogenesis [118].

To observe the expression of sirtuin 1 in this chronic pathology, Taguchi et al. [119] obtained endometriotic stromal cells and exposed them to resveratrol and sirtinol, which are an activator and an inhibitor of sirtinol, respectively. Immunohistochemistry and RT-PCR examined the eutopic endometrial cells, and this study concluded that sirtuin one was identified both in endometriotic stromal and in not affected cells. After the exposure to resveratrol, the authors found that it decreased tumor necrosis factor-α-induced, interleukin-8 release and SIRT1, and increased interleukin-8 release. Therefore, the contrary actions of resveratrol and sirtinol proved that interleukin-8 release is modulated through sirtuin 1. Therefore resveratrol can be used in endometriosis to ameliorate chronic inflammation.

Simvastatin is an inhibitor of 3-hydroxy-3-methylglutaryl-coenzyme A reductase (HMGCR) activity, with intrinsic antioxidant activity [120] that is used in the treatment of endometriosis. In this case, the mechanism of resveratrol does not involve anti-inflammatory pathways. Resveratrol possesses the ability to inhibit HMGCR mRNA expression, whereas both resveratrol and simvastatin inhibit enzymatic activity. HMGCR represent a rate-limiting step of the mevalonate pathway that includes the isoprenoids FPP and GGPP. These isoprenoids are necessary for the isoprenylation of proteins involved in apoptosis, cell proliferation, adhesiveness, and maintenance of cellular functions. Different products of the mevalonate pathway exert negative feedback on HMGCR expression [115]. It is worth mentioning that the effects of resveratrol on the enzymatic activity of HMCGR are independent of the effects on *HMCGR* expression.

So, the addition of resveratrol may potentiate the effect of simvastatin when it is used as a therapeutic agent against endometriosis, through a mechanism that does not involve an anti-inflammatory effect.

To investigate the interactions between simvastatin and resveratrol, focusing on cholesterol biosynthesis and protein activity in cultures of human endometrial stromal cells (HES), Villanueva et al. [121] obtained HES from healthy volunteers. Then, they measured the conversion of acetate to cholesterol and quantified HMGR mRNA transcripts, protein expression, and enzyme activity, by measuring the conversion of 3-hydroxy-3-methyl-glutaryl-coenzyme A to mevalonic acid lactone in HES cells.

The results of this study indicated that resveratrol potentiated the inhibitory effects of simvastatin on cholesterol biosynthesis and the activity of the HMGCR enzyme. It also inhibited the stimulatory effects of statin on protein expression and HMGCR mRNA transcription. Therefore, the combination of resveratrol and Simvastatin may be potentially useful in the development of new management of endometriosis.

Regarding the mechanisms of action of resveratrol, this phytochemical is known to have an anti-inflammatory, anti-angiogenic effect and also to induce apoptosis in various cell types, but its pro-apoptotic role on human endometrial cells remains uncertain.

Given all the presented studies, resveratrol is a promising agent against endometriosis. It has been shown to suppress the expression of various inflammatory biomarkers (TNF-α, COX-2), to activate various transcription factors (NF-kB, PPAR-gamma), and to induce antioxidant enzymes (catalase, superoxide dismutase) [122] and thus it holds promise as a natural therapeutical agent but further studies are necessary in order to establish the doses for human administration.

Table 1. Preclinical studies regarding the effects of resveratrol in endometriosis.

Author	Study Design	Number of Cases	Treatment Regimen/Study Design	Follow-Up	Results
Yavuz et al. [104]	Prospective study, surgically induced lesions of endometriosis	24 female rats	Control group—no treatment Group 1—1 mg/kg/day of resveratrol, injected intraperitoneally Group 2—10 mg/kg/day of resveratrol, injected intraperitoneally	7 days	- Endometriotic implants volume and proliferating cell nuclear antigen expression levels were significantly reduced in treated groups. - Also, the increased activity of superoxide dismutase and glutathione peroxidase in serum and tissue of treated rats was detected.
Tekin et al. [105]	Prospective study, surgically induced lesions of endometriosis	33 female rats	Control group—no treatment Group 1—30 mg/kg resveratrol i.m for 14 days Group 2—1 mg/kg leuprolide acetate s.c. single dose Group 3—30 mg/kg resveratrol i.m. for 14 days and one single dose of 1 mg/kg leuprolide acetate s.c.	14 days	- The volume of endometriotic implants and the histopathological grade were significantly reduced in treated groups. Immunoreactivity to MMP2, MMP9, and VEGF was decreased - Comparing the levels of IL-6, IL-8, and TNF-α in plasma and peritoneal fluid, they were significantly reduced in group 1 and 2 compared to group 3 and the control group
Amaya et al. [106]	Prospective study ovariectomized immunodeficient RAG-2-γ(c) mice with human endometrial tissue implanted	N	Group 1—Subcutaneous pellets of E2 Group 2—Subcutaneous pellets of E2 plus progesterone (P4) Group 3—Subcutaneous pellets E2 plus resveratrol (6, 30, or 60 mg) injected intraperitoneally	30 days	- After the administration of treatments, immunohistochemical expression of ESR1, Ki67, reverse transcriptase polymerase chain reaction of AhR, CYP1A1, and CYP1B1 were analyzed - Decreased expression of ESR1 and proliferative activity (Ki67) was exhibited with 60 mg of resveratrol.
Cenksoy et al. [26]	Prospective study, surgically induced lesions of endometriosis	24 female Wistar–Albino rats	Group 1—resveratrol (7) Group 2—leuprolide acetate (8) Group 3—control group (7)	21 days	- The mean areas of endometriotic implants were reduced after treatment in both group 1 and group 2. - Histopathological scores of the VEGF scores of endometriotic implants and peritoneal fluid levels of VEGF and MCP-1 were decreased in group 1 and 2
Taguchi et al. [109]	Prospective study	Endometriotic tissues collected during surgeries from ovarian endometriosis affected women	Human endometriotic cells were cultured and pretreated with resveratrol in vitro. Then, the cells were incubated with TNF-α-related-apoptosis-inducing ligand		- Resveratrol is not able to induce apoptosis in human endometriotic stromal cells alone - it significantly decreases surviving mRNA expression - enhances TRAIL-induced apoptosis.

155

Table 2. Clinical studies regarding the effects of resveratrol in endometriosis.

Maia Jr. et al. [116]	Prospective Study with Two Arms	Experiment 1: - 12 Patients Treated with Drospirenone Ethinylestradiol 3 mg/30 µg for 6 Months Experiment 2: - 42 patients surgical treatment. - 16 treatment with oral contraceptives - 26 combination with resveratrol	Experiment 1: All the Patients were Switched to a Combination of Drospirenone/Ethinylestradiol /Resveratrol (a Dose of 30 mg/Day) Experiment 2: - 16 patients used drospirenone/ethinylestradiol for at least 2 months before surgery. - 26 patients drospirenone/ethinylestradiol associated with 30 mg of resveratrol.	Experiment 1: 6 Months	Experiment 1: - Decreased Pain Scores after 2 Months of Treatment - 82% of Patients Reported Complete Resolution of Dysmenorrhea and Pelvic Pain Experiment 2: - Expression of both aromatase and cyclooxygenase-2 was reduced in the eutopic endometrium of patients using drospirenone/ ethinylestradiol associated with 30 mg of resveratrol, compared with the endometrium of patients using oral contraceptives alone.
Mendes da Silva et al. [117]	Prospective study, double-blinded trial	44 women with a laparoscopic diagnosis of endometriosis	The patients were randomized to receive oral contraceptives or 40 mg resveratrol/day or placebo pills.	42 days	- In the placebo group, mean pain scores were 5.4 before treatment and in resveratrol group were 5.7. After the procedure, the mean pain scores registered were 3.9 in the placebo group and 3.2 in the resveratrol group.
Villanueva et al. [121]	Prospective study	Endometrial tissue was obtained from 8 patients, undergoing surgeries or healthy volunteers	Cholesterol biosynthesis by human endometrial cells was assessed in vitro by measuring the conversion of [^{14}C] acetate to [^{14}C] cholesterol in the presence of resveratrol (30–100 µM), simvastatin (0.1–10 µM), or resveratrol 30 µM + simvastatin 0.1 µM		- Resveratrol inhibited cholesterol biosynthesis, enzyme activity, and HMGCR mRNA and potentiated the inhibitory effects of simvastatin on cholesterol biosynthesis and HMGCR enzyme activity.

6. Conclusions and Future Perspectives

Endometriosis is a benign gynecological disorder that affects women in the reproductive age worldwide and is characterized mainly by chronic abdominal pain and infertility. Even the pathophysiologic mechanisms of endometriosis are not completely known; chronic inflammation is considered one of the pathways responsible for endometriosis development.

Natural polyphenols are bioactive compounds with multiple beneficial properties that provide new therapeutical perspectives against endometriotic lesions. Polyphenols are known to possess anti-carcinogenic, anti-angiogenic, anti-inflammatory, proapoptotic and anti-oxidative effects. Recently, the anti-inflammatory potential of natural dietary compounds has raised interest for researchers because it might be used in the treatment of endometriosis.

In this article, we summarized some of the epidemiological and clinical research that supports the beneficial effect of resveratrol in endometriosis. Moreover, resveratrol demonstrated its efficiency either alone or associated with other classical therapeutically agents used in endometriosis treatment such as leuprolide acetate or statins.

Knowledge of the precise and more profound mechanisms of how resveratrol can reduce endometriotic lesions is required, and further studies on this topic are crucial. Overall, the role of resveratrol in reducing the volume of endometriotic lesions and chronic abdominal pain is a proven fact.

Author Contributions: D.A.-M., M.A.M., O.G.D., and C.V.A. together initiated, designed, and drafted the manuscript. D.A.-M., G.S., C.V.A., and V.B. contributed to the literature collection. D.A.-M., M.A.M., and C.V.A. drew the figures. All authors revised the manuscript. All authors read and approved the final manuscript.

Funding: This research received no external funding.

Conflicts of Interest: The authors declare no conflict of interest.

Abbreviations

AA	arachidonic acid
AhR	aryl hydrocarbon receptor
AKT	protein kinase B
AP	activator protein
ATF	activating transcription factor
c-Jun	protein encoded by the JUN gene
CO_2	carbon dioxide
CoA	coenzyme A
COX	cyclo-oxygenase
DNA	deoxyribonucleic acid
E2	estradiol
E2F1	transcription factor encoded by the E2F1 gene
ERK-1	extracellular signal-regulated kinase 1
ESR 1	estrogen receptor 1
FOS	protein family of transcription factors
FoxP3+	regulatory T (Treg) cells
FPP	farnesylpyrophosphate
GGPP	geranylgeranylpyrophosphate
GM-CSF	granulocyte macrophage colony-stimulating factor
GnRH	gonadotropin-releasing hormone
H_2O_2	hydrogen peroxide
HES	human endometrial stromal cells
HIF-1	hypoxia-inducible factor 1α
HMGCR	3-hydroxy-3-methylglutaryl-coenzyme A reductase
IL	interleukin

IL-1β	interleukin 1β
JNK	c-Jun N-terminal kinases
LPS	lipopolysaccharide
LTB4	leukotriene B4
MAF	transcription factor
MAPK	mitogen-activated protein kinase
MAPK1/3; ERK1/2	mitogen-activated protein kinase 1/3
MAPK14	mitogen-Activated Protein Kinase 14
MCP-1	monocyte chemoattractant protein 1
MIF	macrophage inhibitory factor
MMP	metalloproteinase
mRNA	messenger ribonucleic acid
NAD	nicotinamide adenine dinucleotide
NFAT	nuclear factor of activated T-cells
NF-kB	nuclear factor-kB
NO	nitric oxide
O_2	oxygen
PG	prostaglandin
PGE2	prostaglandin G2
PPAR	peroxisome proliferator-activated receptors
PGF2α	prostaglandin F2α
PGG2	prostaglandin G2
PGH2	prostaglandin H2
PGI2	prostaglandin I2
RPS6KB2	ribosomal protein S6 kinase beta-2
RT-PCR	reverse transcription polymerase chain reaction
SIRT1	sirtuin 1
STATs	signal transducer and activator of transcription protein family
STAT3	signal transducer and activator of transcription 3
Th17	lymphocytes T helper 17
TNF-α	tumor necrosis factor
TRAIL	TNF-α-related-apoptosis-inducing ligand
UV	ultraviolet
VEGF	vascular endothelial growth factor
VEGFC	vascular endothelial growth factor C
VEGFR	vascular endothelial growth factor receptor
AA	arachidonic acid
AhR	aryl hydrocarbon receptor
AKT	protein kinase B

References

1. Baldi, A.; Campioni, M.; Signorile, P.G. Endometriosis: Pathogenesis, diagnosis, therapy and association with cancer (review). *Oncol. Rep.* **2008**, *19*, 843–846. [CrossRef] [PubMed]
2. Nisolle, M.; Donnez, J. Peritoneal endometriosis, ovarian endometriosis, and adenomyotic nodules of the rectovaginal septum are three different entities. *Fertil. Steril.* **1997**, *68*, 585–596. [CrossRef]
3. Sampson, J.A. Peritoneal endometriosis due to menstrual dissemination of endometrial tissue into the peritoneal cavity. *Am. J. Obstet. Gynecol.* **1927**, *14*, 422–469. [CrossRef]
4. Missmer, S.A.; Cramer, D.W. The epidemiology of endometriosis. *Obstet. Gynecol. Clin. North Am.* **2003**, *301*, 1–19. [CrossRef]
5. Farquar, C. Endometriosis. *BMJ* **2007**, *334*, 249–253. [CrossRef] [PubMed]
6. Fauconnier, A.; Chapron, C. Endometriosis and pelvic pain: Epidemiological evidence of the relationship and implications. *Hum. Reprod. Update* **2005**, *11*, 595–606. [CrossRef] [PubMed]

7. Lousee, J.C.; Van Langendonckt, A.; Defrere, S.; Gonzalez Ramos, R.; Colette, S.; Donnez, J. Peritoneal endometriosis is an inflammatory disease. *Front. Biosci.* **2012**, *4*, 23–40. [CrossRef]
8. Gazvani, R.; Templeton, A. Peritoneal environment, cytokines and angiogenesis in the pathophysiology of endometriosis. *Reproduction* **2002**, *123*, 217–226. [CrossRef] [PubMed]
9. Larosa, M.; Facchini, F.; Leone, M.; Grande, M.; Monica, B. Endometriosis: Aetiopathogenetic basis. *Urologia* **2010**, *77*, 1–11. [CrossRef] [PubMed]
10. Kobayashi, H.; Higashiura, Y.; Shigetomi, H.; Kajihara, H. Pathogenesis of endometriosis: The role of initial infection and subsequent sterile inflammation (Review). *Mol. Med. Rep.* **2014**, *9*, 9–15. [CrossRef] [PubMed]
11. Van Langendonckt, A.; Casanas-Roux, F.; Donnez, J. Oxidative stress and peritoneal endometriosis. *Fertil. Steril.* **2002**, *77*, 861–870. [CrossRef]
12. Howes, M.J.; Simmonds, M.S. The role of phytochemicals as micronutrients in health and disease. *Curr. Opin. Clin. Nutr. Metab. Care* **2014**, *17*, 558–566. [CrossRef] [PubMed]
13. Manach, C.; Williamson, G.; Morand, C.; Scalbert, A.; Remesy, C. Bioavailability and bioefficacy of polyphenols in humans. I. Review of 97 bioavailability studies. *Am. J. Clin. Nutr.* **2005**, *81*, 230S–242S. [CrossRef] [PubMed]
14. Yoon, J.H.; Baek, S.J. Molecular Targets of Dietary Polyphenols with Anti-inflammatory Properties. *Yonsei Med. J.* **2005**, *46*, 585–596. [CrossRef] [PubMed]
15. Rauf, A.; Imran, M.; Butt, M.S.; Nadeem, M.; Peters, D.G.; Mubarak, M.S. Resveratrol as an anti-cancer agent: A review. *Crit. Rev. Food Sci. Nutr.* **2018**, *58*, 1428–1447. [CrossRef] [PubMed]
16. Nakata, R.; Takahashi, S.; Inoue, H. Recent advances in the study on resveratrol. *Biol. Pharm. Bull.* **2012**, *35*, 273–279. [CrossRef] [PubMed]
17. Chu, M.; Almagro, L.; Chen, B.; Burgos, L.; Pedreño, M.A. Recent trends and comprehensive appraisal for the biotechnological production of trans-resveratrol and its derivatives. *Phytochem. Rev.* **2018**, *17*, 1–18. [CrossRef]
18. Bhardwaj, A.; Sethi, G.; Vadhan-Raj, S. Resveratrol inhibits proliferation, induces apoptosis, and overcomes chemoresistance through downregulation of STAT3 and nuclear factor-kappaB regulated antiapoptotic and cell survival gene products in human multiple myeloma cells. *Blood* **2007**, *109*, 2293–2302. [CrossRef] [PubMed]
19. Fremont, L. Biological effects of resveratrol. *Life Sci.* **2000**, *66*, 663–673. [CrossRef]
20. Athar, M.; Back, J.H.; Kopelovich, L.; Bickers, D.R.; Kim, A.L. Multiple molecular targets of resveratrol: Anti-carcinogenic mechanisms. *Arch. Biochem. Biophys.* **2009**, *486*, 95–102. [CrossRef] [PubMed]
21. Brito, P.M.; Devillard, R.; Negre-Salvayre, A.; Almeida, L.M.; Dinis, T.C.; Salvayre, R.; Auge, N. Resveratrol inhibits the mTOR mitogenic signaling evoked by oxidized LDL in smooth muscle cells. *Atherosclerosis* **2009**, *205*, 126–134. [CrossRef] [PubMed]
22. Chan, A.Y.; Dolinsky, V.W.; Soltys, C.L.; Viollet, B.; Baksh, S.; Light, P.E.; Dyck, J.R. Resveratrol inhibits cardiac hypertrophy via AMP-activated protein kinase and Akt. *J. Biol. Chem.* **2008**, *283*, 24194–24201. [CrossRef] [PubMed]
23. Cinar, O.; Seval, Y.; Uz, Y.H.; Cakmak, H.; Ulukus, M.; Kayisli, U.A.; Arici, A. Differential regulation of Akt phosphorylation in endometriosis. *Reprod. Biomed. Online* **2009**, *19*, 864–871. [CrossRef] [PubMed]
24. McKinnon, B.; Bersinger, N.A.; Huber, A.W.; Kuhn, A.; Mueller, M.D. PPAR-gamma expression in peritoneal endometriotic lesions correlates with pain experienced by patients. *Fertil. Steril.* **2010**, *93*, 293–296. [CrossRef] [PubMed]
25. Bruner-Tran, K.L.; Osteen, K.G.; Taylor, H.S.; Sokalska, A.; Haines, K.; Duleba, A.J. Resveratrol inhibits development of experimental endometriosis in vivo and reduces endometrial stromal cell invasiveness in vitro. *Biol. Reprod.* **2011**, *84*, 106–112. [CrossRef] [PubMed]
26. Cenksoy, P.O.; Oktem, M.; Erdem, O.; Karakaya, C.; Cenksoy, C.; Erdem, A.; Guner, H.; Karabacak, O. A potential novel treatment strategy: Inhibition of angiogenesis and inflammation by resveratrol for regression of endometriosis in an experimental rat model. *Gynecol. Endocrinol.* **2015**, *31*, 219–224. [CrossRef] [PubMed]
27. Velmurugan, B.K.; Rathinasamy, B.; Lohanathan, B.P.; Thiyagarajan, V.; Weng, C.F. Neuroprotective role of phytochemicals. *Molecules* **2018**, *23*, 2485. [CrossRef] [PubMed]

28. Anastacio, J.R.; Netto, C.A.; Castro, C.C.; Sanches, E.F.; Ferreira, D.C.; Noschang, C.; Krolow, R.; Dalmaz, C.; Pagnussat, A. Resveratrol treatment has neuroprotective effects and prevents cognitive impairment after chronic cerebral hypoperfusion. *Neurol. Res.* **2014**, *36*, 627–633. [CrossRef]
29. Takaoka, M. Resveratrol, a new phenolic compound, from Veratrum grandiflorum. *Nippon Kagaku Kaishi* **1939**, *60*, 1090–1100. [CrossRef]
30. Catalgol, B.; Batirel, S.; Taga, Y.; Ozer, N.K. Resveratrol: French paradox revisited. *Front. Pharmacol.* **2012**, *3*, 141. [CrossRef]
31. Burns, J.; Yokota, T.; Ashihara, H.; Lean, M.E.J.; Crozier, A. Plant foods and herbal sources of resveratrol. *J. Agric. Food Chem.* **2002**, *50*, 3337–3340. [CrossRef] [PubMed]
32. Sobolev, V.S.; Neff, S.A.; Gloer, J.B. New dimeric stilbenoids from fungal-challenged peanut (Arachis hypogaea) seeds. *J. Agric. Food Chem.* **2010**, *58*, 875–881. [CrossRef] [PubMed]
33. Hurst, W.J.; Glinski, J.A.; Miller, K.B.; Apgar, J.; Davey, M.H.; Stuart, D.A. Survey of the trans-resveratrol and trans-piceid content of cocoa-containing and chocolate products. *J. Agric. Food Chem.* **2008**, *56*, 8374–8378. [CrossRef] [PubMed]
34. Niesen, D.B.; Hessler, C.; Seeram, N.P. Beyond resveratrol: A review of natural stilbenoids identified from 2009–2013. *J. Berry. Res.* **2013**, *3*, 181–196.
35. Bostanghadiri, N.; Pormohammad, A.; Chirani, A.S.; Pouriran, R.; Erfanimanesh, S.; Hashemi, A. Comprehensive review on the antimicrobial potency of the plant polyphenol Resveratrol. *Biomed. Pharmacother.* **2017**, *95*, 1588–1595. [CrossRef] [PubMed]
36. Resveratrol. PubChem Open Chemistry Database. Available online: https://pubchem.ncbi.nlm.nih.gov/compound/resveratrol#section=Top (accessed on 12 November 2018).
37. Delmas, D.; LAncon, A.; Colin, D.; Jannin, B.; Latruffe, N. Resveratrol as a chemopreventive agent: A promising molecule for fighting cancer. *Curr. Drug Targets* **2006**, *7*, 423–442. [CrossRef] [PubMed]
38. Soleas, G.J.; Diamandis, E.P.; Goldberg, D.M. Resveratrol: A molecule whose time has come? And gone? *Clin. Biochem.* **1997**, *30*, 91–113. [CrossRef]
39. Chen, X.; He, H.; Wang, G.; Yang, B.; Ren, W.; Ma, L.; Yu, Q. Stereospecific determination of cis- and trans-resveratrol in rat plasma by HPLC: Application to pharmacokinetic studies. *Biomed. Chromatogr.* **2007**, *21*, 257–265. [CrossRef] [PubMed]
40. Camont, L.; Cottart, C.H.; Rhayem, Y.; Nivet-Antoine, V.; Djelidi, R.; Collin, F.; Beaudeaux, J.L.; Bonnefont-Rousselot, D. Simple spectrophotometric assessment of the trans-/cis-resveratrol ratio in aqueous solutions. *Anal. Chim. Acta* **2009**, *634*, 121–128. [CrossRef]
41. Sang, S.; Yang, I.; Buckley, B.; Ho, C.T.; Chung, S.Y. Autoxidative quinone formation in vitro and metabolite formation in vivo from tea polyphenol (-)-epigallocatechin-3-gallate: Studied by real–time mass spectrometry combined with tandem mass ion mapping. *Free Radic. Biol. Med.* **2007**, *43*, 362–371. [CrossRef]
42. Jensen, J.S.; Wertz, C.F.; O'Neill, V.A. Preformulation Stability of trans-Resveratrol and trans–Resveratrol Glucoside (Piceid). *J. Agric. Food Chem.* **2010**, *58*, 1685–1690. [CrossRef]
43. King, R.E.; Bomser, J.A.; Min, D.B. Bioactivity of Resveratrol. *Comprehens Rev. Food Sci. Food Safe* **2006**, *5*, 65–70. [CrossRef]
44. Huang, K.S.; Lin, M.; Cheng, G.F. Anti-inflammatory tetramers of resveratrol from the roots of Vitis amurensis and the conformations of the seven-membered ring in some oligostilbenes. *Phytochem.* **2001**, *58*, 357–362. [CrossRef]
45. Berkley, K.J.; Rapkin, A.J.; Papka, R.E. The pains of endometriosis. *Science* **2005**, *308*, 1587–1589. [CrossRef]
46. Marki, G.; Bokor, A.; Rigo, J.; Rigo, A. Physical pain and emotion regulation as the main predictive factors of health-related quality of life in women living with endometriosis. *Hum. Reprod.* **2017**, *32*, 1432–1438. [CrossRef]
47. Lagana, A.S.; La Rosa, V.L.; Rapisarda, A.M.C. Anxiety and depression in patients with endometriosis: Impact and management challenges. *Int. J. Women Health* **2017**, 323–330. [CrossRef]
48. Zheng, W.; Cao, L.; Zheng, X.; Yuanyuan, M.; Liang, X. Anti-Angiogenic Alternative and Complementary Medicines for the Treatment of Endometriosis: A Review of Potential Molecular Mechanisms. *Evid. Based Complement. Alternat. Med.* **2018**, *4128984*, 1–28. [CrossRef]
49. Attar, E. Aromatase and other steroidogenic genes in endometriosis. Translational aspects. *Hum. Reprod. Update* **2006**, *12*, 49–56. [CrossRef]

50. Casoy, M.H.; Valente, J.; Filho, J. Is aromatase expression in the endometrium the cause of endometriosis and its related infertility? *Gynecol. Endocrinol.* **2009**, *25*, 253–257.
51. Guo, S.W. Nuclear factor-kappa B (NF-kappaB): An unsuspected major culprit in the pathogenesis of endometriosis that is still at large? *Gynecol. Obstet. Invest.* **2007**, *63*, 71–97. [CrossRef]
52. Maia, H., Jr.; Haddad, C.; Coelho, G.; Casoy, J. Role of inflammation and aromatase expression in the eutopic endometrium and its relationship with the development of endometriosis. *Women's Health* **2012**, *8*, 647–658. [CrossRef] [PubMed]
53. Maia, H., Jr.; Haddad, C.; Maia, R.; Casoy, J. Nuclear factor kappa B (NF-kappa B) expression in the endometrium of normal and pathological uterus. *Giorn. It. Ost. Gin.* **2012**, *34*, 236–638.
54. Sugino, N.; Karube-Harada, A.; Taketani, T.; Sakata, A.; Nakamura, Y. Withdrawal of ovarian steroids stimulates prostaglandin F2-alpha production through nuclear factor-kappaB activation via oxygen radicals in human endometrial stromal cells: Potential relevance to menstruation. *J. Reprod. Dev.* **2004**, *50*, 215–225. [CrossRef] [PubMed]
55. Asante, A.; Taylor, R.N. Endometriosis: The role of neuroangiogenesis. *Ann. Rev. Physiol.* **2011**, *73*, 163–182. [CrossRef] [PubMed]
56. Risau, W. Mechanisms of angiogenesis. *Nature* **1997**, *386*, 671–674. [CrossRef] [PubMed]
57. Hey-Cunningham, A.J.; Peters, K.M.; Zevallos, H.B.V.; Berbic, M.; Markham, R.; Fraser, I. Angiogenesis, lymphangiogenesis and neurogenesis in endometriosis. *Front. Biosci. Elite.* **2013**, *5*, 1033–1056. [CrossRef]
58. Hanahan, D.; Folkman, J. Patterns and emerging mechanisms of the angiogenic switch during tumorigenesis. *Cell* **1996**, *86*, 353–364. [CrossRef]
59. Gagne, D.; Page, M.; Robitaille, G.; Hugo, P.; Gosselin, D. Levels of vascular endothelial growth factor (VEGF) in serum of patients with endometriosis. *Hum. Reprod.* **2003**, *18*, 1674–1680. [CrossRef] [PubMed]
60. Song, W.W.; Lu, H.; Hou, W.J.; Guang-Xu, X.; Ji-Hong, Z.; Sheng, Y.H.; Cheng, M.J.; Zhang, R. Expression of vascular endothelial growth factor C and anti-angiogenesis therapy in endometriosis. *Int. J. Clin. Exp. Pathol.* **2014**, *7*, 7752–7759. [PubMed]
61. Yang, H.; Liu, J.; Fan, Y. Associations between various possible promoter polymorphisms of MMPs genes and endometriosis risk: A meta-analysis. *Eur. J. Obstet. Gynecol. Reprod. Biol.* **2016**, *205*, 174–188. [CrossRef]
62. Abutorabi, R.; Baradaran, A.; Mostafavi, F.S.; Zarrin, Y.; Mardanian, F. Evaluation of tumor necrosis factor alpha polymorphism frequencies in endometriosis. *Int. J. Fertil. Steril.* **2015**, *9*, 329–337. [PubMed]
63. Chishima, F.; Hayakawa, S.; Sugita, K. Increased expression of cyclooxygenase-2 in local lesions of endometriosis patients. *Am. J. Reprod. Immunol.* **2002**, *48*, 50–56. [CrossRef] [PubMed]
64. Jana, S.; Chatterjee, K.; Ray, A.K.; Das Mahapatra, P.; Swarnakar, S.; Ramchandran, R. Regulation of Matrix Metalloproteinase 2 Activity by COX-2-PGE2-pAKT Axis Promotes Angiogenesis in Endometriosis. *PLoSONE* **2016**, *11*, 0163540. [CrossRef] [PubMed]
65. Sakamoto, Y.; Harada, T.; Horie, S. Tumor necrosis factorα-induced interleukin-8 (IL-8) expression in endometriotic stromal cells, probably through nuclear factor-κB activation: Gonadotropin-Releasing Hormone Agonist Treatment Reduced IL-8 Expression. *J. Clin. Endocrinol. Metab.* **2003**, *88*, 730–735. [CrossRef] [PubMed]
66. Capobianco, A.; Rovere-Querini, P. Endometriosis, a disease of the macrophage. *Front. Immunol.* **2013**, *4*, 9. [CrossRef] [PubMed]
67. Harris, T.; Vlass, A.M. Can Herbal Medicines Improve Cellular Immunity Patterns in Endometriosis? *Med. Aromat. Plants* **2015**, *4*, 2. [CrossRef]
68. Soares, S.R.; Martinez-Varea, A.; Hidalgo-Mora, J.J.; Pellicer, A. Pharmacologic therapies in endometriosis: A systematic review. *Fertil. Steril.* **2012**, *98*, 529–555. [CrossRef] [PubMed]
69. Grund, E.M.; Kagan, D.; Tran, C.A.; Zeitvogel, A.; Strazinski-Powitz, A.; Nataraja, S. Tumor necrosis factor-α regulates inflammatory and mesenchymal responses via mitogen-activated protein kinase, p38, and nuclear factor-kB in human endometriotic epithelial cells. *Mol. Pharm.* **2008**, *73*, 1394–1404. [CrossRef] [PubMed]
70. Zhang, H.; Li, M.; Wang, F.; Liu, S.; Li, J.; Wen, Z. Endometriotic epithelial cells induce MMPs expression in endometrial stromal cells via NF-kB-dependent pathway. *Gynecol. Endocrinol.* **2010**, *26*, 456–467. [CrossRef] [PubMed]
71. Donnez, J.; Binda, M.M.; Donnez, O.; Dolmans, M.M. Oxidative stress in the pelvic cavity and its role in the pathogenesis of endometriosis. *Fertil. Steril.* **2016**, *106*, 1011–1017. [CrossRef] [PubMed]

72. Khanapure, S.P.; Garvey, D.S.; Janero, D.R.; Letts, L.G. Eicosanoids in inflammation: Biosynthesis, pharmacology, and therapeutic frontiers. *Curr. Topics Med. Chem.* **2007**, *7*, 311–340. [CrossRef]
73. Gonzalez-Ramos, R.; Van Langendonckt, A.; Defrere, S.; Lousse, J.C.; Colette, S.; Devoto, L.; Donnez, J. Involvement of the nuclear factor-kB pathway in the pathogenesis of endometriosis. *Fertil. Steril.* **2010**, *94*, 1985–1994. [CrossRef] [PubMed]
74. Klemmt, P.A.; Starzinski-Powitz, A. Molecular and Cellular Pathogenesis of Endometriosis. *Curr. Women's Health Rev.* **2018**, *14*, 106–116. [CrossRef] [PubMed]
75. Giudice, L.C.; Kao, L.C. Endometriosis. *Lancet* **2004**, *364*, 1789–1799. [CrossRef]
76. Subbaramaiah, K.; Chung, W.J.; Michaluart, P. Resveratrol inhibits cyclooxygenase-2 transcription and activity in phorbol ester-treated human mammary epithelial cells. *J. Biol. Chem.* **1998**, *273*, 21875–21882. [CrossRef] [PubMed]
77. Xie, W.; Herschman, H.R. v-src induces prostaglandin synthase 2 gene expression by activation of the c-Jun N-terminal kinase and the c-Jun transcription factor. *J. Biol. Chem.* **1995**, *270*, 27622–27628. [CrossRef]
78. Schecter, A.; Birnbaum, L.; Ryan, J.J.; Constable, J.D. Dioxins: An overview. *Environ. Res.* **2006**, *101*, 419–428. [CrossRef]
79. Esser, C.; Rannug, A.; Stockinger, B. The aryl hydrocarbon receptor in immunity. *Trends Immunol.* **2009**, *30*, 447–454. [CrossRef]
80. Casper, R.F.; Quesne, M.; Rogers, I.M.; Shirota, T.; Jolivet, A.; Milgrom, E.; Savouret, J.F. Resveratrol has antagonist activity on the aryl hydrocarbon receptor: Implications for prevention of dioxin toxicity. *Mol. Pharmacol.* **1999**, *56*, 784–790.
81. Ciolino, H.P.; Yeh, G.C. Inhibition of aryl hydrocarbon-induced cytochrome P-450 1A1 enzyme activity and CYP1A1 expression by resveratrol. *Mol. Pharmacol.* **1999**, *56*, 760–767.
82. Quintana, F.J.; Basso, A.S.; Iglesias, A.H.; Korn, T.; Farez, M.F.; Bettelli, E.; Weiner, H.L. Control of T(reg) and T(H)17 cell differentiation by the aryl hydrocarbon receptor. *Nature* **2008**, *453*, 65–71. [CrossRef]
83. Bettelli, E.; Carrier, Y.; Gao, W.; Korn, T.; Strom, T.B.; Oukka, M.; Kuchroo, V.K. Reciprocal developmental pathways for the generation of pathogenic effector TH17 and regulatory T cells. *Nature* **2006**, *441*, 235–238. [CrossRef] [PubMed]
84. Lanzilli, G.; Cottarelli, A.; Nicotera, G.; Guida, S.; Ravagnan, G.; Fuggetta, M.P. Anti-inflammatory effect of resveratrol and polydatin by in vitro IL-17 modulation. *Inflammation* **2011**, *35*, 240–248. [CrossRef] [PubMed]
85. Švajger, U.; Jeras, M. Anti-inflammatory effects of resveratrol and its potential use in therapy of immune-mediated diseases. *Int. Rev. Immunol.* **2012**, *31*, 202–222. [CrossRef]
86. Wang, Z.Y.; Sato, H.; Kusam, S.; Sehra, S.; Toney, L.M.; Dent, A.L. Regulation of IL-10 gene expression in Th2 cells by Jun proteins. *J. Immunol.* **2005**, *174*, 2098–2105. [CrossRef] [PubMed]
87. Meixner, A.; Karreth, F.; Kenner, L.; Wagner, E.F. JunD regulates lymphocyte proliferation and T helper cell cytokine expression. *EMBO J.* **2004**, *23*, 1325–1335. [CrossRef]
88. Chun, K.S.; Kim, S.H.; Song, Y.S.; Surh, Y.J. Celecoxib inhibits phorbol ester-induced expression of COX2 and activation of AP-1 and p38 MAP kinase in mouse skin. *Carcinogenesis* **2004**, *25*, 713–722. [CrossRef] [PubMed]
89. Kim, A.L.; Zhu, Y.; Zhu, H.; Han, L.; Kopelovich, L.; Bickers, D.R.; Athar, M. Resveratrol inhibits proliferation of human epidermoid carcinoma A431 cells by modulating MEK1 and AP-1 signalling pathways. *Exp. Dermatol.* **2006**, *15*, 538–546. [CrossRef]
90. Ghosh, S.; May, M.J.; Kopp, E.B. NF-kappa B and Rel proteins: Evolutionarily conserved mediators of immune responses. *Ann. Rev. Immunol.* **1998**, *16*, 225–260. [CrossRef]
91. Ghosh, S.; Karin, M. Missing pieces in the NF-kappaB puzzle. *Cell* **2002**, *109*, S81–S96. [CrossRef]
92. Manna, S.K.; Mukhopadhyay, A.; Aggarwal, B.B. Resveratrol suppresses TNF-induced activation of nuclear transcription factors NF-kappa B, activator protein-1, and apoptosis: Potential role of reactive oxygen intermediates and lipid peroxidation. *J. Immunol.* **2000**, *164*, 6509–6519. [CrossRef] [PubMed]
93. Estrov, Z.; Shishodia, S.; Faderl, S.; Harris, D.; Van, Q.; Kantarjian, H.M.; Aggarwal, B.B. Resveratrol blocks interleukin-1beta-induced activation of the nuclear transcription factor NF-kappaB, inhibits proliferation, causes S-phase arrest, and induces apoptosis of acute myeloid leukemia cells. *Blood* **2003**, *102*, 987–995. [CrossRef] [PubMed]
94. Soleas, G.J.; Diamandis, E.P.; Goldberg, D.M. Wine as a biological fluid: History, production, and role in disease prevention. *J. Clin. Lab. Anal.* **1997**, *11*, 287–313. [CrossRef]

95. Baur, J.A.; Sinclair, D.A. Therapeutic potential of resveratrol: The in vivo evidence. *Nat. Rev. Drug Discov.* **2006**, *5*, 493–506. [CrossRef]
96. Jang, M.; Cai, L.; Udeani, G.O.; Slowing, K.V.; Thomas, C.F.; Beecher, C.W. Cancer chemopreventive activity of resveratrol, a natural product derived from grapes. *Science* **1997**, *275*, 218–220. [CrossRef]
97. Vignali, M.; Infantino, M.; Matrone, R. Endometriosis: Novel etiopathogenetic concepts and clinical perspectives. *Fertil. Steril.* **2002**, *78*, 665–678. [CrossRef]
98. Murphy, A.A.; Santanam, N.; Parthasarathy, S. Endometriosis: A disease of oxidative stress? *Semin. Reprod. Endocrinol.* **1998**, *16*, 263–273. [CrossRef]
99. Murphy, A.A.; Palinski, W.; Rankin, S.; Morales, A.J.; Parthasarathy, S. Macrophage scavenger receptor (s) and oxidatively modified proteins in endometriosis. *Fertil. Steril.* **1998**, *69*, 1085–1091. [CrossRef]
100. Polak, G.; Mazurek, D.; Rogala, E.; Nowicka, A.; Derewianka-Polak, M.; Kotarski, J. Increased oxidized LDL cholesterol levels in peritoneal fluid of women with advanced-stage endometriosis. *Ginekol. Pol.* **2011**, *82*, 191–194. [PubMed]
101. Liu, Y.; Luo, L.; Zhao, H. Levels of lipid peroxides and superoxide dismutase in peritoneal fluid of patients with endometriosis. *J. Tongji Med. Univ.* **2001**, *21*, 166–167. [PubMed]
102. Szczepanska, M.; Koz'lik, J.; Skrzypczak, J.; Mikoajczyk, M. Oxidative stress may be a piece in the endometriosis puzzle. *Fertil. Steril.* **2003**, *79*, 1288–1293. [CrossRef]
103. Chen, Z.H.; Hurh, Y.J.; Na, H.K. Resveratrol inhibits TCDD induced expression of CYP1A1 and CYP1B1 and catechol estrogen-mediated oxidative DNA damage in cultured human mammary epithelial cells. *Carcinogenesis* **2004**, *25*, 2005–2013. [CrossRef] [PubMed]
104. Yavuz, S.; Aydin, N.E.; Celik, O.; Yilmaz, E.; Ozerol, E.; Tanbek, K. Resveratrol successfully treats experimental endometriosis through modulation of oxidative stress and lipid peroxidation. *J. Cancer Res. Therapeut.* **2014**, *10*, 324–329. [CrossRef] [PubMed]
105. Tekin, B.Y.; Guven, S.; Kirbas, A.; Kalkan, Y.; Tumkaya, L.; Guvendag Guven, E.S. Is resveratrol a potential substitute for leuprolide acetate in experimental endometriosis? *Eur. J. Obstet. Gynecol. Reprod. Biol.* **2015**, *184*, 1–6. [CrossRef] [PubMed]
106. Amaya, S.C.; Savaris, R.F.; Filipovic, C.J.; Wise, J.D.; Hestermann, E.; Young, S.L.; Lessey, B.A. Resveratrol and Endometrium. A Closer Look at an Active Ingredient of Red Wine Using In Vivo and In Vitro Models. *Reprod. Sci.* **2014**, *21*, 1362–1369. [CrossRef] [PubMed]
107. Ergenoglu, A.M.; Yeniel, A.O.; Erbas, O. Regression of endometrial implants by resveratrol in an experimentally induced endometriosis model in rats. *Reprod. Sci.* **2013**, *20*, 1230–1236. [CrossRef] [PubMed]
108. Henry, L.A.; Witt, D.M. Resveratrol: Phytoestrogen effects on reproductive physiology and behavior in female rats. *Hormones Behav.* **2002**, *41*, 220–228. [CrossRef] [PubMed]
109. Taguchi, A.; Koga, K.; Kawana, K.; Makabe, T.; Sue, F.; Miyashita, M. Resveratrol enhances apoptosis in endometriotic stromal cells. *Am. J. Reprod. Immunol.* **2016**, *75*, 486–492. [CrossRef] [PubMed]
110. Flower, A.; Andrew, F.; Liu, J.P.; Lewith, G.; Little, P.; Li, Q. Chinese herbal medicine for endometriosis. *Cochrane Database Syst. Rev.* **2012**, *5*, CD006568. [CrossRef] [PubMed]
111. Shakibaei, M.; Buhrmann, C.; Mobasheri, A. Resveratrol-mediated SIRT-1 interactions with p300 modulate receptor activator of NF-kappaB ligand (RANKL) activation of NF-kappaB signaling and inhibit osteoclastogenesis in bone-derived cells. *J. Biol. Chem.* **2011**, *286*, 11492–11505. [CrossRef] [PubMed]
112. Ryu, J.; Ku, B.M.; Lee, Y.K. Resveratrol reduces TNF-α-induced U373M human glioma cell invasion through regulating NF-κB activation and uPA/uPAR expression. *Anticancer Res.* **2011**, *31*, 4223–4230. [PubMed]
113. Kitawaki, J.; Kado, N.; Ishihara, H.; Koshiba, H.; Kitaoka, Y.; Honjo, H. Endometriosis: The pathophysiology as estrogen-dependent diseases. *J. Steroid Biochem. Mol. Biol.* **2002**, *83*, 149–155. [CrossRef]
114. Maia, H., Jr.; Casoy, J.; Correia, T. Activation of NF-KappaB and Cox-2 expression is associated with breakthrough bleeding in patients using oral contraceptives in extended regimens. *Gynecol. Endocrinol.* **2010**, *26*, 265–269. [CrossRef] [PubMed]
115. Edwards, P.A.; Lan, S.F.; Tanaka, R.D.; Fogelman, A.M. Mevalonolactone inhibits the rate of synthesis and enhances the rate of degradation of 3-hydroxy-3-methylglutaryl coenzyme A reductase in rat hepatocytes. *J. Biol. Chem.* **1983**, *258*, 7272–7275. [PubMed]
116. Maia, H., Jr.; Haddad, C.; Pinheiro, N.; Casoy, J. Advantages of the association of resveratrol with oral contraceptives for management of endometriosis-related pain. *Int. J. Women's Health* **2012**, *4*, 543–549. [CrossRef]

117. Mendes da Silva, D.; Gross, L.A.; De Paula Guedes Neto, E.; Lessey, B.A.; Francalacci Savaris, R. The Use of Resveratrol as an Adjuvant Treatment of Pain in Endometriosis: A Randomized Clinical Trial. *J. Endocrine Soc.* **2017**, 359–369. [CrossRef]
118. Ford, J.; Jiang, M.; Milner, J. Cancer-specifific functions of SIRT1 enable Human epithelial cancer cell growth and survival. *Cancer Res.* **2005**, *65*, 10457–10463. [CrossRef]
119. Taguchi, A.; Wada-Hiraike, O.; Kawana, K.; Koga, K.; Yamashita, A.; Shirane, A.; Urata, Y.; Kozuma, S.; Osuga, Y.; Fujii, T. Resveratrol suppresses inflammatory responses in endometrial stromal cells derived from endometriosis: A possible role of the sirtuin 1 pathway. *J. Obstet. Gynaecol. Res.* **2014**, *40*, 770–778. [CrossRef]
120. Franzoni, F.; Quinones-Galvan, A.; Regoli, F. A comparative study of the in vitro antioxidant activity of statins. *Int. J. Cardiol.* **2003**, *90*, 317–321. [CrossRef]
121. Villanueva, J.A.; Sokalska, A.; Cress, A.B.; Ortega, I.; Bruner-Tran, K.L.; Osteen, K.G.; Duleba, A.J. Resveratrol Potentiates Effect of Simvastatin on Inhibition of Mevalonate Pathway in Human Endometrial Stromal Cells. *J. Clin. Endocrinol. Metab.* **2013**, *98*, E455–E462. [CrossRef]
122. Harikumar, K.B.; Aggarwal, B.B. Resveratrol: A multitargeted agent for age-associated chronic diseases. *Cell Cycle* **2008**, *7*, 1020–1035. [CrossRef] [PubMed]

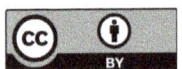

© 2019 by the authors. Licensee MDPI, Basel, Switzerland. This article is an open access article distributed under the terms and conditions of the Creative Commons Attribution (CC BY) license (http://creativecommons.org/licenses/by/4.0/).

MDPI
St. Alban-Anlage 66
4052 Basel
Switzerland
Tel. +41 61 683 77 34
Fax +41 61 302 89 18
www.mdpi.com

Molecules Editorial Office
E-mail: molecules@mdpi.com
www.mdpi.com/journal/molecules

www.ingramcontent.com/pod-product-compliance
Lightning Source LLC
LaVergne TN
LVHW071951080526
838202LV00064B/6725